Selected Topics in Cardiac Arrhythmias

Editor: Benjamin Befeler, M.D.
Associate Professor of Medicine
University of Miami School of Medicine
Chief of Cardiology
Hialeah Hospital
Hialeah, Florida

Associate Editors: Ralph Lazzara, M.D.
Professor of Medicine
Chief of Cardiology
University of Oklahoma Health Sciences Center
Oklahoma City, Oklahoma

Benjamin J. Scherlag, Ph.D.
Professor of Medicine and Physiology
University of Oklahoma Health Sciences Center
Oklahoma City, Oklahoma

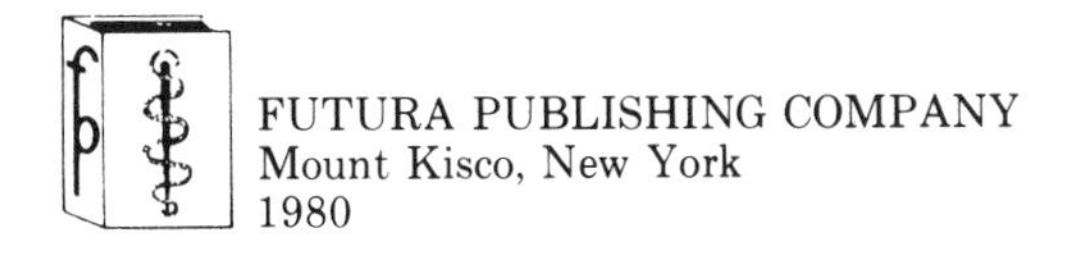
FUTURA PUBLISHING COMPANY
Mount Kisco, New York
1980

Dedication

We dedicate this book to our families
for the many hours that we spent away from them
in the preparation of this work

B.B.
R.L.
B.J.S.

Published by
Futura Publishing Company, Inc.
P.O. Box 330, 295 Main Street
Mount Kisco, New York 10549

LC #: 79-93092
ISBN #: 0-87993-139-6

Contributors

Victor A. Alatriste, M.D.
Division of Cardiology, Department of Medicine, University of Miami School of Medicine, Miami, Florida and the Instituto Nacional de Cardiologia, Mexico City, Mexico

Pierre Atlas, M.D.
Israel Heart Institute, The Chaim Sheba Medical Center, Tel-Hashomer and the Tel-Aviv University, Tel-Aviv, Israel

Frits W. Bar, M.D.
University of Limburg Section of Cardiology, Annadal Hospital, Maastricht, The Netherlands

Benjamin Befeler, M.D.
Chief of Cardiology, Hialeah Hospital; Associate Professor of Medicine, University of Miami School of Medicine, Miami, Florida

Ing. Barouh V. Berkovits, E.E.
Director, New England Research Program, Medtronics, Inc., Wellesley, Massachusetts

Agustin Castellanos, Jr., M.D.
Professor of Medicine, University of Miami School of Medicine; Director, Clinical Electrophysiology, Jackson Memorial Hospital, Miami, Florida

Pablo A. Chiale, M.D.
Section of Cardiology, Hospital Ramos Mejias, Buenos Aires, Argentina

Philippe Coumel, M.D.
Professeur Agrégé de la Faculté, Hôpital Lariboisiere, Paris, France

Leonard S. Dreifus, M.D.
Professor of Medicine, Department of Medicine of the Lankenau Hospital and Jefferson Medical College of the Thomas Jefferson University, Philadelphia, Pennsylvania

D. Durrer, M.D.
Chief of Cardiology and Professor, Department of Cardiology and Clinical Physiology, the Inter-University Institute of Cardiology, Amsterdam, The Netherlands

Marcelo Elizari, M.D.
Section of Cardiology, Hospital Ramos Mejias, Buenos Aires, Argentina
Jeronimo Farré, M.D.
Department of Cardiology, Annadal Hospital and the University of Limburg, Maastricht, The Netherlands; Department of Cardiology Service Fundación Jimenez Diaz, Madrid, Spain
Charles Fisch, M.D.
Distinguished Professor of Medicine and Director, Cardiovascular Division, Indiana University School of Medicine, Indianapolis, Indiana
Daniel Flammang, M.D.
Hopitaux de Paris, Paris, France
Guy Fontaine, M.D.
University of Paris and the Hopitaux de Paris, Paris, France
Dietmar Gann, M.D.
Division of Cardiology, Mount Sinai Medical Center, Miami Beach, Florida and the Department of Medicine, University of Miami School of Medicine, Miami, Florida
M. Susana Halpern, M.D.
Section of Cardiology, Hospital Ramos Mejias, Buenos Aires, Argentina
Marion Hefer, M.D.
Israel Heart Institute, The Chaim Sheba Medical Center, Tel-Hashomer, and the Tel-Aviv University Medical School, Tel-Aviv, Israel
Ronald R. Hope, M.D.
Associate Professor of Medicine, University of Oklahoma Health Sciences Center, Oklahoma City, Oklahoma
Elieser Kaplinsky, M.D.
Professor of Medicine, Lankenau Hospital and Jefferson Medical College of Thomas Jefferson University, Philadelphia, Pennsylvania; Meir Hospital Kfan Saba, the Tel-Aviv University Medical School, Tel-Aviv, Israel
Yehezkiel Kishon, M.D.
Israel Heart Institute, The Chaim Sheba Medical Center, Tel-Hashomer, and the Tel-Aviv University Medical School, Tel-Aviv, Israel
Michael D. Klein, M.D.
Associate Professor of Medicine, Section of Cardiology, Boston University School of Medicine and the University Hospital, Boston, Massachusetts
Henri E. Kulbertus, M.D.
Associate Professor of Medicine and Chief, Cardiology Section, University of Liege, Liege, Belgium
Ralph Lazzara, M.D.
Chief of Cardiology, Professor of Medicine, University of Oklahoma Health Sciences Center, Oklahoma City, Oklahoma

Julio O. Lazzari, M.D.
Section of Cardiology, Hospital Ramos Mejias, Buenos Aires, Argentina
Raul J. Levi, M.D.
Section of Cardiology, Hospital Ramos Mejias, Buenos Aires, Argentina
Paul A. Levine, M.D.
Cardiology Section, Boston University School of Medicine and University Hospital, Boston, Massachusetts
K. I. Lie, M.D.
Department of Cardiology and Clinical Physiology and the Inter-University Institute of Cardiology, Amsterdam, The Netherlands
Gerardo J. Nau, M.D.
Section of Cardiology, Hospital Ramos Mejias, Buenos Aires, Argentina
Henry N. Neufeld, M.D.
Director, Israel Heart Institute and Professor of Medicine, Chaim Sheba Medical Center, Tel-Hashomer, and the Tel-Aviv University Medical School, Tel-Aviv, Israel
Julio Przybylski, M.D.
Section of Cardiology, Hospital Ramos Mejias, Buenos Aires, Argentina
David L. Ross, M.B., B.S., F.R.A.C.P.
Department of Cardiology, Annadal Hospital and the University of Limburg, Maastricht, The Netherlands
Mauricio B. Rosenbaum, M.D.
Chief, Cardiology Section, Hospital Ramos Mejias; Professor of Medicine, Buenos Aires, Argentina
Michael Rosengarten, M.D.
Cardiology Section, Hôpital Lariboisiere, Paris, France
Lino Rossi, M.D.
Section of Pathology, University of Milan, Milan, Italy
Philip Samet, M.D.
Chief of Cardiology, Mount Sinai Medical Center; Professor of Medicine, University of Miami School of Medicine, Miami, Florida
Benjamin J. Scherlag, Ph.D.
Professor of Medicine and Physiology, University of Oklahoma Health Sciences Center, Oklahoma City, Oklahoma
Libi Sherf, M.D.
Associate Professor of Cardiology, Heart Institute, Chaim Sheba Medical Center, Tel-Hashomer and Tel-Aviv University Medical School, Tel-Aviv, Israel
Shlomo Stern, M.D.
Professor of Medicine, Hadassah Medical School and the General Hospital Bikur Cholim, Jerusalem, Israel
Zvi Stern, M.D.
Section of Cardiology, the General Hospital Bikur Cholim, Jerusalem, Israel

Ruey J. Sung, M.D.
Associate Professor of Medicine, Division of Cardiology, Department of Medicine, University of Miami School of Medicine, Miami, Florida
Paul Touboul, M.D.
Professeur Agrégé, Hôpital Cardiovasculaire et Pneumologique, University of Lyon, Lyon, France
Zvi Vered, M.D.
Israel Heart Institute, and the Chaim Sheba Medical Center, Tel-Hashomer, and the Tel-Aviv University Medical School, Tel-Aviv, Israel
Hein J. J. Wellens, M.D.
Professor of Cardiology, University of Limburg; Head, Section of Cardiology, Annadal Hospital, Maastricht, The Netherlands
Isaac Wiener, M.D.
Department of Cardiology, Annadal Hospital and the University of Limburg, Maastricht, The Netherlands
Joseph H. Yahini, M.D.
Associate Director, Israel Heart Institute; Professor of Medicine, Tel-Aviv, University Medical School, Tel-Aviv, Israel

Foreword

The preparation of this book began several years ago simultaneously with the development of a group of young cardiologists who devoted their time to teaching, research, and care of patients in an environment of mutual cooperation and support. This group assembled at the Veterans Administration Hospital in Miami and for a number of years worked as a productive and cohesive team in the academic setting of the University of Miami. Among the activities we developed was a yearly arrhythmia conference which attracted physicians from various states of the Union who found it attractive to come to Miami during the winter and brush up on their information on cardiac arrhythmias. Eventually this course produced an offshoot which was an international venture; the first such conference took place in Tel-Aviv, Israel, at the end of October 1978. The local Co-Chairman of this conference was Dr. Libi Sherf, and we are grateful to him for his assistance.

This volume presents the edited proceedings of that conference in Israel, as well as a few other topics which were added in order to cover some material which was not part of the conference and would make the book a more balanced and didactic text.

It is the desire of the editors that the book will present up-to-date and clinically relevant information on various topics in cardiac arrhythmias and that the book will become a vehicle for learning and the dissemination of concepts and ideas in this area.

As we plan to continue our arrhythmia conference on a regular basis, even though our original group has now divided into several new groups in various cities and hospitals, we hope that the book will eventually represent the written vehicle of the information exchange of these conferences which will be held regularly and it can be so updated after each conference.

The international tone of the book will definitely provide ideas from various parts of the world and will attest to the fact that human knowledge knows no frontiers and that progress is being made throughout the world which enriches our knowledge of heart disease. It is a tribute to human cooperation and understanding that chapters in this book have been written from faraway places such as Buenos Aires, Argentina and Tel-Aviv, Israel, with stops in various European countries and various cities in the United States.

The book is organized into sections which follow pretty close the program of the conference. As mentioned, some chapters have been added to make the book more complete.

The book does not pretend to be encyclopedic, that is, to be a textbook of arrhythmias. There are several books which cover cardiac arrhythmias in a systematic manner. We rather intend to present topics which are of current interest and in areas where new concepts have been introduced in recent years. The book is directed to a wide audience of cardiologists and internists and other physicians with an interest in cardiac rhythm disturbances.

I want to take this opportunity to thank a number of people who over the years have provided significant assistance in our work and have been a vital part of our original group. The following list does not pretend to be a catalog of all those people who have helped us in various ways, and probably contains many omissions. Those people are: Abraham A. Embi, Marisa Gonzalez, Teresa Vallone, Edward Berbari, Audrey Magid, Marcelino Obaya, Jorge Rodriguez, and Miguel Soto.

To Futura Publishing Company we are grateful for their editorial support and for the promptness with which the entire process of putting the book together has been carried out.

Benjamin Befeler, M.D.
Miami, Florida

Preface

It is indeed a pleasure—but more than a pleasure, an honor—to write the necessary introduction to this book. Although most prefaces are written with the specific purpose of exalting the relevance of the publication, I must confess that this monograph is unique, since its claim to greatness lies in the fact that it had its genesis precisely in the land of Genesis. The majority of the articles included (one notable exception being that from our own department) were based on data presented in a meeting held in the fall of 1978, in Tel Aviv, Israel. Because much information was given verbally and visually to a large and receptive audience, the participants agreed to prepare manuscripts and make the material available for publication. We all do this at the end of any meeting, while still influenced by the enthusiasm generated by it, but this flaming desire is cooled when, on returning home, we find the considerable amount of work accumulated during our absence.

Hence, it appeared at first glance unexpected that the authors met their deadline earlier than usual. But this reaction did not surprise me, for I have no doubt whatsoever that it was related to the long-lasting after-effects of the impact caused by the exposure to the legendary place where the seminar took place. Perhaps miracles do exist after all!

However, credit must be given to the efforts performed by the one individual who masterminded and, more important, carried out the mechanics of this meeting against apparently overwhelming odds, and who (last to be mentioned but not least among his accomplishments) also edited the book.

Of course, this is not to say that the participant-authors played no role. Obviously, without them there could have been no meeting, and consequently no book. Indeed, the list of names is impressive. No one doubts that the authors have contributed significantly to the advancement of experimental and clinical electrophysiology. So instead of mentioning their names individually, it appears better if I let them present their own worth through their own work.

Agustin Castellanos, M.D.
Miami, Florida

Contents

Part III: New Developments in the Treatment of Cardiac Arrhythmias

Part IV: Sudden Death Due to Cardiac Arrhythmias

Part V: Chronic Conduction System Disease

Part VI: Pre-excitation Syndrome

Part VII: Selected Topics in Arrhythmias with Clinical Relevance

1

Cardiac Cellular Electrophysiology: Its Contribution to the Understanding of Arrhythmias

Ralph Lazzara, M.D.

The introduction of the microelectrode to cardiac electrophysiology nearly 30 years ago[1] has produced a bounty of observations, ideas, and questions. Unquestionably much of the information obtained from intracellular recordings simply affirmed preexisting conclusions. Investigators rediscovered electrophysiological concepts with the new technology. Yet, certain information has come exclusively from intracellular recordings; certain concepts arose uniquely because of the microelectrode technique. During this period of avid application of intracellular recording, techniques for extracellular recording have been refined and extended. All in all the result has been a heartening growth of understanding of cardiac electrophysiology. Throughout this time numerous comprehensive critical reviews have summed up the state of knowledge. It will not be the purpose of this paper to present yet another comprehensive review, but to present and to discuss certain recent findings and ideas that are of current interest in relation to mechanisms of generation of cardiac arrhythmias.

THE PROCESS OF ACTIVATION AND CONDUCTION

The proposal by Weidmann[2] that cardiac cells generate upstrokes by a rapid, voltage-dependent, transient inflow of sodium ions, i.e., that the Hodgkin-Huxley hypothesis[3] applies to cardiac cells, has been accepted with little reservation or modification until recently. The discovery that there is slow inward current predominately of calcium ions during the plateau of the action potential of cardiac cells[4] has engendered the idea that the slow inward current may be the mechanism for the action potential upstroke of certain specialized normal cells, e.g., sinus (SA) node and A-V node cells, and of some abnormal cells operating at low resting potentials![5-7] The conduit for this slow current has been termed the "slow channel" to distinguish it from the "rapid channel" for sodium inflow. Whether it is a channel in any physical sense is unknown. The term "slow" is applied because the kinetics of activation, inactivation, and reactivation of the current are considerably slower than those for the inward sodium current which generates the upstroke of most normal cardiac cells. The rapid channel is normally inactivated at membrane potentials more positive than approximately −60 mv, but the slow channel may be activated at more positive levels. The slow channel is not only slow to "open" and "close" but the current admitted is relatively weak. Because of these characteristics the slow channel has been implicated as in the normal sinus and A-V nodes, and in abnormally depressed regions containing markedly depolarized cells. Blockers of the slow channel, e.g., verapamil, severely depress conduction in the SA and A-V nodes,[8-9] whereas tetrodotoxin, a blocker of the rapid channel, has comparatively little effect. This finding and others give plausibility to the idea that slow current is a major factor in the activation of A-V nodal cells. SA nodal cells may operate with a mixed dependence on rapid and slow currents.[5]

There has been keen interest in the role of the slow channel in conduction in abnormally depolarized cells. It has been suggested that the slow kinetics and low intensity of slow current would result in very slow conduction and great propensity for block and reentry. Under certain experimental conditions in vitro,[10-11] reentry occurs readily in depolarized cardiac cells generating action potentials by means of slow current. Whether this mechanism commonly produces clinical arrhythmias remains uncertain. Thus far, it has not been possible to implicate the slow current in the activation process of ischemic cells. Both in vitro and in vivo, slow channel blockers have little effect on depressed conduction in ischemic cells. Indeed the most consistent effect is improvement in ischemia-induced depression. On the other hand, cardiac cells depressed by ischemia are quite sensitive to blockers of the rapid channel. The effects of tetrodotoxin on cardiac cells depressed by ischemia are shown in Figure 1-1. These findings indicate that depression of the rapid channel may be the mechanism for slow conduction and reentry in ischemia.

Recently there has been increasing interest in intercellular junctions and their influence on conduction. Normally cell to cell junctions (tight junctions) have low electrical resistance and allow relatively free current flow between the cells. Increase in resistance of these junctions would

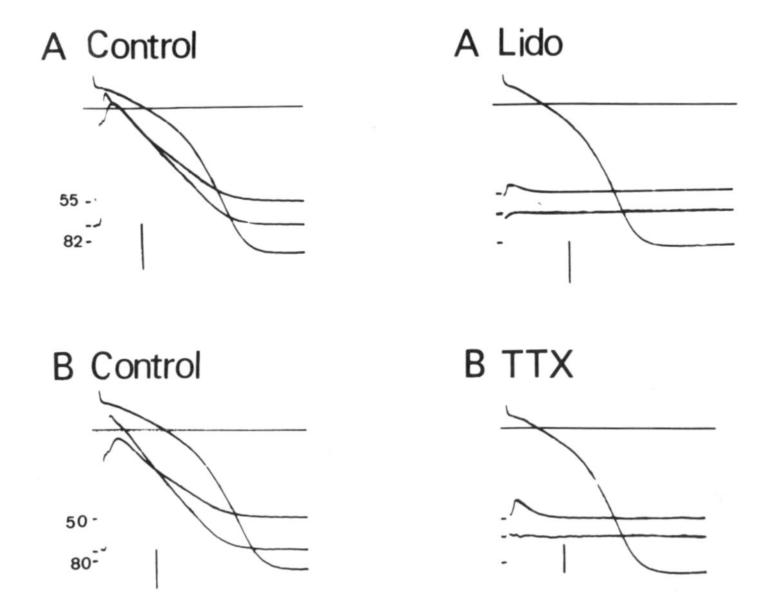

Figure 1-1. Depressed rapid channel in ischemic cells. Recordings from two ischemic myocardial cells and one normal Purkinje fiber are shown before (*A* and *B* Control) and after treatment with lidocaine (*A* Lido) and tetrodotoxin (*B* TTX). Note that one cell has a resting potential of approximately −50 mv, the other −80 mv. There is a modest effect on the upstroke velocity of the normal Purkinje fiber, which is represented by the vertical bar but the depressed cells become unresponsive. The upstroke velocity in *A* Control is 420 v/sec.

impair the flow of current and the process of propagation. It has been shown that the resistance of these junctions are sensitive to the intracellular concentrations of sodium and calcium ions.[12,13] It is likely that abnormal cardiac cells, especially in ischemia, may have higher than normal concentrations of sodium and calcium ions in the sarcoplasm.[14] The resultant increase in resistance of tight junctions may be a factor in slow and irregular propagation and reentry.

AUTOMATICITY

There has been encouraging progress in the elucidation of the mechanisms for automaticity. The application of voltage clamping to cardiac cells has greatly helped this progress. It is agreed that inactivation of a potassium current which is activated during the action potential is a major factor in the positive drift of the membrane potential of automatic fibers during diastole (i.e., the pacemaker potential).[15] It is also agreed that a resting inward current carried mainly by sodium ions is also important. These two factors combine to produce the pacemaker potentials of automatic Purkinje fibers.

The processes for pacemaker potentials in the sinus node may differ qualitatively and quantitatively from those described for Purkinje fibers. Unfortunately, voltage clamping techniques have not been applied to sinus node cells as successfully or as extensively as to Purkinje fibers. Pacemaker cells in the sinus node operate at considerably more positive levels of membrane potential than Purkinje fibers.[5] The maximum diastolic potential of sinus node cells is about −60 mv as compared to −90 mv for Purkinje fibers. The threshold potential for sinus node cells is approximately −40 mv but for Purkinje fibers it is approximately −60 mv. Some investigators are persuaded that deactivation of the potassium current may also play a role in sinus node pacemaking but the background inward current may be the slow calcium current rather than a sodium current. Sensitivity of sinus node fibers to slow channel blocking agents[16] supports this idea.

The discovery that digitalis compounds produce afterpotentials in Purkinje fibers[17,18] has rekindled interest in anomalous forms of automaticity,[19] especially those forms of automatic firing that ensue from early or late afterpotentials. Because these forms of automaticity depend on prior action potentials, they have been termed "triggerable" automaticity. Since normal automatic mechanisms also depend on prior action potentials (which activate the potassium current) this terminology presents a false distinction. Yet there is a difference in the responses of afterpotentials and of normal pacemaker potentials to preceding cycle length. Afterpotentials, especially delayed afterpotentials may be enhanced by decreasing cycle lengths over a wide range of cycle lengths, but normal diastolic depolarization is uniformly depressed by decreasing cycle lengths (overdrive depression). In that sense, the appellation of "triggerable" automaticity is apt. Because triggerable automaticity may be instigated or terminated by premature beats there may be problems distinguishing this automatic process from reentrant process in vivo.

Afterpotentials have been produced under a wide variety of experimental circumstances. Conditions which promote the slow current such as high concentrations of calcium or intense beta-adrenergic activity, enhance delayed after-potentials, but blockers of slow channel depress both early and delayed afterpotential.[19]

Normal ventricular myocardial cells,[20] coronary sinus cells, and cardiac cells in the atrioventricular valves develop afterpotentials and automatic firing with beta-adrenergic stimulation.[19] These findings suggest that afterpotentials may occur under physiological conditions and may be a mechanism for premature atrial contractions, premature ventricular contractions, and atrial and ventricular tachyarrythmias in man. Induction of afterpotentials in normal canine ventricular myocardial cells by norepinephrine is shown in Figure 1-2.

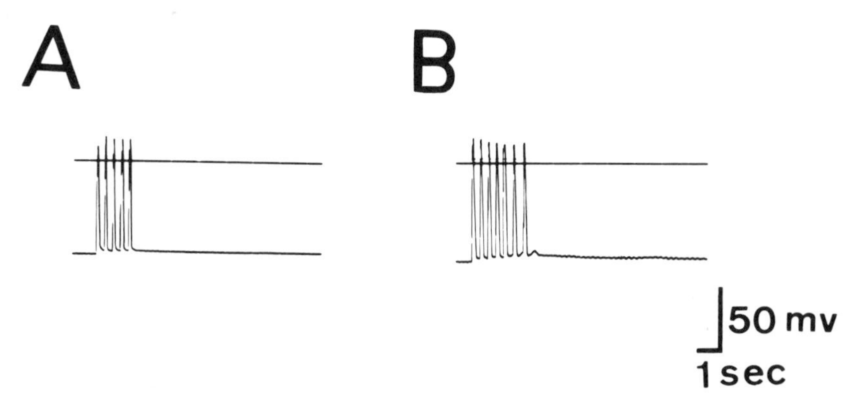

Figure 1-2. Induction of afterpotentials in normal canine ventricular myocardial cells. The action potentials are shown both before (*A*) and after treatment with norepinephrine (10^{-6}M). The last two action potentials in *B* are spontaneous.

REFRACTORINESS

In most normal cardiac cells the refractory periods are determined by the membrane potential levels during the action potential. The absolute refractory period coincides with that portion of the action potential which is more positive than approximately −60 mv and the relative refractory period coincides with the terminal phase of repolarization between −60 mv and the resting potential. This strong dependence on the repolarizing membrane potential is the consequence of the rapid kinetics of reactivation of the rapid sodium channel. As the membrane repolarizes, reactivation of the rapid sodium channel lags behind the membrane potential by only a few milliseconds. For normal cardiac cells behaving in this way, changes in the refractory periods come about because of changes in configuration and duration of the action potential. Examples of such changes are shown in Figure 1-3.

In certain types of normal cardiac cells, for example SA nodal cells and A-V nodal cells,[5,21] refractoriness is not closely related to the membrane potential and the refractory periods outlast the action potential duration. The persistence of refractoriness even after full repolarization reflects slow reactivation of the "channels" for the excitatory current. In the case of A-V nodal cells, it is probable that the channels are slow

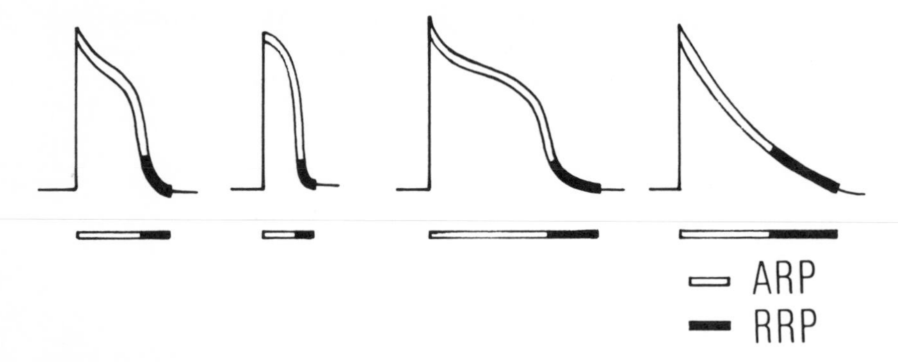

Figure 1-3. The influence of action potential shape on the durations of absolute (ARP) and relative (RRP) refractory periods in cells in which refractoriness is dependent on membrane potential.

channels, known to have relatively slow kinetics of activation, inactivation, and reactivation. It also appears that the rapid sodium channel may exhibit slow kinetics under certain abnormal conditions, e.g., ischemia.[22] An illustration constructed from an ischemic cell with pronounced "postrepolarization refractoriness" is shown in Figure 1-4.

This refractoriness is probably important in the generation of reentrant activation because very long relative refractory periods result in markedly depressed and slowly propagated responses throughout much of the cardiac cycle. The marked spatial heterogeneity of postrepolarization refractoriness in depressed regions contributes to reentry by

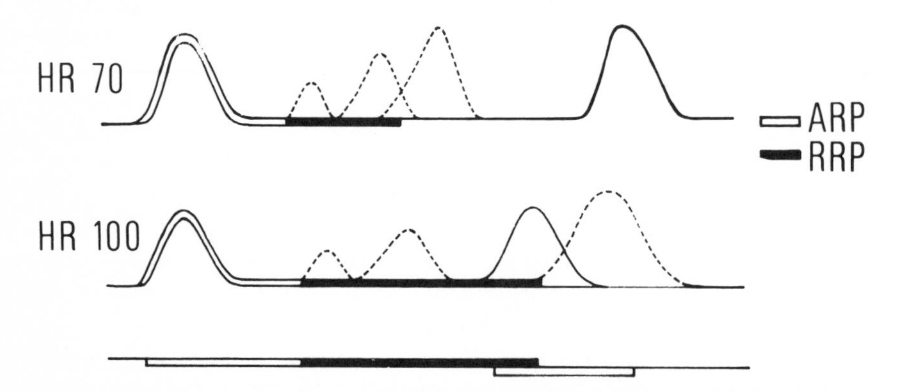

Figure 1-4. Postrepolarization refractoriness in a depressed ischemic cell. The absolute (ARP) and relative (RRP) refractory periods outlast the action potential. At a heart rate (HR) of 100 (lower trace) the refractory period exceeds the duration of the basic cycle.

fostering irregular activation wavefronts and local block as the impulse seeks routes of lesser refractoriness. Local block that depends on refractoriness is time-dependent. With the recession of the refractory state a site of local block could conduct a later returning impulse. As a result, "unidirectional block" could occur because of temporal and not spatial factors. The strong relationship between reentry and cycle length in ischemic tissues makes this mechanism plausible.

SUMMARY

The investigation of cardiac cellular electrophysiology in recent years has been more preoccupied with the anomalous and the abnormal, because it has become evident that the understanding of arrhythmias and the mechanisms of therapy cannot be completely clarified by observing the behavior of normal cells. Focus on phenomena such as afterpotentials, calcium-dependent upstrokes, time-dependent refractoriness, and depression of the rapid channel, is enriching the bank of information that will be the basis for the understanding of clinical arrhythmias and the development of a rational therapy.

REFERENCES

1. Draper, M.H., and Weidmann, S.: Cardiac resting and action potentials recorded with an intracellular electrode. *J. Physiol.* **115**:74–94, 1957.
2. Weidmann, S.: The effect of the cardiac membrane potential on rapid availability of the sodium-carrying system. *J. Physiol.* **127**:213–224, 1955.
3. Hodgkin, A.L., and Huxley, A.F.: A quantitative description of membrane current and its application to conduction and excitation in nerve. *J. Physiol.* **117**:500–544, 1952.
4. Reuter, H.: The dependence of slow inward current in Purkinje fibers on the extracellular calcium concentration. *J. Physiol.* **192**:479–92, 1967.
5. Strauss, H.C., Prystowsky, E.N., and Scheinman, M.M.: Sino-atrial and atrial electrogenesis. *Prog. Cardiovasc. Dis.* **19**:385–404, 1977.
6. Zipes, D.P., Lesch, H.R., and Watanabe, A.M.: Role of the slow current in cardiac electrophysiology. *Circulation* **51**:761–766, 1975.
7. Cranefield, P.F.: *The Conduction of the Cardiac Impulse.* Mt. Kisco, N.Y., Futura Publishing Co., 1975.
8. Wit, A.L., and Cranefield, P.F.: Effect of verapamil on the sino-atrial and atrioventricular nodes of the rabbit and the mechanism by which it arrest reentrant atrioventricular nodul tachycardia. *Circ. Res.* **35**:413–425, 1974.
9. Zipes, D.P., and Mendez, C.: Action of manganese ions and tetrodotoxin on A-V nodal transmembrane potentials in isolated rabbit hearts. *Circ. Res.* **32**:447–454, 1973.

10. Wit, A.L., Cranefield, P.F., and Hoffman, B.F.: Slow conduction and reentry in the ventricular conducting system: II: Single sustained circus movement in networks of canine and bovine Purkinje fibers. *Circ. Res.* **30**:11–22, 1972.
11. Wit, A.L., Hoffman, B.F., and Cranefield, P.F.: Slow conduction and reentry in the ventricular conducting system: I. Return extrasystole in canine Purkinje fibers. *Circ. Res.* **30**:1–10, 1972.
12. DeMello, W.C.: Effect of intracellular injection of calcium and strontium on cell communications in heart. *J. Physiol.* **250**:231–246, 1975.
13. DeMello, W.C.: Sodium pump. Its importance to intercellular communication in heart fibers. *Experientia* **32**:355, 1976.
14. Russel, R.A., Crafoord, J., and Harris, A.S.: Changes in myocardial composition after coronary artery ligation. *Am. J. Physiol.* **200**:995–998, 1961.
15. McAllister, R.E., Noble, D., and Tsien, R.W.: Reconstruction of the electrical activity of cardiac Purkinje fibers. *J. Physiol.* **251**:1–59, 1975.
16. Zipes, D.P., and Fischer, J.C.: Effects of agents which inhibit the slow channel on sinus node automaticity and atrioventricular induction in the dog. *Circ. Res.* **34**:184–192, 1974.
17. Ferrier, G.R., Saunders, J.H., and Mendez, C.: A cellular mechanism for the generation of ventricular arrhythmias by acetystrophanthidin. *Circ. Res.,* **32**:600–609, 1973.
18. Rosen, M.R., Gelband, H., and Hoffman, B.F.: Correlation between effects of ouabain on the canine electrocardiogram and transmembrane potentials of isolated Purkinje fibers. *Circulation* **47**:65–72, 1973.
19. Cranefield, P.F.: Action potentials, afterpotentials, and arrhythmias. *Circ. Res.* **41**:415–423, 1977.
20. Lazzara, R., Hope, R.R., and Yeh B.K.: Implication of cAMP and calcium as mediators of automaticity included in working myocardium. *Am. J. Cardiol.* **41**:417, 1978.
21. Merideth, J., Mendez, C., Mueller, W.J., and Moe, G.K.: Electrical excitability of atrioventricular nodal cells. *Circ. Res.* **23**:69–85, 1968.
22. Lazzara, R., El-Sherif, N., Hope, R.R., and Scherlag, B.J.: Ventricular arrhythmias and electrophysiological consequences of myocardial ischemia and infarction. *Circ. Res.* **42**:740–749, 1978.

2

The Contribution of New Intracardiac Techniques to the Understanding of Human Electrophysiology

Benjamin J. Scherlag, Ph.D.

The standard electrocardiogram has been an invaluable tool in the analysis of the electrical properties of the normal and diseased heart. During its inception and development in the first third of the 20th century, the ECG remained a noninvasive procedure from which much diagnostic information could be deduced, e.g., the anatomic position of the heart, site and degree of hypertrophy or myocardial injury. In the 1940s and early 1950s deductive analysis of the electrocardiogram reached its zenith with the brilliant arrhythmia analyses of Katz and Pick.[1] In the last two decades electrocardiography began to wane, electrocardiographic studies became more esoteric and arrhythmia analysis became the purview of smaller and smaller numbers of interested cardiologists and investigators.

In the 1960s Hoffman and his co-workers [2,3] began a series of studies designed to directly record from the specialized tissues of the heart by placing electrodes on the endocardial surface during cardiotomy and cardiopulmonary bypass. These studies formulated the realization that much of the electrical activation of the heart was silent, i.e., not represented by waveforms on the standard ECG.[4] For example, the depolarization of the sinoatrial or atrioventricular node and His-Purkinje system occurs during the isoelectric segment preceding or following the P wave.

In 1969 a right heart catheterization technique was introduced by Scherlag et al.[5] which allowed the consistent recording of the His bundle's electrical activation by an electrode catheter placed near the A-V junction. Using three or more standard ECG leads and the His bundle electrogram, the P-R interval can now be divided into three component parts (Fig. 2-1):

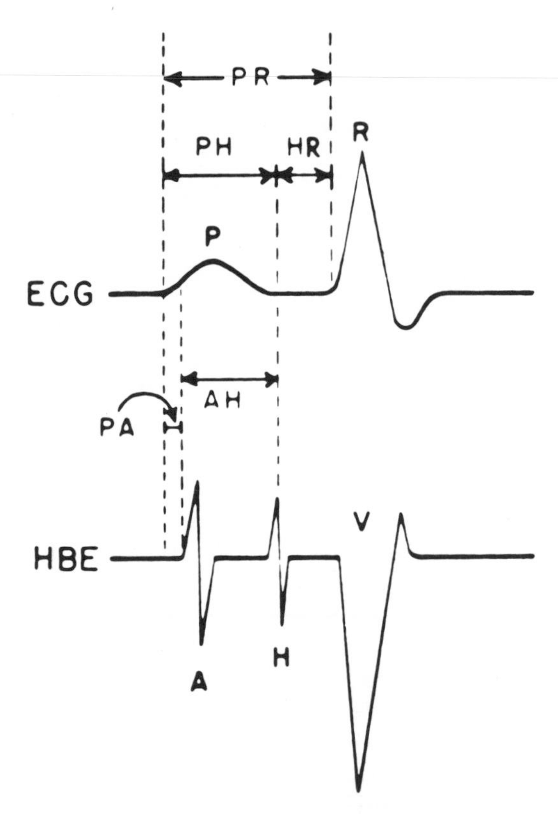

Figure 2-1. A breakdown of the PR interval into component portions using standard electrocardiogram and His bundle electrogram. (After Hecht et al., *Am. J. Cardiol.* **31**: 232–244, 1973.)

P-A Interval—from the beginning of the P-wave (activation of the sinus node area) to the onset of atrial activity in the His bundle electrogram (activation of the A-V nodal area). This interval is a measure of intra-atrial conduction and averages 44 msec in the normal human heart.

A-H Interval—from the onset of atrial activity in the His bundle electrogram to the beginning of the His bundle potential. This interval is a measure of the conduction time through the A-V node. In the normal heart the A-H interval ranges from 50 to 120 msec; average 94 msec.

H-V Interval —from the onset of the His bundle potential to the earliest time of ventricular activation recorded in any of the extra- or intracardiac leads. The H-V interval is a measure of conduction through the His-Purkinje or ventricular specialized conduction system. The normal range is 35 to 55 msec; average 41 msec.

The uses of the His bundle recording technique have been myriad. In less than 10 years, there have been more than 600 citations of the original paper describing the clinical technique for His bundle recordings. Moreover, the number of basic reports using a similarly described technique in the dog[6] has not been enumerated. Initially, in the clinical setting the technique was used to establish and validate the site of block in the cardiac conduction system which had been previously deduced from standard ECG recordings. For example, the site of block in Wenckebach (type I) periodicity was assumed to be the A-V node whereas type II A-V block (also known as Mobitz type II) was assumed to be infranodal. With His bundle recordings these deductions could be verified.[7–9] However, in many cases infranodal Wenckebach (type I) has been reported.[8–10]

The use of His bundle recordings has been a significant key in unlocking the mechanism underlying various forms of the pre-excitation syndrome.[11] The understanding of the function of bypass or accessory pathways between the atria and ventricles has led to a more effective therapeutic approach—both medical and surgical—for patients with pre-excitation syndrome and associated supraventricular tachycardias that were symptomatic or potentially lethal.

Perhaps the area of earliest and most intense interest which developed with the advent of the His bundle recording technique was that of identifying those at risk for impending complete heart block. In Table 2-1, taken from Narula et al.,[12] of 131 patients with right bundle branch block and left axis deviation or left anterior hemiblock, 72 percent showed H-V prolongation. This conduction delay existed not only in the right bundle branch and left anterior division of the left bundle branch but also in the posterior division of the left bundle as well.*

---

*Of interest is the high percentage of H-V prolongation, 79 percent in the 123 patients with left bundle branch block pattern on the ECG. In these cases there must be right bundle branch block to a lesser degree or intra-His bundle block coexisting with the left bundle branch block. The H-V prolongation for other forms of intraventricular conduction defects indicate that the electrocardiogram was not a specific indicator of the degree and site(s) of lesion in the ventricular conduction system.

TABLE 2-1. H-V ABNORMALITIES AND IVCD IN PATIENTS WITH PRIMARY CONDUCTION SYSTEM DISEASE.

Number	Conduction Defect	Prolonged H-V
123	LBBB	79%
8	Int. LBBB	63%
5	RAD	40%
76	LAD	30%
62	RBBB	32%
131	RBBB+LAD	72%
30	RBBB+RAD	87%
16	IVCD	87%

Reproduced with permission from Narula, O.S., Gann, D., and Samet, P.: Prognostic value of H-V intervals. In Narula, O.S. (ed.): *His Bundle-Electrocardiography and Clinical Electrophysiology.* Philadelphia, F.A. Davis Co., 1975, Ch. 20.

Recent studies [12-15] have shown that H-V prolongation is observed in a high percentage of patients with a suspicious electrocardiographic pattern, i.e., right bundle branch block plus left anterior hemiblock. These patients were symptomatic and exhibited dizziness and syncope not related to neurological disorders. In Figure 2-2, taken from Narula et al.,[12] 24 symptomatic patients with right bundle branch block and left axis deviation or left anterior hemiblock had prolonged H-V intervals and were treated by pacemaker implantation. These patients were followed for a year up to six years. The average annual mortality was 13 percent. Of the 34 who were symptomatic (without pacemakers) the average yearly mortality was almost three times as great, 36 percent. These findings have been confirmed in a recent prospective study by Altschuler et al.[16] Thus these investigators found that the H-V interval has considerable prognostic significance in terms of mortality, supposedly from A-V block, and in determining the method of management, i.e., whether to implant a permanent pacemaker or not.

On the other hand, another study by Denes et al.[17] of 119 asymptomatic patients with right bundle branch block and left anterior hemiblock, followed for up to two years, did not show any marked differences in the incidence of A-V block or mortality (see Fig. 2-3). The differences between the studies outlined in Figures 2-2 and 2-3 may be explained by two important factors in regard to the etiology of A-V heart block. First, the average age of the patients in the Narula study[12] was 72 and in the study by Altchuler et al.,[16] 69. On the other hand, the average age in the study by Denes et al.[17] was 62. Thus it would be expected that the older patients would represent a population showing a higher incidence of primary conduction system disease and a greater tendency, due to age, for the conduction system disease to go on to complete heart block. Indeed, in the study by Narula et al.[12] it was noted that almost 30 percent of the patients studied were diagnosed as exhibiting primary conduction system disease as the major, if not the sole, disease entity.

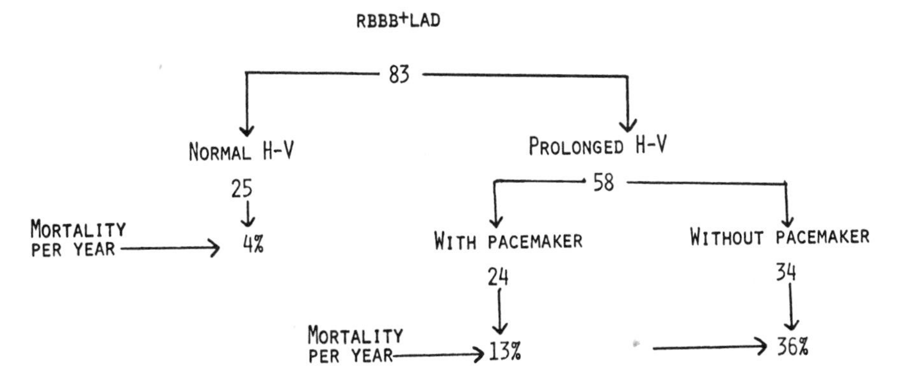

Figure 2-2. Schematic diagram showing disposition of 83 patients with right bundle branch block and left axis deviation in a prospective study by Narula, O.S., et al., 1975. (Reproduced with permission from Narula, O.S. (ed.): *His Bundle-Electrocardiography and Clinical Electrophysiology.* Philadelphia, F.A. Davis Co., 1975, Ch. 20.)

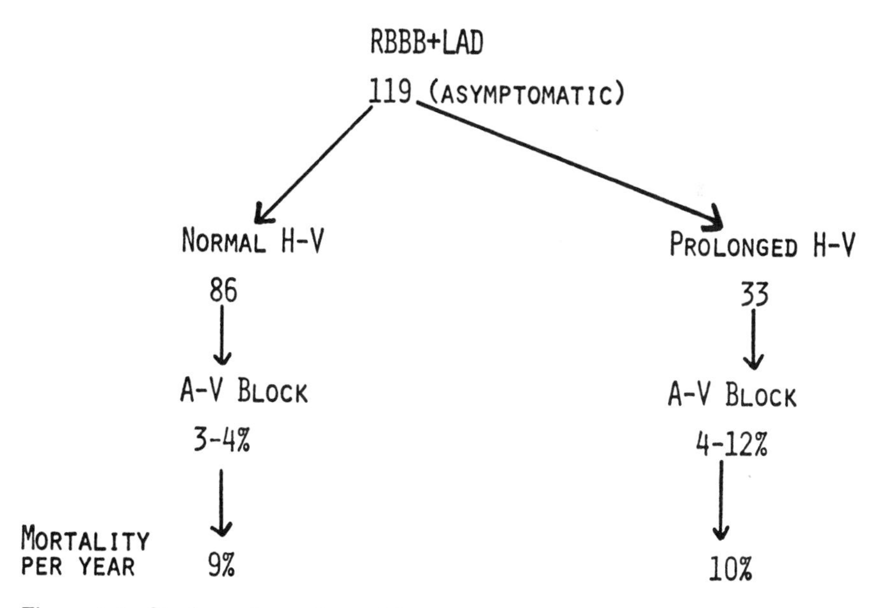

Figure 2-3. Similar schematic as Figure 2-2 of a prospective study by Denes et al., 1975. (Reproduced with permission from *Am. J. Cardiol.* 35: 23–28, 1975.)

Moreover, in the population study by Denes et al.[17] the majority of patients showed moderate to severe coronary artery disease as reflected by a high incidence of cardiomegaly, functional class III and class IV status and the presence of third heart sounds and other indications of severe hemodynamic impairment. Thus, even in those cases showing prolonged H-V intervals, overriding coronary artery disease would provide a lethal factor preventing these patients from reaching an age at which the primary conduction system disease would manifest as complete A-V heart block. In fact, the annual mortality of 10 percent in the 33 asymptomatic patients would preclude the large majority of them reaching the average age represented in the studies by Narula et al.[12] and Altschuler et al.[16] The differences in patient population can also be seen in recent studies of patients with electrocardiographic patterns of right bundle branch block and left anterior hemiblock induced by acute myocardial infarction. Lie et al. [18] found that prolongation of H-V intervals in these patients was associated with a high mortality and that permanent pacemaker implantation in a comparable group significantly decreased mortality. Similar findings were reported by Lichstein et al.[19]

On the other hand, Ginks et al.[20] followed 25 patients for an average of 49 months who survived acute myocardial infarction and transient A-V block. The majority, 14, had bifascicular block on the electrocardiogram. At the end of the follow-up period, ten of the 14 were alive. Of four in whom permanent pacing was established, two died. These authors concluded that "long term pacing is not justified in patients, otherwise asymptomatic, (with bifascicular) block persisting after . . . anterior myocardial infarction." Unfortunately only eight patients were studied using His bundle electrocardiography and no apparent relationship between H-V and outcome was evidenced. Further studies are required to determine the long-term prognostic value of H-V intervals in patients with bifascicular block resulting from acute anterior wall myocardial infarction. It is important to recognize the severe malignant potential of the hemodynamic dysfunction, i.e., congestive heart failure and conduction failure, in complete A-V heart block caused by coronary artery disease. Indeed, Lie et al. in their study[18] did not include patients with pulmonary edema or shock. It is probable that the high mortality associated with the development of bundle branch block in acute anterior wall myocardial infarction [21,22] is mainly the result of pump failure and much less attributable to cardiac conduction disorders.

NEW APPROACHES TO DETECTION OF IMPENDING COMPLETE HEART BLOCK

Both the electrocardiographic patterns and the measurements of H-V intervals in patients with partial A-V heart block are limited in determining those persons at risk for impending complete block. The limitations are based on the chronic course of primary conduction system disease generally, and the variable nature of the disease process in any given individual.[14,15] It is controversial whether a single determination of an abnormal H-V interval in a patient with right bundle branch block and left anterior hemiblock is indicative of impending complete heart block even if the value is greater than 65 msec.[12,15,23] Under these circumstances it would be important to follow such patients to ascertain progressive changes in the electrocardiogram and H-V interval. Although the electrocardiogram is noninvasive, the His bundle recording requires catheterization, thus precluding its use in a serial fashion. Recently, a noninvasive procedure to record His-Purkinje system activation has been reported by several groups.[24-28] This technique is based on signal averaging.

The small mass of the His-Purkinje tissue precludes the registration of its electrical depolarization in the standard electrocardiogram. However, if the standard electrocardiogram (Fig. 2-4*A*) is amplified considerably and displayed on an oscilloscope at a rapid sweep speed, the terminal portion of the P wave would appear at one end of the screen and the beginning of the greatly amplified QRS complex at the other end (Fig. 2-4*B*). Unfortunately, the signal of interest, the His-Purkinje system, occurring during the P-R segment would be obscured by the electrical "noise," i.e., 60 Hz and its harmonics. Such noise is inherent in all electrical equipment including the recording apparatus to detect the ECG. However, signal averaging can be used to extract the signal from the noise. If many cardiac cycles are superimposed or added to each other and divided by the total number of cycles, the periodic signals during the P-R segment i.e., the His-Purkinje activation, will be undiminished. However, the electrical noise which is aperiodic with the cardiac cycle will decrease toward zero as troughs and peaks of the sine waves composing the noise are alphabetically added and averaged (Fig. 2-4*B*). After many cycles, depending on the level of the noise, the desired signal will emerge (Fig. 2-4*C*).

The concept was initially tested in anesthetized dogs using bipolar chest leads. Figure 2-5*A* shows the amplified and averaged electrocardiogram at the top with the end of the P wave and the beginning of the QRS complex on the other side of the tracing. The three traces below represent the separate signal averaged leads (SAL). Each of these was markedly amplified (100,000 to 200,000 times) and averaged over 100 cardiac cycles. Note that there is a reproducible waveform (G) prior to the onset of ventricular activation (V). By increasing the heart rate with atrial pacing from 185 to 225-240/min, conduction through the A-V node is prolonged; however, the configuration and duration (30 msec) of

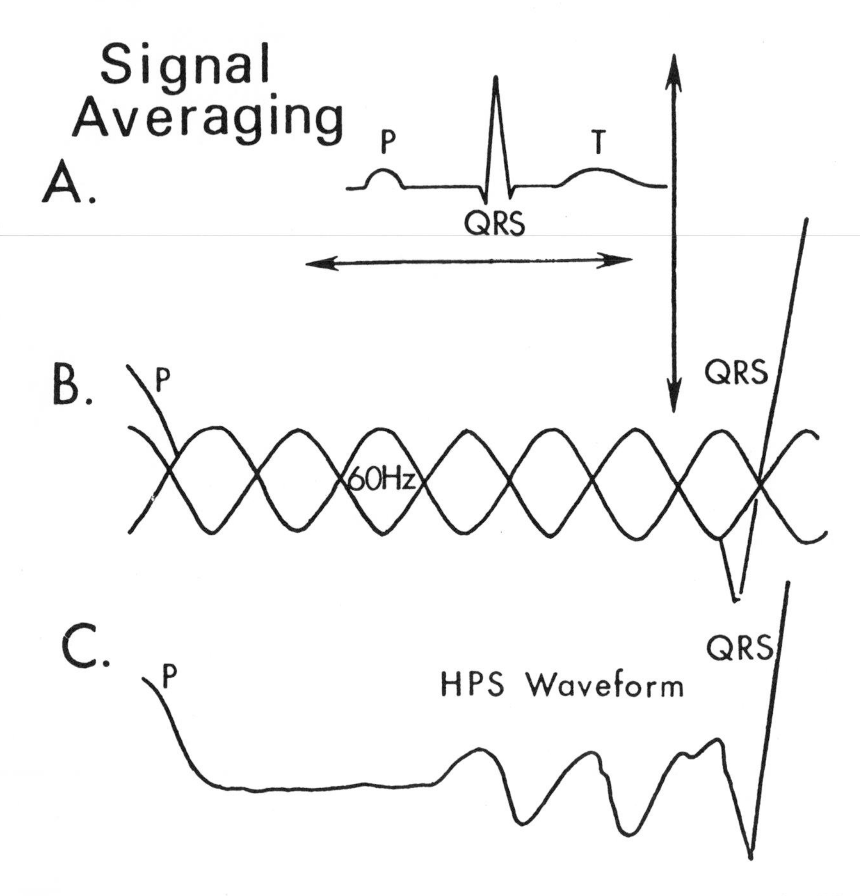

Figure 2-4. Illustration of the principles of signal averaging applied to the PR segment of the standard electrocardiogram. See text for details.

the reproducible waveform is constant, suggesting that it represents the His-Purkinje system activation. The H-V interval in the normal dog heart averages 33 msec.[29]

Further validation of signal average recordings from the body surface provided positive confirmation that these waveforms emanated from the His-Purkinje system.[30] Figure 2-6 was taken from a study which applied signal averaging techniques to patients.[31] In this report a His bundle recording was made before or after the noninvasive signal averaging recordings were performed. In Figure 2-6*A* His bundle-electrocardiography established that the first-degree heart block in this patient was due to an abnormal A-V nodal (A-H) conduction as well as the prolonged H-V interval, 60 msec. Three signal averaged leads (SAL) made from a bipolar chest lead showed a reproducible waveform whose duration matched the H-V interval, 60 msec (Fig. 2-6*B*).

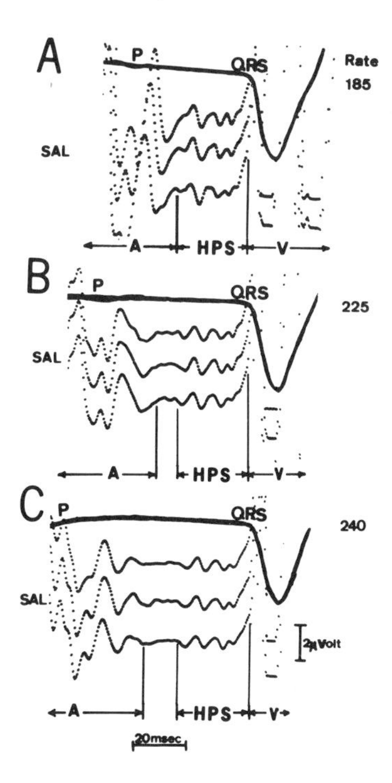

Figure 2-5. Reproducibility of the HPS complex in repeat averages and at different heart rates. Three separate averages of the surface averaged lead (SAL) are shown at three different heart rates: 185 (*A*), 225 (*B*), and 240 (*C*). Also displayed is the ECG showing portions of the P and QRS waves. When A-V conduction prolonged, at the higher rates, the HPS complex retained its temporal relationship with ventricular deflections (V) and moved away from the atrial deflections (A), leaving a longer period of relative inactivity preceding the HPS complex. The configuration of the HPS complex remained quite similar for each average and for each heart rate. (Reproduced with permission from Berbari, E.J., et al., *Circulation* 48: 1005–1013, 1973.)

Figure 2-7*A* through *E*, presents signal average recordings from five different patients in each of whom three consecutive 100 averages were made to determine reproducibility of the onset of such reproducibility. The arrow on each trace indicates the onset of the reproducible His-Purkinje system waveform. The duration of these waveforms (from the arrow to the onset of ventricular activation) in traces *A* to *E* was 39, 43, 55, 60, and 72 msec, respectively. A plot of these values against the measured H-V intervals obtained by His bundle recording provides a line of identity with an excellent correlation coefficient, r = 0.95 (Fig. 2-8).

Before the technique of signal averaging can be generally useful in the clinical setting, at least one important technical problem must be overcome. At normal heart rates, atrial activation may obscure the initial

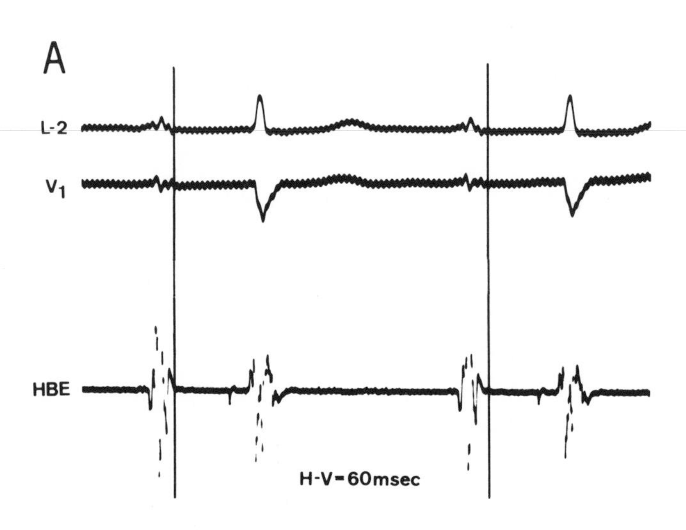

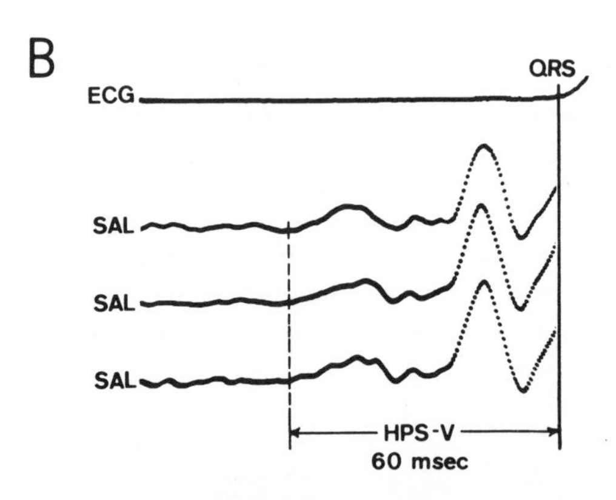

Figure 2–6. Patient with an abnormal H-V and HPS-V time. Panel *A* shows the results of the His bundle catheterization procedure. The timelines are 1 sec apart and the H-V time is 60 msec. Panel *B* shows the ECG and three SAL recordings. (Reproduced with permission from Berbari, E.J., et al.: The His-Purkinje electrocardiogram in man: An initial assessment of its uses and limitations. *Circulation* **54**: 219–224, 1976.)

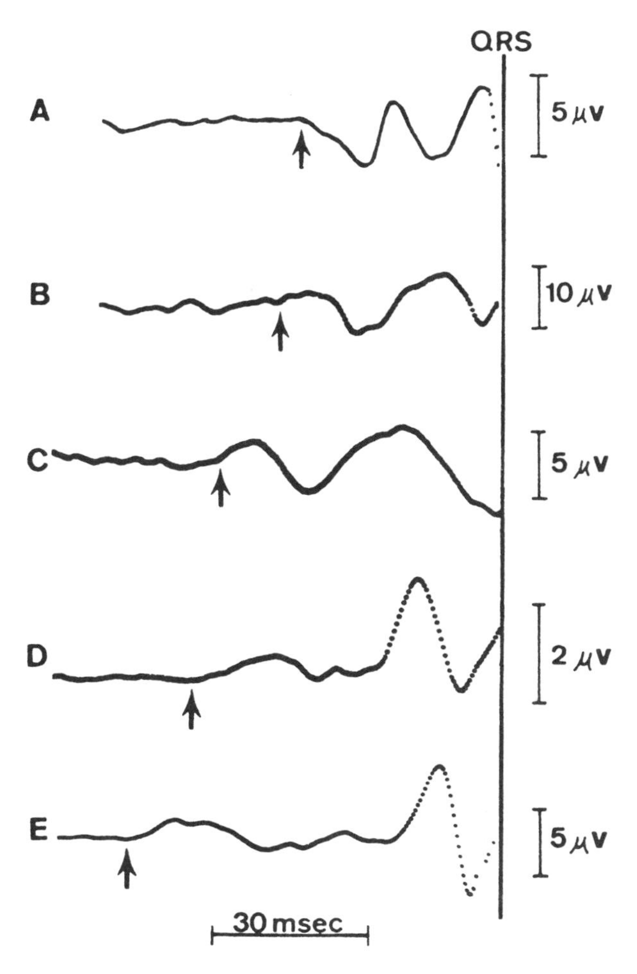

Figure 2-7. *SAL* recordings from five different patients. Each trace is aligned so that the onset of the *QRS* occurs at the solid vertical line on the right. Each recording is the result of averaging 300 cardiac cycles. The arrow points to a more clearly defined onset of the His-Purkinje system (*HPS*) waveform. The duration of the *HPS* waveform in traces *A*-*E* is 39, 43, 55, 60 and 72 msec, respectively. Panel *B* was obtained from a patient with atrial fibrillation, while the others are all from patients with first degree heart block. The voltage scale for each trace is shown opposite itself. (Reproduced with permission from Berbari, E.J., et al.: The His-Purkinje electrocardiogram in man: An initial assessment of its uses and limitations. *Circulation* 54: 219–224, 1976.)

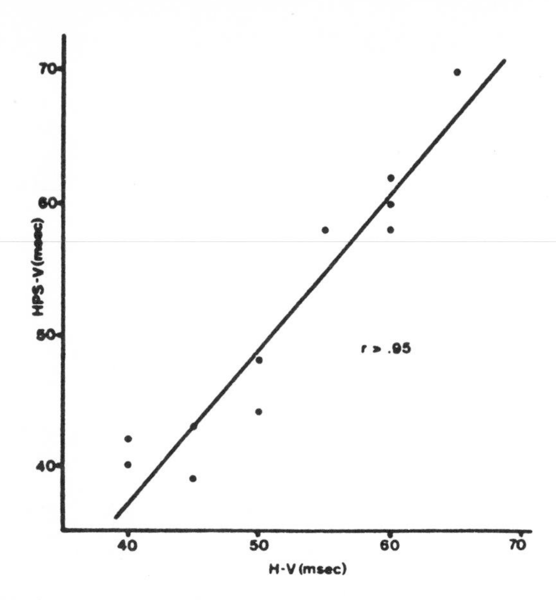

Figure 2-8. Graph comparing the *H-V* time and duration of the HPS waveform (HPS-V) from 11 patients. Each is a measure of ventricular conduction times. The correlation coefficient equals 0.953 and the regression line equation is $Y = 1.16\ X - 8.75$. (Reproduced with permission from *Proceedings of IEEE*, May 1977.)

portion of the His-Purkinje waveform. It should be noted in the patients described above that all were selected because of the presence of first degree heart block on the electrocardiogram. The selection was made to avoid the possible overlap and His-Purkinje system activity. Some method such as transesophageal atrial pacing may be required in order to solve this problem.

SUMMARY

The ability to detect those at risk for impending complete heart block has been aided with the establishment of the concept of biphasicular block and the application of invasive techniques to monitor the cardiac conduction time, specifically H-V intervals. The use of noninvasive techniques such as ambulatory monitoring, exercise stress tests and signal averaging may provide further diagnostic capabilities. With whatever means, the goal still remains to prevent Stokes-Adams attacks and sudden death due to paroxysmal A-V heart block.

REFERENCES

1. Katz, L.N., and Pick, A.: *Clinical Electrocardiography,* Part I. The Arrhythmias. Philadelphia, Lea and Febriger, 1956.
2. Hoffman, B.F., Amer, N.S., Stuckey, J.H., et al.: Activation of the interventricular septal myocardium studied during cardiopulmonary bypass. *Am. Heart J.* **59**: 224–237, 1960.
3. Hoffman, B.F., Cranefield, P.F., Stuckey, J.H., and Bagdonas, A.A.: Electrical activity during the P-R interval. *Circ. Res.* 8: 1200–1211, 1960.
4. Cranefield, P.F., and Hoffman, B.F.: The electrical activity of the heart and the electrocardiogram. *J. Electrocard.* **1**: 2–4, 1968.
5. Scherlag, B.J., Lau, S.H., Helfant, R.H., et al.: Catheter techniques for recording His bundle activity in man. *Circulation* **39**: 13–18, 1969.
6. Scherlag, B.J., Helfant, R.H., and Damato, A.N.,: Catheterization technique for His bundle stimulation and recording in the intact dog. *J. Appl. Physiol.* **25**: 425–428, 1968.
7. Damato, A.N., Lau, S.H., Helfant, R.H., et al.: Study of A-V conduction in man using electrode catheter recordings of His bundle activity. *Circulation* **39**: 287–296, 1969.
8. Narula, O.S., Scherlag, B.J., Javier, R.P., et al.: Analysis of the A-V conduction defect in complete heart block utilizing His bundle electrograms. *Circulation* **41**: 437, 1970.
9. Narula, O.S., Scherlag, B.J., Samet, P., and Javier, R.P.: A-V block: Localization and classification by His bundle recordings. *Am. J. Med.* **50**: 146–166, 1971.
10. El-Sherif, N., Scherlag, B.J., Lazzara, R., et al.: The pathophysiology of tachycardia-dependent paroxysmal A-V block after acute myocardial ischemia. Experimental and clinical observations. *Circulation* **50**:515–528, 1974.
11. Gallagher, J.J., Gilbert, M., Svenson, R.H., et al.: Wolff-Parkinson-White syndrome. The problem, evaluation and surgical correction. *Circulation* **51**: 83, 1975.
12. Narula, O.S., Gann, D., and Samet, P.: Prognostic value of H-V intervals. In Narula, O.S. (ed.): *His Bundle-Electrocardiography and Clinical Electrophysiology.* Philadelphia, F.A. Davis Co., 1975, Chapt. 20.
13. Scheinman, M., Weiss, A., and Kunkel, F.: His bundle recordings in patients with bundle branch block and transient neurological symptoms. *Circulation* **48**: 322, 1973.
14. Ranganathan, N., Dhurandhar, R., Phillips, J.H., and Wigle, E.D.: His bundle electrogram in bundle branch block. *Circulation* **48**: 282, 1972.
15. Vera, Z., Mason, D.T., Fletcher, R.D., et al.: Prolonged His-Q interval in chronic bifascicular block: Relation to impending complete heart block. *Circulation* **53**: 46–55, 1976.
16. Altschuler, H., Fisher, J.D., and Furman, S.: Prolonged H-V interval. Preventable early mortality in symptomatic patients without documented heart block. *Clin. Res.* **25**: 203A, 1977 (Abstr).
17. Denes, P., Dhingra, R.G., Wu, D., et al.: H-V interval in patients with bifascicular block (Right bundle branch block and left anterior hemiblock). *Am. J. Cardiol.* **35**: 23–28, 1975.

18. Lie, K.I., Wellens, H.J., Schuilenberg, R.M., et al.: Factors influencing prognosis of bundle branch block complicating acute anteroseptal infarction. *Circulation* **50**: 935–941, 1974.
19. Lichstein, E., Gupta, K.D., Chadda, H., et al.: Findings of prognostic value in patients with incomplete bilateral bundle branch block complicating acute myocardial infarction. *Am. J. Cardiol.* **32**: 913, 1977.
20. Ginks, W.R., Sutton, R., Winston, O.H, and Leatham, A.: Long-term prognosis after acute anterior infarction with atrioventricular block. *Br. Heart J.* **39**: 186–189, 1977.
21. Norris, R.M., Mercer, C.J., and Croxson, M.S.: Conduction disturbances due to anteroseptal myocardial infarction and their treatment by endocardial pacing. *Am. Heart J.* **81**: 560, 1972.
22. Godman, M.J., Lasser, W.D., and Julian, D.J.: Complete bundle branch block complicating acute myocardial infarction. *N. Eng. J. Med.* **282**: 237, 1970.
23. Dreifus, L.S.: Clinical judgement is sufficient for the management of conduction defects. In Corday, E. (ed.): *Controversies in Cardiology.* Philadelphia, F.A. Davis Co., 1977, pp. 195–201.
24. Berbari, E.J., Lazzara, R., and Scherlag, B.J.: Surface recording technique for detecting electrical activity during the P-R segment. *Am. J. Cardiol.* **31**: 120, 1973.
25. Flowers, N.C., Hand, R.C., Orander, P.C., et al.: Surface recording of electrical activity from the region of the bundle of His. *Am. J. Cardiol.* **33**: 384, 1974.
26. Stopozyk, M.J., Kopec, J., Zochowski, R.J., and Pieniak, M.: Surface recording of electrical heart activity during the P-R segment in man by a computer averaging technique. *Proc. World Cong. Cardiol.* **#162**, 1974 (Abstr).
27. Furness, A., Sharratt, G.P., and Carson, P.: The feasibility of detecting His bundle activity from the body surface. *Cardiovasc. Res.* **9**: 390, 1975.
28. Hishmoto, Y., and Sawayama, T.: Non-invasive recording of His bundle potential in man. *Br. Heart J.* **37**: 635, 1975.
29. Scherlag, B.J., Abelleira, J.L., and Samet, P.: Electrode catheter recording from the His bundle and left bundle in the intact dog. In Kao, F.F., Koizumi, K., and Vassalle, M. (eds.): *Research in Physiology.* Bologna, Italy, Aulo Gaggi, Editore, 1971, pp. 223–238.
30. Berbari, E.J., Lazzara, R., El-Sherif, N., and Scherlag, B.J.: Extracardiac recordings of His-Purkinje activity during conduction disorders and junctional rhythms. *Circulation* **51**: 802–810, 1975.
31. Berbari, E.J., Scherlag, B.J., El-Sherif, N., et al.: The His-Purkinje electrocardiogram in man: An initial assessment of its uses and limitations. *Circulation* **54**: 219–224, 1976.

3

Anatomic Basis of Cardiac Arrhythmias

Lino Rossi, M.D.

The current approach to pathophysiology of cardiac arrhythmias attempts to overcome a sharp differentiation between disturbances in impulse formation and conduction.[1]

The mechanism of decremental conduction and unidirectional block in single or groups of myocardial fibers results in re-entry which could be responsible for arrhythmias which were formerly regarded as due to increased automaticity. The classical debate of mechanisms of ectopic automatic focus and local impulse re-entry might become just a different way to look at the same phenomenon.

Newer trends in cardiac electrophysiology may have a bearing on histopathology of arrhythmias. At the site of the traditional focal lesion, responsible for disturbances in impulse formation or conduction (or both), local inhomogenity of cardiac muscle in areas of junction may play a role in arrhythmia production. In homogeneous myocardial structures, normal or pathological, seem to correlate with electrophysiological inhomogeneity of cardiac tissue, by asynchronous repolarization or asymmetrical depression of conductivity, that are basic mechanisms for dysrhythmias, namely, re-entry. The products of abnormal muscular connections between atria and ventricles, within and outside the conducting system, deserve the utmost attention as a possible background for re-entrant arrhythmias, and not only for classical ventricular pre-excitation.

The importance of morphologic studies for a better understanding of arrhythmias has been stressed by the author for a long time.[2–5]

MATERIAL AND METHODS

One hundred hearts were examined from necropsies of subjects who had exhibited disturbances in impulse formation and/or conduction grouped according to electrocardiographic diagnosis of arrhythmias. The histologic evaluation included serial section of the conducting system, together with evaluation of other tissues within the heart.[5]

Although the classification follows current criteria,[6] a discussion of questions in nomenclature of cardiac arrhythmias is beyond this presentation.

Regarding the anatomoclinical correlation between tissue damage and dysrhythmias, conduction disturbances in particular, the only sound criterion was total and irreversible anatomic interruption versus complete and permanent functional impairment. Whenever partial, irreversible tissue lesions are correlated with complete or incomplete functional block such as in a case of reversible lesions with transient dysfunction, a close clinicopathological correlation becomes difficult. Sophisticated histo-statistical techniques[7,8] can help if the lesions are well delineated, such as sclerosis or atrophy. In case of widespread, reversible changes (degenerative, inflammatory, or necrotic) only conjectural arguments can be made in relation to arrhythmias.

Dealing with neuropathological evidence (collected on the sinoatrial [SA] node's plexus, mostly), one cannot expect anatomoclinical comparisons as comprehensive and precise as those one is accustomed to in the domain of conducting system and blocks. This evidence, nevertheless, allows for some anatomic information available on abnormalities of the sinoatrial node.[2–4]

Rate Disturbances

Sinus tachycardia (two cases) is influenced by neural abnormalities involving the perinodal ganglionated plexus, but sparing the sinoatrial node and the inner nerve network. In pronounced sinus bradycardia (two cases), changes of the sinoatrial node and atrial connections are prominent, as seen in other sinoatrial disorders such as sick sinus node syndrome. This disorder is manifested by extensive homogeneous disruption of the atrial subepicardial nerve plexuses. Sinus tachycardia seems to show comparatively milder abnormalities than those recorded in cases of focal inhomogeneous damage to the sinoatrial node nerve supply. Asymmetric abnormalities of neural autonomic control of heart action may play a role in serious rhythm disturbances.[2]

ECTOPIC RHYTHMS

Neuromyocardial lesions inside and around the sinoatrial node and its approaches have been found in the present 12 cases of AV junctional rhythm or escape and other multifocal rhythms. Some of the abnormalities mentioned can also be found in more complex disturbances in atrial impulse formation and conduction; namely, the sick sinus node syndrome.[25]

Specific myocardial and intrinsic nervous lesions have been observed in five cases of supraventricular and in four of ventricular paroxysmal tachycardias. The finding of normal and pathologic inhomogeneity (AV nodal type "star cells" and inflammatory focus) in the common bundle in one case, and of an accessory septo-septal AV bundle in another case shows morphologically that re-entry in paroxysmal tachycardias, by either junctional or bundle-branch circus movement, can occur. In one case of right atrial ectopic tachycardia (prolonged), operated upon, it was demonstrated that a focus of abnormally heightened automaticity had taken over pacemaking and provoked continuous tachycardia, despite a normal sinoatrial node. These spontaneously firing "pacemaker" myocells[9,10] in this focus, close to but not coincident with an inflammatory nodule, were morphologically identical with common atrial myocardium.

Automatic and re-entrant impulses should be regarded as basically different mechanisms for tachydysrhythmias. The common anatomic bases (accessory AV pathways) of some re-entrant tachycardia and pre-excitation, and the existence of cases of "concealed pre-excitation syndrome" that only exhibit bouts of supraventricular tachyarrhythmias can be demonstrated histologically [11] (Fig. 3-1). Ventricular tachycardia (four cases) seems to accompany severe impairments in impulse formation and conduction (multiple blocking lesions of the AV pathway).[12] In torsade de pointes, the typical QRS axis coiling might imply septal re-entry encompassing part of the bundle branches;[13] moreover, recent findings of torsades-like patterns of ventricular dysrhythmias from an autonomic neural mechanism[14] with or without QT interval prolongation, have been published.

ATRIAL AND VENTRICULAR FIBRILLATION (AND FLUTTER)

The pathologic features of atrial fibrillation seem to vary from case to case, independently of onset and duration. In our 23 cases, the incidence of severe changes of the sinoatrial nodal cells was not as high as one could expect,[16,17] and that of local neuroganglionic abnormalities averaged 50 percent. Pericardial and subepicardial inflammation, from chronic rheumatic heart disease mostly in the region of the sinoatrial node, crista

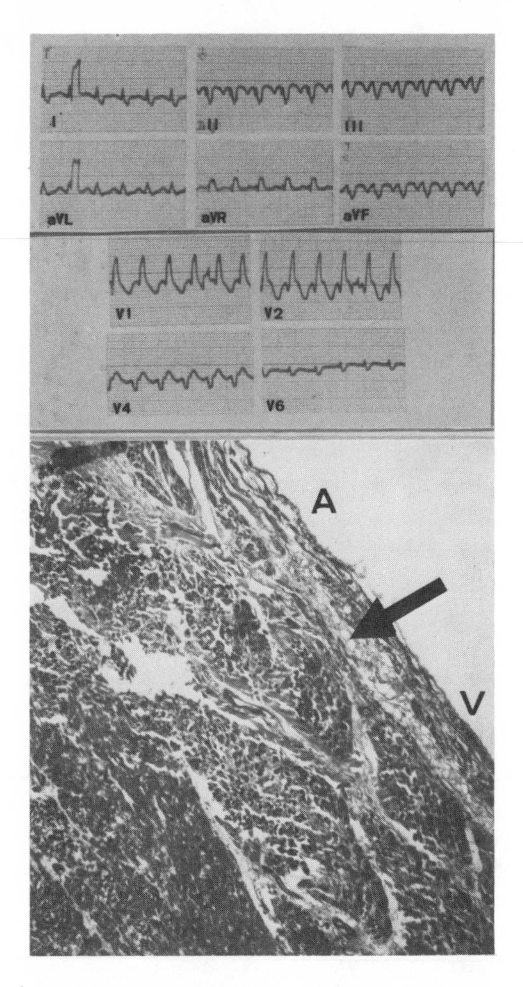

Figure 3-1. Supraventricular paroxysmal tachycardia, without pre-excitation syndrome: an AV septo-septal accessory bundle of Kent (arrow). (Haematoxylin-eosin; x 25)

terminalis and intercaval bridge have been noted. Reciprocating (circus movement) atrial fibrillation has been seen in a case of pre-excitation syndrome, with a lateral accessory AV connection; likewise, the re-entry mechanism of atrial flutter has been suggested.[18] Ventricular fibrillation was associated with extremely severe injury of the conducting and working myocardium, such as early infarction, massive sarcoidosis, etc. Patchy myofibrillar degeneration with contraction bands was seen, occasionally, in common myocardium on acute infarction, but never in adjacent specific fibers (Fig. 3-2). The inference that a sympathetic (catecholamine-induced) mechanism for producing this type of degeneration is capable of producing ventricular fibrillation in experimental cardiac ischemia [19,20] has opened a promising trend in anatomoclinical study of arrhythmias.

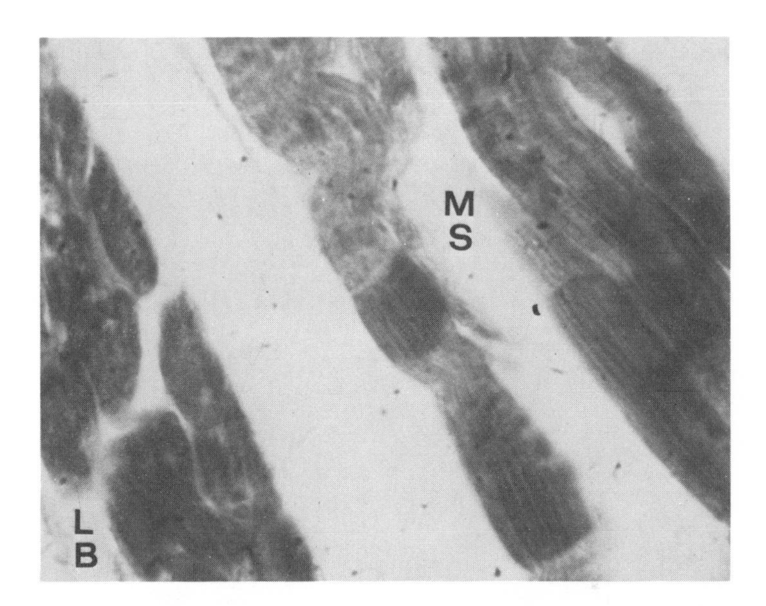

Figure 3-2. Ventricular fibrillation in early myocardial infarction: myofibrillar degeneration with contraction bands in common myocardium of the ventricular septum (MS), alongside well preserved fibres of the left bundle branch (LB). (Azan; x 500)

SINOATRIAL BLOCK AND SICK SINUS SYNDROME

Sinoatrial block and/or bradycardia alternating with bursts of ectopic tachycardias merge into the composite features of so-called "sick sinus syndrome"[21] or sinoatrial disorder[22] (Fig. 3-3). The diagnostic aspects have been widely discussed.[23,24] Similar pathological involvement can underlie several types of atrial arrhythmias; in sick sinus syndrome, however, an ischemic background tends to be less common[22] and is usually associated with abnormalities of other parts of the conduction system.

In five cases studied, lesions other than those of the specific myocardium of the sinus node, underlying so-called sick sinus syndrome, have occurred; they are neural changes of the perinodal ganglionated plexus (Fig. 3-4) and/or damage to the atrial approaches to the sinoatrial node.

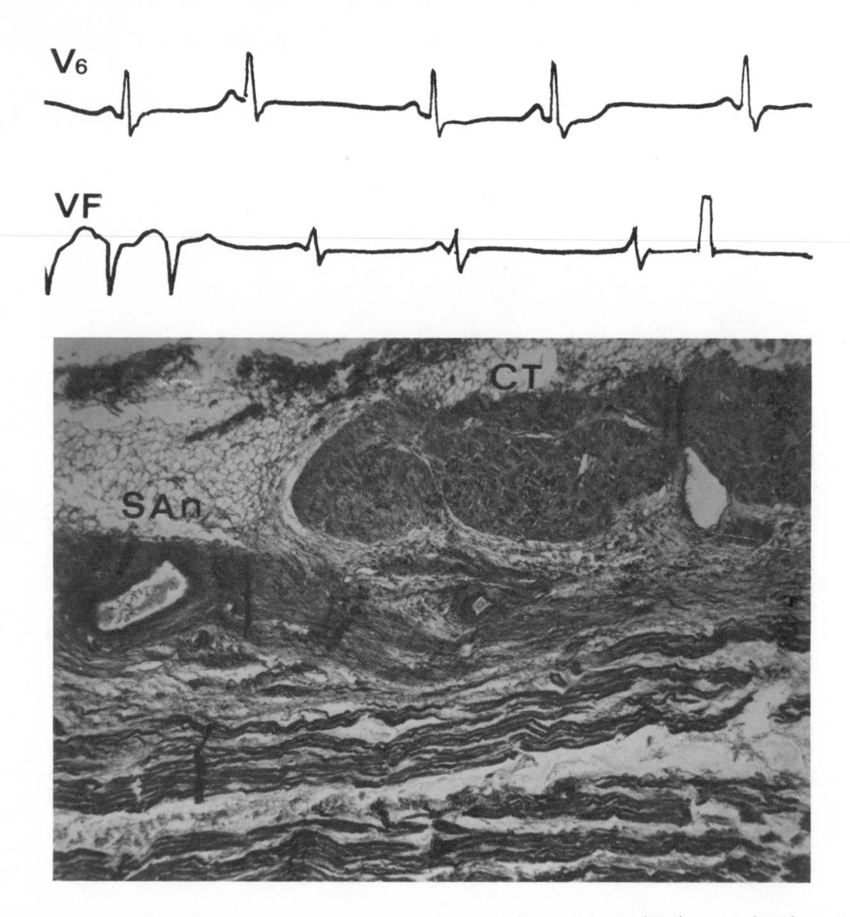

Figure 3-3. Sick Sinus Syndrome with sinoatrial 2:1 block (V6), and (VF) end of a burst of supraventricular tachycardia followed by junctional beats: hypotrophic sinoatrial node (SAn), with pronounced sclerosis of crista terminalis (CT) and atrial approaches. (Azan; x 12)

The involvement of crista terminalis in sinoatrial disorders has also been found. The crista terminalis not only correlates anatomically with Thorel's posterior internodal tract, but also exhibits, in experimental neurophysiology, peculiar effects from sympathetic stimulation.[26] Hence, the sick sinus syndrome may show juxta-nodal nervous and/or myocardial lesions,[27] and not only on disease of sinoatrial node-specific tissue. In general, intrinsic sinoatrial node dysfunction is accompanied by disturbances in neural regulation of sinoatrial node function.[28]

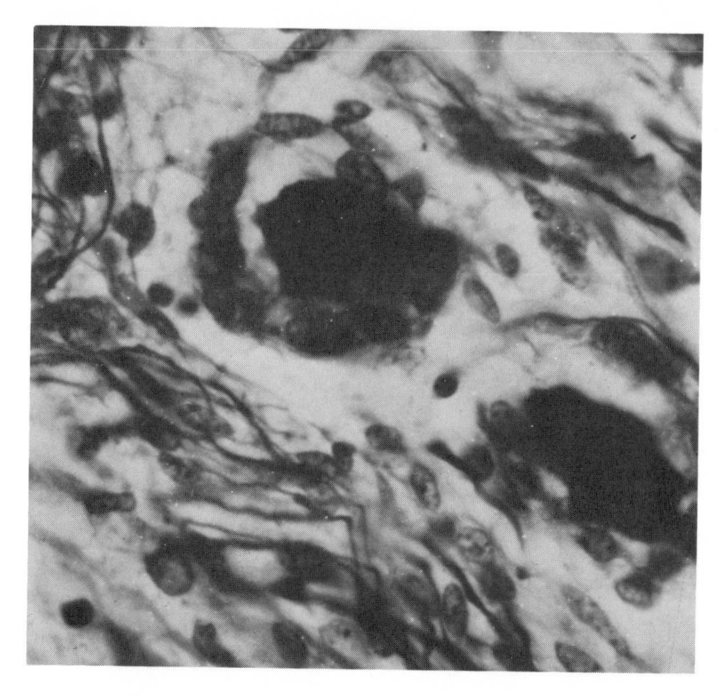

Figure 3-4. Pathological proliferation of capsular cells close to the neuronal body, in a ganglion of the sinoatrial plexus, from a case of Sick Sinus Syndrome. (Bielschowsky; x 850)

ATRIOVENTRICULAR BLOCK

Anatomoclinical correlation in cases of AV block are focused upon two major problems: The etiology draws a high incidence of a "primary or idiopathic" disease of the conducting system (Fig. 3-5) and the clinical diagnosis can demonstrate the location and severity of the blocking lesions by new catheter recording techniques which can locate the block at levels above, within, and below the bundle of His and by standard electrocardiography as Mobitz-Wenckebach type I and II. As far as etiology is concerned, Davies[29] endorses Lenegre-Lev's thesis of a frequent "primary" nonatherosclerotic conduction system disease[30,31] in sharp contrast with Knieriem-Finke's data,[32] which support the traditional concept of the frequent ischemic-dystrophic cause of conducting system blockage. Besides these opposing viewpoints, the hypothesis was recently put forward[33] that senile coronary arteriosclerosis can easily bring about atrophy and sclerocalcification of the myocardium of the ventricular septum crest (Fig. 3-5). Since the vascularity of the latter is

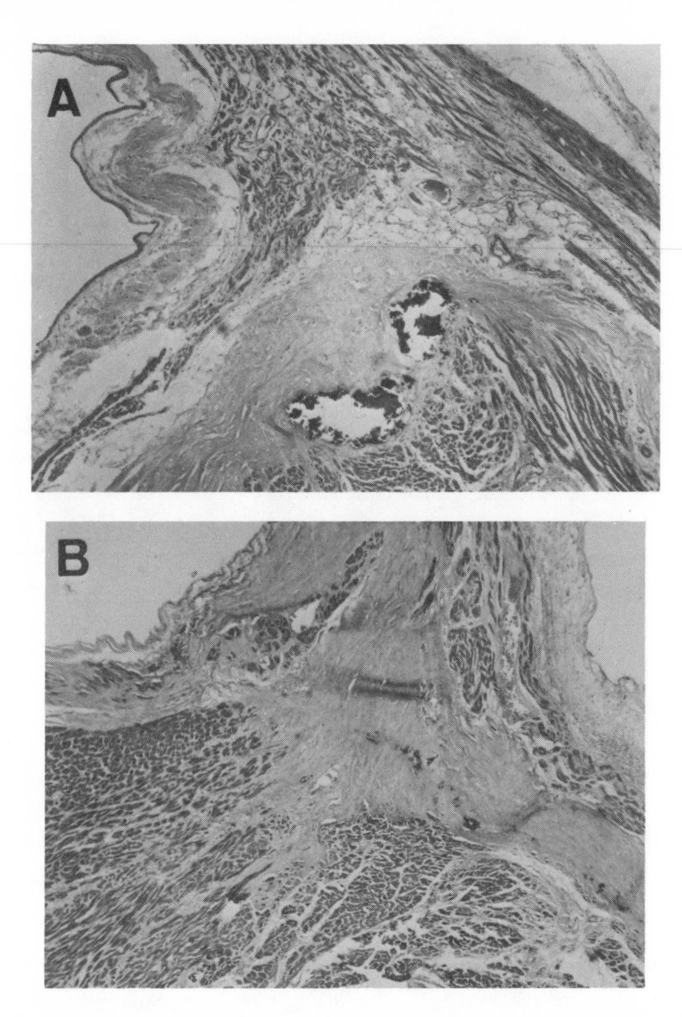

Figure 3–5. So-called "idiopathic or primary disease" affecting the conducting system: sclerocalcification of the upper ventricular septum, either sparing (*A*) or involving (*B*) the branching portion of His bundle, with AV block. (Haematoxylin-eosin; x 25)

normally very poor,[34] stretch and compression of the AV bundle, bifurcation and upper bundle branches against the hardened septal spur can result in local atrophy of specific myofibers ("tertiary in nature"). In our 40 cases, coronary atherosclerosis was significant in 17.5 percent.[5] In a series of 400 clinicopathological correlations from the literatue,[18] heart block from primary idiopathic and/or coronary disease was found in 65 percent. In Knieriem-Finke's 100 cases[32] the ratio between primary and coronary disease was about 1 to 77. In the whole group of 400 cases (besides the above mentioned 65 percent of primary ischemic AV block) the following incidence was found: cardiomyopathy 4 percent, tumors (cardiac epitheliome in particular) 4 percent, valvular disease 10 percent, endomyocarditis 4 percent, congenital abnormalities 4 percent, surgery 3 percent, syphillis 1 percent, amyloidosis 1 percent, collagen disease (lupus erythematosus[35] and panarteritis nodosa[36] in particular) 3 percent, and miscellaneous disease groups of 2 percent including diphtheria, sarcoidosis, tuberculosis, tetanus, lymphangitis, siderosis, etc.

As far as location of the lesions, the frequency of AV block-producing lesions seems to increase in a downward direction along the conducting system; the quoted 400 observations showed lesions of both bundle branches and/or bifurcation in about 70 percent of cases, of the common His bundle in 15 percent, of the AV node in 10 percent and of atrio-AV nodal approach in 5 percent. In our series, the incidence of proximal damage was slightly higher (atrio-AV nodal approaches 11 percent, AV node 14 percent). Among AV blocks from supraventricular origin, those showing disruption of atrio-AV nodal connections, or higher up, deserve attention. In rare cases either no blocking lesions were found, or the left bundle branch alone was altered.[5,30,32] Also in some cases apparently established AV block disappeared despite the presence of significant lesions of the AV pathway.[5,37,38]

Clinicopathological correlations of severity of lesions in incomplete AV block, judged by surface electrocardiograms, were not revealing in as much as second and first degree AV blocks often fail to exhibit any substantial differences in conducting tissue damage. Neither could histology account for the current belief [1,39] that Wenckebach-Mobitz type I, second-degree AV block should be due to milder changes of the AV pathway than type II.

Regarding correlations between histopathological findings and His bundle electrographic recording of AV blocks (three cases in our series), doubts can be cast upon the correlation between intra-hisian conduction impairment and the so-called "split His potential" which have been recorded in one case with normal His bundle and partially fibrotic bifurcation. In another case, prolonged A-H interval (with Wenckebach phenomenon) was present, showing pronounced atrophy of His bundle and bifurcation. A reduction in number of specific fibers of the His bundle is, apparently, not well correlated with "split His", and with intra-hisian block, as suggested by some.[40] Something still escapes a clearcut correlation between physiologic recordings and histologic findings.

BUNDLE BRANCH BLOCK

The morphological background of bundle branch block (BBB) is more difficult to assess than that of AV block, although the etiological factors seem to be fairly similar. The electrocardiographic-anatomic correlation between diagnostic patterns of unilateral BBB and histologic disruption of the homologous bundle branch is clinically poorly correlated pathologically. In the present 20 cases, as well as in cases from the literature,[5] it is difficult to equate the amount of disease in both branches underlying the ECG patterns of conduction impairment in a single branch alone.[41]

When significant lesions are found, in chronic complete right bundle branch block (RBBB) fibroelastic replacement of the specific myocardium in the second portion of the right bundle prevails in comparison with lesions of the first or third part of it. In chronic complete left bundle branch block, the damage quite often consists of a fine fibrosing atrophy of the individual fibers of the root of the left bundle which can be related to pathology of the so-called "primary disease" of the conducting system. Lesions of the common bundle have been suggested to bring about unilateral bundle branch block whenever a precocious partition can be demonstrated, in the proximal AV junction of specific fibers destined to each bundle branch.[42] Finally, cases of complete bundle branch block on standard electrocardiograms can reveal incomplete block in electrical stimulation studies.[43]

The modern outlook of bundle branch block encompasses the concept of Rosenbaum,[44] based upon the assumption of a "trifascicular" nature of what has been hitherto considered the Tawarin "bifurcation", by constant splitting of the left bundle branch into two main ramifications, at the side of the undivided segment. Along with this thesis, eleven different types of blocks can occur by isolated or combined conduction impairments in the "trifurcated" branchings of the AV system. Out of these varieties of block, which are an interesting matter of clinical electrophysiology, only the so-called left bundle branch hemiblocks or fascicular blocks are relevant to histopathological discussion.

HEMI- (OR FASCICULAR) BLOCKS; BILATERAL BUNDLE BRANCH BLOCK

The concept and term of left hemiblock, either anterior (LAH) or posterior (LPH), rely on the anatomofunctional assumption of a bifurcation of the left bundle branch into anterior and posterior fascicles, and on the inferred "trilaterality" of the conducting system.[44] By postulating isolated blockade of the anterior or of the posterior "half" of the left branch (LAH and LPH, respectively), whether or not combined with

RBBB (bilateral BBB), quick and easy answers can be given to debated questions in intraventricular conduction impairments and axis deviations.[44–46]

Heavy doubts on the alleged organic basis of hemiblocks were cast by three main arguments: (1) Anatomically, a definite bifurcation of the LBB, in man, is uncommon; the branch is known to fan out, mostly, into three distal strands (anterior, middle, and posterior)[47–49] that are richly anastomosed to one another, making it difficult to draw any exact anatomofunctional delimitation.[46] (2) Physiologically, in the human heart, left ventricular activation initiates simultaneously in three septoparaseptal areas,[50] which suggests a tri- and not a bipartitioned impulse distribution. (3) Clinicophysiological studies[51] also suggest the possibility of sorting out conduction disturbances of the midseptal group of LBB fibers. From the pathological viewpoint, the changes of the left bundle in left anterior hemiblock and left posterior hemiblock with or without RBBB[42,52] histologically do not correlate with lesions found. Eleven such cases were studied in this series.

However, until better anatomoclinical correlations can be established, the diagnosis of hemi- or fascicular block can well be retained for practical purposes with a caution that further histologic studies are necessary.

REFERENCES

1. Katz, A.M.: *Physiology of the Heart*. New York, Raven Press, 1977.
2. James, T.N.: De subitaneis mortibus XXVIII. Apoplexy of the heart. *Circulation* **57**: 385, 1978.
3. Randall, W.C.: *Neural Regulation of the Heart*. New York, Oxford University Press, 1977.
4. Coumel, P., Attuel, P., Lavellée, J., et al.: Syndrome d'arythmie auriculaire d'origine vagale. *Arch. Mal. Coeur* **71**: 645, 1978.
5. Rossi, L.: *Histopathologic Features of Cardiac Arrhythmias*. Milan, Casa Editrice Ambrosiana, 1969.
6. WHO/ISC Task Force: Definition of terms related to cardiac rhythm. *Am. Heart J.* **95**: 796, 1978.
7. Davies, M.J., and Pomerance, A.: Quantitative study of ageing changes in the human sinuatrial node and internodal tracts. *Br. Heart J.* **34**: 150, 1972.
8. Demoulin J.C., Simar L.J., and Kulbertus H.E.: Quantitative study of left bundle branch fibrosis in left anterior hemiblock: a stereologic approach. *Am. J. Cardiol.* **36**: 751, 1975.
9. Ferroni, A.: *Le basi biologiche della medicina moderna*, 2nd vol., Torino, Ed. Medico-Scientifiche, 1976, p. 265.
10. Salerno, J.A., Chimienti, M., Viganò M., Ferroni A., Tavazzi L., Rossi L., and Bobba P.: Atrial tachycardia: surgical ablation of the ectopic focus

after epicardial mapping. 1st Joint Meeting of the working groups E.S.C., Brighton, June, 1978 (in press).

11. Barold, S.S., and Coumel, P.: Mechanism of atrioventricular junctional tachycardia. Role of re-entry and concealed accessory bypass tracts. *Am. J. Cardiol.* **39**: 97, 1977.
12. Krikler, D.M., and Curry, P.V.L.: Torsade de pointes, an atypical ventricular tachycardia. *Br. Heart J.* **38**: 117, 1976.
13. Rossi, L., and Matturri, L.: Histopathological findings in two cases of torsade de pointes with conduction disturbances. *Br. Heart J.* **38**: 1312, 1976.
14. Coumel, P., Fidelle, J., Lucet, V., et al.: Catecholamine induced severe ventricular arrhythmias with Adams-Stokes syndrome in children: report of four cases. *Br. Heart J.* **40 (Suppl.)**: 28, 1978.
15. Schwartz, P.J., and Malliani, A.: Electrical alteration of the T wave: clinical and experimental evidence of its relationship with the sympathetic nervous system and with the long Q-T syndrome. *Am. Heart J.* **89**: 45, 1975.
16. Hudson, R.E.B.: The human pacemaker and its pathology. *Br. Heart J.* **22**: 153, 1960.
17. Davies, M.J., and Pomerance, A.: Pathology of atrial fibrillation in man. *Br. Heart J.* **34**: 520, 1972.
18. Rossi, L.: *Histopathology of Cardiac Arrhythmias,* 2nd ed. Milan, Casa Editrice Ambrosiana, 1978.
19. Reichenbach, D.D., and Moss, N.S.: Myocardial cell necrosis and sudden death in humans. *Circulation* **52 (Suppl. III)**: 60, 1975.
20. Lazzara, R., El-Sherif, N., and Scherlag, B.J.: Electrophysiological properties of canine Purkinje cells in one-day-old myocardial infarction. *Circ. Res.* **33**: 722, 1973.
21. Ferrer, I.: The sick sinus syndrome in atrial disease. *J.A.M.A.* **206**: 645, 1968.
22. Evans, R., and Shaw, D.B.: Pathological background of sinoatrial disorder (Sick Sinus Syndrome). *Br. Heart J.* **39**: 778, 1977.
23. Breithardt, G.: Funktionsanalyse des Sinusknotens. In Seipel, L.: *His Bündel-Elektrographie und intrakardiale Stimulation.* Stuttgart, Thieme, 1978.
24. Lotto, A., and Finzi, A.: La malattia atriale. In *Le emergenze in cardiologia.* Roma, Pozzi, 1975, p. 87.
25. Rasmussesn, K.: Chronic sinoatrial heart block. *Am. Heart J.* **81**: 38, 1971.
26. Hoffman, B.F.: Neural influences on cardiac electrical excitability and rhythm. In Randall, W.C. (ed.): *Neural Regulation of the Heart,* New York, Oxford University Press, 1977, p. 289 ff.
27. Kulbertus, H.E., and Demoulin, J.C.: The conduction system: Anatomical and pathological aspects. In Krikler, D.M., and Goodwin, J.F. (eds.): *Cardiac Arrhythmias.* London, W.B. Saunders Co., 1975, p. 16 ff.
28. Jordan, J.J., Yamaguchi, I., and Mandel, W.J.,: Studies on the mechanism of sinus node dysfunction in the Sick Sinus Syndrome. *Circulation* **57**: 217, 1978.
29. Davies, M.J.: The conduction system in permanent acquired conduction disturbances. In Pomerance, A., and Davies, M.J. (eds.): *Pathology of the Heart.* Oxford, Blackwell, 1975, p. 392 ff.

30. Lenègre, J.: Les blocs auriculo-ventriculaires complets chroniques. Etude des causes et des lesions à propos de 37 cas. *Mal. Cadiovas.* 3: 311, 1962.
31. Lev, M.: Anatomic basis for atrioventricular block. *Am. J. Med.* 37: 742, 1964.
32. Knieriem, H.J, and Finke, E.: *Morphologie und Aetiologie des totalen A.V. Blocks.* München, Urban & Schwarzenberg, 1974.
33. Demoulin, J.C., Rossi, L., and Kulbertus, H.E.: In Krikler, B.M., and Goodwin, J.F. (eds.): *Cardiac Arrhythmias. The Modern Electrophysiological Approach.* edited by Krikler B.M., and Goodwin J.F. London, W.B. Saunders Co., 1975, p. 28.
34. Van der Hauwaert, L.G., Stroombandt, R., and Werhaege, L.: Arterial blood supply of the atrioventricular node and main bundle. *Br. Heart J.* 34: 1045, 1972.
35. Lev, M.: The pathogenesis of atrioventricular block. In Dreifus L.S., and Likoff, W. (eds.): *Cardiac Arrhythmias.* New York, Grune & Stratton, 1973, pp. 253 ff.
36. Thiene, G., Valente, M.L., and Rossi, L.: Involvement of the conducting system in panarteritis nodosa. *Am. Heart J.* 95: 716, 1978.
37. Rosen, K.M. Wu, D., Kanakis, C., et al.: Return of normal conduction after paroxysmal heart block: report of a case with major discordance of electrophysiological and pathological findings. *Circulation* 51: 197, 1975.
38. Reid, J.M., Coleman, E.N., and Doig, W.: Reversion to sinus rhythm 11 years after surgically induced heart block. *Br. Heart J.* 38: 1217, 1976.
39. Narula, O.S.: *His Bundle Electrocardiography and Clinical Electrophysiology.* Philadelphia, F.A. Davis, 1975.
40. Puech, P.: Atrioventricular block: value of intracardiac recordings. In Krickler, D.M., and Goodwin, J.F. (eds.): *Cardiac Arrhythmias: The Modern Electrophysiological Approach.* London, W.B. Saunders, 1975, p. 81 ff.
41. Lev, M., Unger, P.N., Rosen, K.M., and Bharati S.: The anatomic substrate of complete left bundle branch block. *Circulation* 50: 479, 1974.
42. Sciacca, A.: *Le basi anatomiche dei blocchi atrioventricolari.* Atti 25° Congr. Soc. Ital. Cardiol., vol. II, Roma, 1964.
43. Seipel, L., Breithardt, G., and Kuhn, H.: Left bundle branch block in patients with and without cardiomyopathy. In Kaltenbach, M., Loogen, F., and Olsen, E.G.J. (eds.): *Cardiomyopathy and Myocardial Biopsy.* Berlin, Springer Verlag, 1978, p. 237 ff.
44. Rosenbaum, M.B.: The hemiblocks: diagnostic criteria and clinical significance. *Mod. Concept. Cardiovasc. Dis.* 39: 141, 1970.
45. Watt, T.B., Jr., Murao, S., and Pruitt, R.D.: Left axis deviation induced experimentally in a primate heart. *Am. Heart J.* 70: 381, 1965.
46. Blondeau, M., and Lenègre, J.: *Bloc atypique de la branche droite.* Paris. Masson, 1970.
47. Rossi, L.: Histopathology of conducting system in left anterior hemiblock. *Br. Heart J.* 38: 1304, 1976.
48. Rizzon, P., Rossi, L., Baissus, C., et al.: Left posterior hemiblock in acute myocardial infarction *Br. Heart J.* 37: 711, 1975.

49. Hecht, H.H., Kossmann, C.E., Childers, C.E., Atrioventricular and intraventricular conduction. Revised nomenclature and concepts. *Am. J. Cardiol.* **31**: 232, 1973.
50. Durrer, D., van Dam, R.T., Freud, G.E., et al.: Total excitation of the isolated human heart. *Circulation* **41**: 899, 1970.
51. Kulbertus, H.: Contribution à l'etude des blocs segmentaires de la branche gauche du faisceau de His et de leurs associations avec le bloc de branche droite. Thèse, Université de Liège, 1972.
52. Rossi, L.: The anatomical basis of hemiblock. *Cardiology Today* **6** n.3: 5, 1978.

4

Mode of Action of Antiarrhythmic Agents

Henri E. Kulbertus, M.D.

Vaughan-Williams'[1] widely accepted classification of antiarrhythmic agents[1] is based upon experimental electrophysiological observations made on isolated cardiac muscle. In this symposium, Touboul[2] presents another approach and divides drugs according to their electrophysiological effects studied in man by intracardiac electrocardiography and programmed electrical stimulation of the heart.

In spite of the existence of these classifications, one must admit that it is extremely difficult in a given case to decide the exact mechanism by which a drug can terminate an arrhythmia or prevent its recurrence. At present, antiarrhythmic drug therapy remains almost entirely empirical and cannot yet become scientifically rational.[3]

In the following paragraphs, we should like to indicate how complex the situation is, at least on a theoretical basis. The genesis of arrhythmias is generally considered to be due either to (1) enhanced automaticity (i.e., increase in the rate of phase 4 depolarization) or to (2) reentry.

ENHANCED AUTOMATICITY

An antiarrhythmic agent can influence a focus of enhanced automaticity in different ways: (1) The drug may suppress or decrease the slope of phase 4 depolarization and thus suppress the arrhythmia or reduce the rate of firing of the automatic focus. This is produced by class I antiarrhythmic agents.

(2) The drug may, in addition to a slowing of phase 4, displace the threshold potential towards zero, thus making it more difficult for the automatic focus to manifest its presence. This effect is also obtained with class I agents.

(3) The drug may, finally, in addition to its effects on phase 4, increase the resting membrane potential of the cell which, in fact, produces the same results as a slowing of diastolic depolarization. This effect has, for example, been observed with diphenylhydantoin at low potassium concentrations. Thus, even with this very simple model, it appears that the mechanism of action of antiarrhythmic drugs may be multifaceted.

REENTRY

The situation is still more complex in the presence of reentry (Fig. 4-1). A review of the problem has recently been published by M. Rosen.[4] We shall summarize it as follows. Reentry depends on a fine balance between abnormal conduction and refractoriness. The theoretical means for abolishing it are several. For successful pharmacotherapy, it is necessary (1) to improve antegrade conduction through a depressed segment of the conduction system so as to permit its effective participation in antegrade activation; (2) or to further depress conduction to produce bidirectional block and failure of both antegrade and retrograde conduction; (3) or to prolong refractoriness in some segments of the reentrant loop so as to interrupt the propagation of impulses along the circuit.

Improving Conduction

To improve conduction a drug would have, for example, to hyperpolarize depressed cardiac fibers with low resting membrane potential. By hyperpolarizing such fibers, their action potential could develop increased amplitude and upstroke velocity and thus be better conducted. Hyperpolarization of depressed cardiac fibers has been observed with epinephrine, lidocaine, diphenylhydantoin and digitalis.

Depressed conduction in cells of the His-Purkinje system can also result from initiation of the action potential at a low level of resting membrane potential due to marked phase 4 depolarization. By slowing the slope of phase 4 (lidocaine, quinidine, procaine-amide, diphenylhydantoin, beta-blockers), the action potential may be initiated at a higher level of membrane potential than before and may thus have better amplitude and upstroke velocity. This would improve conduction.

Conduction blockade can finally be the result of an abnormally long duration of the action potential in cells of a segment of the His-Purkinje system. Premature beats falling before the end of the refractory period may not be transmitted through this segment. Drugs producing shortening of action potential duration (lidocaine, diphenylhydantoin, propranolol) may thus improve conduction through this segment.

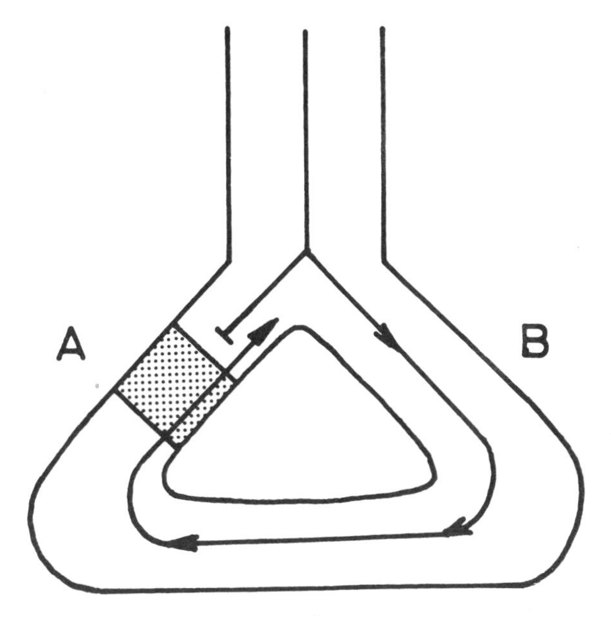

Figure 4-1. Schematic representation of a reentrant loop.
This represents a distal portion of the His-Purkinje system. The dotted area is depressed and the site of unidirectional block. The impulse can only proceed along segment B. When it reaches the distal end of segment A, the latter is excitable and thus a reentrant circuit can be initiated.

Depressing Conduction

Bidirectional block in a depressed segment can be obtained by drugs which either further depolarize the cells or lengthen the duration of their action potential (quinidine, procaine-amide).

Action on Refractoriness

Pharmacological agents used for the treatment of cardiac arrhythmias might, in some cases, act by prolonging refractoriness in some fibers (normal or depressed) of the reentrant loop.

Therapy of Arrhythmias

Unrelated to Enhanced Automaticity or Reentry

It has recently been hypothesized that mechanisms other than focal automaticity and reentry may play a role in the genesis of cardiac arrhythmias. In particular experimental conditions, the action potential of some cardiac fibers may be followed by an early after-hyperpolarization which is itself followed by a delayed after-depolarization.[5] If this after-depolarization reaches a threshold, it may give rise to another action potential. The delayed after-depolarization which follows this action potential may in turn induce another action potential and thus, sustained rhythmic activity can be initiated. Whether such a mechanism may by operative in clinical situations still remains to be further investigated. Let us mention that verapamil can terminate this type of rhythmic activity.[6]

Janse and co-workers[7] have introduced yet another possible mechanism which applies to the early stages of myocardial infarction and relates to the local current circuits between ischemic and nonischemic cells. In this situation, primarily because of delayed activation within the ischemic zone, repolarization of the ischemic area may outlast repolarization in the normal zone. This results in an electrical current flowing towards the normal zone where excitability has already recovered. Reexcitation by these currents of injury may be a factor in the genesis of the arrhythmias occurring within the first minutes of ischemia. It is difficult to speculate which pharmacological agents might show efficacy on such a mechanism. On theoretical grounds, however, one can suggest that a mild increase in extracellular potassium concentration might be beneficial.[7]

SUMMARY

This brief review indicates that the mode of action of antiarrhythmic drugs is a very complex matter. Most classifications of these pharmacological agents may be intellectually satisfactory; on practical grounds, they are of limited significance. At the present time, drug therapy of cardiac arrhythmias remains, in most cases, entirely empirical.[3] Rather than considering electrophysiological properties, we believe that a classification based upon pharmacokinetic characteristics might at times be more helpful to the clinician.

REFERENCES

1. Vaughan-Williams, E.M.: Classification of antiarrhythmic drugs. In Sandoe, E., Flensted-Jensen, E., and Olesen, K.H. (eds.): *Symposium on Cardiac Arrhythmias*. Sweden, Astra AB, 1970, p. 499.
2. Touboul, P.: Classification of antiarrhythmic drugs. In Sandoe, E., Flensted-Jensen, E., and Olesen, K.H. (eds.): *Symposium on Cardiac Arrhythmias*. Sweden, Astra AB, 1970.
3. Jewitt, D.E.: Limitations of present drug therapy of cardiac arrhythmias: A review. *Postgrad. Med. J.* **53** (**Suppl. 1**): 12, 1977.

4. Rosen, M.R.: Effects of pharmacological agents on mechanisms responsible for reentry. In Kulbertus, H. (ed.): *Reentrant Arrhythmias: Mechanisms and Treatment.* Lancaster, MTP Press, 1977.
5. Cranefield, P.F.: Action potentials, after-potentials and arrhythmias. *Circ. Res.* 41: 415, 1977.
6. Mary-Rabine, L., Kulbertus, H., and Rosen, M.: Sustained rhythmicity in human atria. *Trans. Europ. Soc. Cardiol.* 1: 95, 1978.
7. Janse, M.J., Morena, H., Cinca, J., et al.: Role of reentry and currents of injury in early ischemic ventricular tachyarrhythmias: which properties should theoretically make a drug effective in the management of these arrhythmias. In Sandoe, E., Julian, D.G., and Bell, J.W. (eds.): *Management of Ventricular Tachycardia: Role of Mexiletine.* Amsterdam, Exerpta Medica, 1978.

5

The Early Arrhythmic Phase of Myocardial Ischemia

Benjamin J. Scherlag, Ph.D.

In the past decade there have been important modifications of previously established concepts of ectopic impulse formation in myocardial ischemia and infarction. For 30 years the prevailing view was that sudden, severe myocardial ischemia enhanced the automaticity of ventricular ectopic foci causing ventricular premature beats, ventricular tachycardia and fibrillation.[1] It was long recognized in experimental animal studies that the ventricular arrhythmias caused by acute myocardial ischemia and infarction showed two phases. The initial phase occurred during the first few minutes after major coronary artery ligation. If the animal survived this early phase, a later phase of ventricular arrhythmias was seen 24 to 48 hours after coronary artery ligation. This idea of two phases of ventricular arrhythmias secondary to myocardial infarction was attractive to clinicians because the pre-hospital phase of ventricular tachycardia and fibrillation in acute myocardial infarction seems to be closely analogous to the early phase seen in the experimental studies. Similarly, the ventricular arrhythmias seen in the coronary care unit were comparable to the later phase of the experimental studies. Harris, on the basis of many animal studies postulated that the mechanism and site of origin of both early and later ventricular arrhythmias were related to rapidly discharging, automatic foci arising at the borders of the ischemic or infarcted myocardium and normal tissue.[2]

He arrived at this view, whose wide acceptance held firm for more than three decades, mainly by a process of elimination. Harris and his coworker in their initial studies[1] recorded multiple electrograms from the surface of the heart before and after coronary artery occlusion. They reasoned that the mechanism of the ventricular arrhythmia occurring after coronary artery occlusion could be due to slow conduction through the ischemic zone and reentry into normal myocardium or could result from enhanced ventricular automaticity. If it were reentry (Fig. 5-1) it should be possible to detect delay or slow conduction in local electrograms throughout the ischemic zone. Delay of the electrical activity of these local electrograms would exceed the time required for repolarization of the rest of the heart, i.e., the normal myocardium. When the delayed activation extended beyond the QT interval, reentry of the impulse into the recovered normal tissue could cause ventricular premature beats. These ectopic beats could in themselves move through the same circuit leading to ventricular tachycardia and ventricular fibrillation. If a sufficient number of sites was recorded in the ischemic zone,

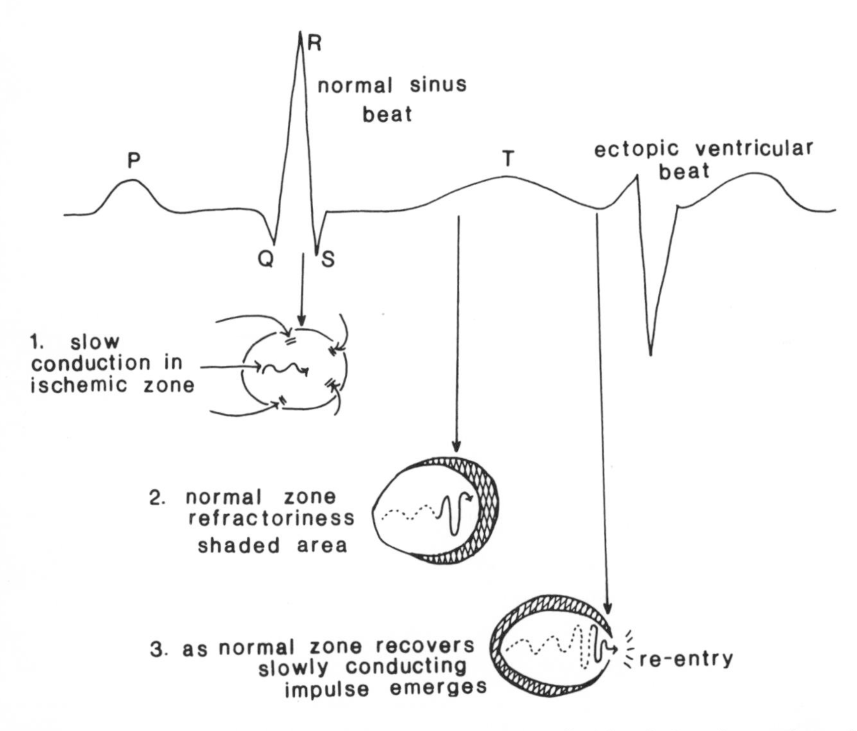

Figure 5-1. Schematic representation of reentry. In the ischemic portion of the heart, the impulse approaches from all sides, but blocks at the border except in one area through which it enters but conducts slowly (one-way conduction, #1). Conduction of the impulse through the ischemic zone continues during the S-T segment and T wave, during which time the rest of the heart is refractory (shaded borders in #2 and 3). As the normal zone recovers, the slowly conducting impulse emerges from the ischemic tissue and reenters the normal zone to induce one or more ventricular ectopic beats.

Harris and Rojas postulated that it should be possible to detect continuous electrical activity of the circuit connecting the normal sinus beat and the first ventricular ectopic beat and successive ventricular beats. However, the lack of adequate amplification of electrograms recorded on the heart surface during ischemia, was the cause of these workers' inability to demonstrate such continuous electrical activity prior to and during continuous reentry. As a result, enhanced automaticity was designated as the mechanism of these early arrhythmias. Recent studies have clearly shown that during this early phase, enhanced ventricular automaticity cannot be demonstrated.[3–5]

It was only in the past 10 years that evidence began to accumulate favoring reentry as the mechanism of the early stage arrhythmias.[6–9] Figure 5-2 is an illustration of the continuous electrical activity which

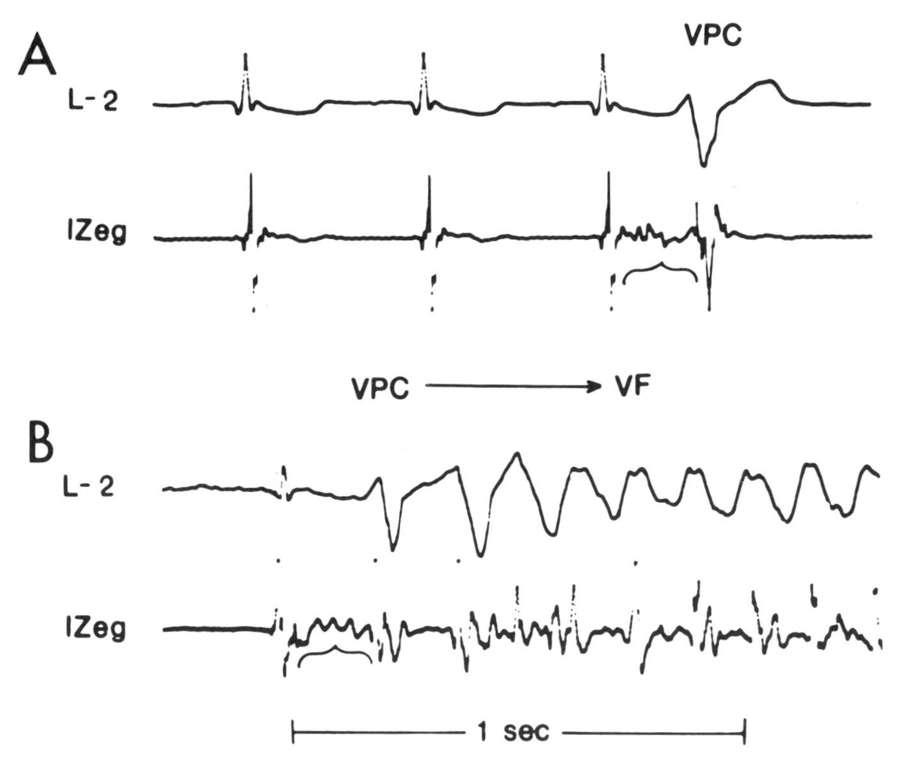

Figure 5–2. Recording of continuous electrical activity bridging the diastolic interval (bracket) between a supraventricular beat and a ventricular premature contraction (VPC). In panel *B* another episode of continuous activity (bracket) leads to ventricular fibrillation (VF). L-2 = a standard lead II electrogram; IZeg = a composite electrogram recording electrical activity from the ischemic zone (epicardium).

can be recorded bridging the diastolic interval between a normal sinus beat and a ventricular ectopic beat (Fig. 5-2*A*) and between successive ectopic beats (Fig. 5-2*B*). In this dog heart acute myocardial ischemia caused by coronary artery ligation proceeded to ventricular fibrillation as the terminal event. These recordings of bridging diastolic activity represent strong presumptive evidence for reentry. Such recordings can now be consistently made by the use of specially constructed multiple-contact bipolar recordings, i.e., "composite" electrodes[10-12] applied to the epicardial surface overlying the ischemic or infarcted zone.

It would thus appear that in acute myocardial ischemia corresponding to the pre-hospital phase clinically, ventricular arrhythmias have a reentrant mechanism as their basis and these arrhythmias carry with them a high mortality due to ventricular fibrillation. However, enhanced automaticity of ectopic ventricular pacemakers does appear to play a primary role as a source of ventricular ectopic beats and ventricular tachycardia which appear within 24 hours after the onset of acute myocardial ischemia. This phase is comparable to the clinical coronary care phase. Basic studies have shown that ventricular ectopic beats and ventricular tachycardia are the result of enhanced automaticity arising in sick Purkinje fibers that survive within the infarcted endocardium.[13,14]

The postulations of Harris have thus been modified so that the initial or immediate phase of ventricular arrhythmias induced by coronary artery occlusion is due to a reentrant mechanism. The area of slow conduction has been identified as the ventricular myocardium which has been made ischemic rather than a "border" zone postulated by Harris and Rojas.[1] On the other hand, 24 to 48 hours after the onset of ischemia, enhanced ventricular automaticity in sickened Purkinje fiber has been reported by several investigators.

THE LATE ARRHYTHMIC PHASE OF MYOCARDIAL INFARCTION

The healing phase of myocardial infarction is not devoid of arrhythmias. Clinically it has been reported that 30 percent of patients who leave the coronary care unit show ventricular arrhythmias within three days to two weeks of discharge.[15] Correspondingly, recent experimental studies have documented ventricular arrhythmias in the infarcted dog heart 3 to 10 days after coronary artery occlusion. Marked slowing of the heart rate indicates that ventricular automaticity enhanced in the 24 to 48 hour period has returned toward preligation levels. However, during spontaneous sinus rhythm or by increasing the heart rate with atrial or ventricular pacing, ectopic ventricular beats can be commonly observed. Figure 5-3 shows recordings taken from a dog four days after coronary artery ligation. During sinus rhythm at a rate of 75/min (panel A) note that electrical recordings from two sites in the epicardium overlying the infarct zone (IZ) are coincident with activation of the QRS complex in the electrocardiogram (L-2). In panel B at a rate of 200/min, induced by atrial pacing, both electrograms in the infarct zone show fractionation; however, the last trace actually shows fractionated activation which forms a link between beats. At the middle of the trace the reentrant beats become manifest, initially as fusion beats then as a regular bi-

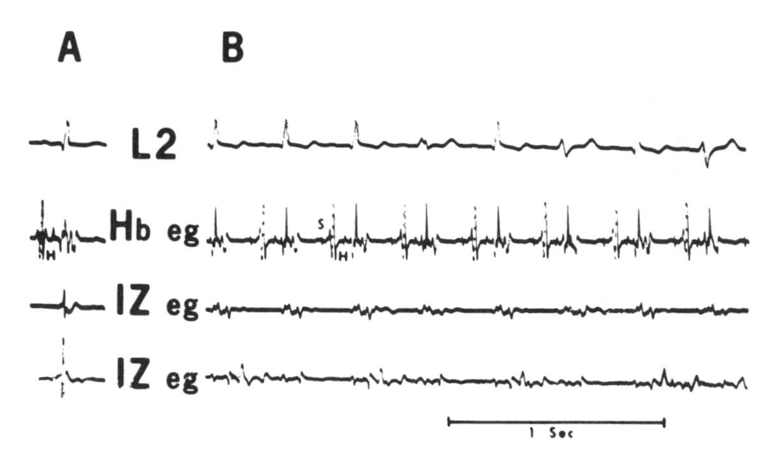

Figure 5-3 Bigeminal rhythm in a dog heart four days after the induction of myocardial infarction. *A*, Electrocardiogram, L II (L-2), His bundle electrogram (Hbeg) and two electrograms from the epicardium overlying the infarction zone (IZeg). This record was obtained during a relatively slow rate (75/min). *B*, Same recordings during atrial pacing at 200/min. Note the continuous activity every other beat which gradually manifests as ventricular bigeminy in the ECG toward the end of the tracing (Reproduced from Hope, R.R., et al.: *Am. J. Cardio.* **40**: 733–737, 1977. Used with permission.)

geminal rhythm. The occurrence of coupled extrasystoles, i.e., bigeminy or extrasystolic groups such as tri-, quadri-, and pentageminies were easily induced or occurred spontaneously in the 3 to 9 day period following the onset of myocardial infarction.[16–19] The occurrence of these coupled extrasystoles are seldom life-threatening. However, on occasion a potentially lethal arrhythmia can be demonstrated to occur spontaneously. Figure 5-4 illustrates the sequential fractionation and delay of activation recorded in a dog four days after the onset of acute myocardial infarction. In the last trace a composite electrogram recorded a

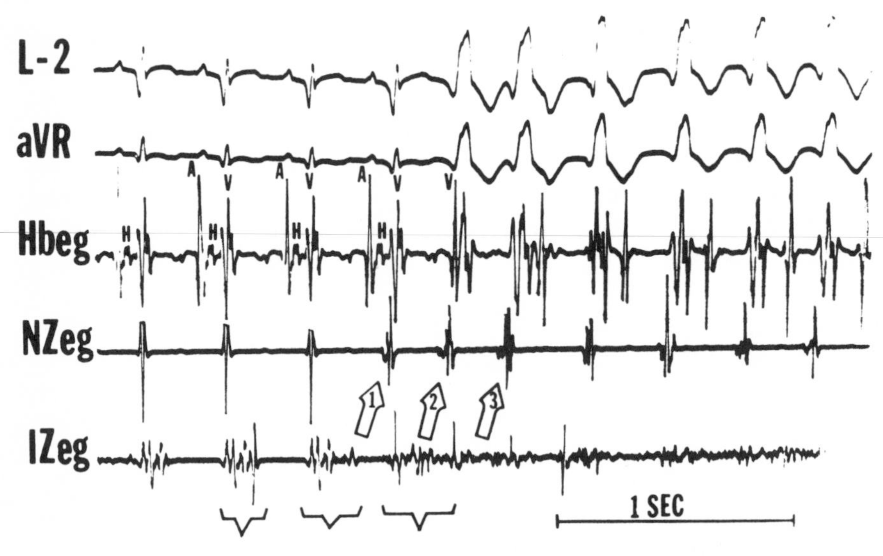

Figure 5-4 In a dog heart four days afer the induction of myocardial infarction, a spontaneous increase in heart rate to 170/min induces fractionation in the infarct zone (IZ). The next beat causes further fractionation and delay of the IZ potentials. The following beat shows complete fractionation through the entire cardiac cycle. The fractionated activity results in early depolarization of adjacent normal zone (NZ) leading to ventricular tachycardia. L-2, ECG, lead II and AVR; Hbeg = His bundle electrogram; NZeg = composite electrogram recording from normal tissue; IZeg = composite electrogram obtained from the epicardium overlying the infarction zone.

Wenckebach-like delay of portions of the electrogram (indicated by the brackets) until there is continuous electrical activity across the diastolic interval leading to the first ectopic beat. The subsequent ventricular tachycardia shows continuous activity in the interectopic intervals. Also note that the paroxysmal ventricular tachycardia starts with a late-coupled ectopic beat. This coincides with recent clinical reports on the initiation of many episodes of paroxysmal ventricular tachycardia.[20,21]

CHRONIC ISCHEMIA

The question that persistently plagues the basic scientist is how comparable are animal models with induced coronary artery lesions to the naturally occurring atherosclerosis in the clinical setting. In particular, are the mechanisms and pathophysiological conditions comparable in the clinical arrhythmias due to long-standing coronary artery disease and those arising from short-term ischemia and infarction in essentially normal animal hearts?

Only recently have investigators sought to establish models of chronic infarction which show either spontaneous[22] or induced[23] ventricular arrhythmias. In addition, other models have been described of infarction with chronic ischemia designed to simulate clinical conditions such as ventricular aneurysms.[24] It is evident even at this time, that much insight into mechanisms of arrhythmias has been gained from the use of experimental induction of ischemia and infarction for varying periods of time. Such studies which attempt to more closely simulate clinical conditions are gathering momentum. The study of appropriate animal counterparts of clinical conditions such as multiple vessel disease and coronary artery spasm, will aid in determining the underlying pathophysiology for lethal arrhythmias and establishing modes of prevention of sudden death.

REFERENCES

1. Harris, A.S., and Rojas, A.G.: The initiation of ventricular fibrillation due to coronary occlusion. *Exper. Med. Surg.* **1**: 105–121, 1943.
2. Harris, A.S.: Delayed development of ventricular ectopic rhythm following experimental coronary occlusion. *Circulation* **1**: 1318–1328, 1950.
3. Scherlag, B.J., Helfant, R.H., Haft, J.I., and Damato, A.N.: Electrophysiology underlying ventricular arrhythmias due to coronary ligation. *Am. J. Physiol.* **219**: 1665–1671, 1970.
4. Kerzner, J., Wolf, M., Kosowsky, B.D., and Lown, B.: Ventricular ectopic rhythms following vagal stimulation in dogs with acute myocardial infarction. *Circulation* **47**: 44–50, 1973.
5. Kaplinsky, E., Horowitz, A., and Neufeld, H.N.: Ventricular reentry and automaticity in myocardial infarction. *Chest* **74**; 66–71, 1978.
6. Han, J.: Mechanisms of ventricular arrhythmias associated with myocardial infarction. *Am. J. Cardiol.* **24**: 800–812, 1969.
7. Durrer, D., VanDam, R.T., Freud, G.E., and Janse, M.J.: Re-entry and ventricular arrhythmias in local ischemia and infarction of the intact dog heart. *Proc. Kon. Nedrl. Akad. Wet.* **C73**: 321–334, 1971.
8. Boineau, J.P., and Cox, J.L.: Slow ventricular activation in acute myocardial infarction: A source of reentrant premature ventricular contraction. *Circulation* **48**: 702–713, 1973.
9. Waldo, A.L., and Kaiser, G.A.: Study of ventricular arrhythmias associated with acute myocardial infarction in the canine heart. *Circulation* **41**: 1222–1228, 1973.
10. Williams, D.O., Scherlag, B.J., Hope, R.R., et al.: The pathophysiology of malignant ventricular arrhythmias during acute myocardial infarction. *Circulation* **50**: 1163–1172, 1974.
11. Hope, R.R., Williams, D.O., El-Sherif, N., et al.: The efficacy of anti-arrhythmic agents during acute myocardial ischemia and the role of heart rate. *Circulation* **50**: 507–514, 1974.

12. El-Sherif, N., Scherlag, B.J., Lazzara, R., and Hope, R.R. Reentrant ventricular arrhythmias in the late myocardial infarction period. I. Conduction characteristics in the infarction zone. *Circulation* **55**: 686–702, 1977.
13. Friedman, P.L., Stewart, J.R., and Wit, A.L. Spontaneous and induced cardiac arrhythmias in subendocardial Purkinje fibers surviving extensive myocardial infarction in dogs. *Circ. Res.* **33**: 612–625. 1973.
14. Lazzara, R., El-Sherif, N., and Scherlag, B.J.: Electrophysiological properties of canine Purkinje cells in 1-day-old myocardial infarction. *Circ. Res.* **33**: 722–734, 1973.
15. Grace, W.J.: The mobile coronary care unit and the intermediate coronary care unit in the total systems approach to coronary care. *Chest* **58**: 363–368, 1970.
16. Hope, R.R., Scherlag, B.J., El-Sherif, N., and Lazzara, R.: Continuous concealed ventricular arrhythmias. *Am. J. Cardiol.* **40**: 733–738, 1977.
17. Hope, R.R., Scherlag, B.J., El-Sherif, N., and Lazzara, R.: Ventricular arrhythmias in healing myocardial infarction: Role of rhythm vs. rate in reentrant activation. *J. Thorac. Cardiovasc. Surg.* **75**: 458–466, 1978.
18. El-Sherif, N., Scherlag, B.J., and Lazzara, R.: Conduction disorders in the canine proximal His-Purkinje system following acute myocardial ischemia. I. The pathophysiology of intra-His bundle block. *Circulation* **49**: 837–847, 1974.
19. El-Sherif, N., Lazzara, R., Hope, R.R., and Scherlag, B.J.: Reentrant ventricular arrhythmias in the late myocardial infarction period. III. Manifest and concealed extrasystolic grouping. *Circulation* **56**: 225–234, 1977.
20. DeSoyza, N., Bisset, J.K., Kane, J.J., et al.: Ectopic ventricular prematurity and its relationship to ventricular tachycardia in acute myocardial infarction in man. *Circulation* **50**: 529–533, 1974.
21. Rothfeld, E.L., Zucker, I.R., Parsonnet, V., et al.: Idioventricular rhythm in acute myocardial infarction. *Circulation* **37**: 203–209, 1968.
22. Bassett, A.L., Gelband, H., Nilsson, K., et al: Electrophysiology following heald experimental myocardial infarction. In Kulbertus, H.E. (ed.): *Reentrant Arrhythmias.* Baltimore, University Park Press, 1976.
23. Garan, H., and Ruskin, J.N.: Demonstration of inducible sustained ventricular tachycardia in dogs with chronic myocardial infarction. *Clin. Res.* **27**: 168A, 1979 (Abstr).

6

Mechanism of Ventricular Arrhythmias Associated With Acute Ischemia

Elieser Kaplinsky, M.D., and Leonard S. Dreifus, M.D.

The association of severe and fatal ventricular arrhythmias with acute myocardial ischemia in the experimental animal has been known now for more than a century.[1,2] Wilson and Harris have tried to elucidate the origin of these arrhythmias by direct recordings from the ischemic zone and concluded that any activity within the zone of injury is unrelated to the rhythm disorders.[3,4] However, it is important to note that Harris did observe delay and fragmentation of the activation of the epicardial ischemic zone and the concomitant appearance of ectopic rhythm.[4]

In later years Harris classified the experimental arrhythmias into two distinct phases: an early phase lasting for 20 to 30 minutes after ligation, and a late phase beginning 8 to 16 hours after ligation and lasting for 24 to 72 hours.[5]

Extensive studies during the last decade have elucidated many of the electrophysiological mechanisms involved in the experimental post ligation arrhythmias. The early Phase 1 arrhythmias were demonstrated to be associated with reentry, while those of the late phase were found to be due to increased automaticity of the surviving Purkinje fibers within the infarction.[5-10]

Scherlag[6-9] has summarized the pertinent developments in the electrophysiology of ventricular arrhythmias associated with myocardial ischemia. This chapter will summarize some newer aspects of the ischemic arrhythmias.

Experiments were performed on open chest dogs anesthetized with 25 mg/kg of Nembutal. Local electrograms from various sites of the ischemic, border and normal zones were recorded through close bipolar stainless steel wire plunge electrodes. The distance between the electrode tips was less than 0.5 mm. All electrograms were recorded with a band width of 50 to 1000 cycles per second. The proximal left anterior descending coronary artery was exposed and ligated in one stage. In the animals that survived for 30 minutes, the artery was abruptly reperfused.

The results of these studies have contributed to the understanding of the arrhythmias associated with acute ischemia in the following four aspects:

1. Classification of the Harris Phase 1 arrhythmias
2. Patterns of activation during the early post ligation arrhythmias
3. Significance of "right" versus "left" ventricular arrhythmias
4. Reperfusion arrhythmias

CLASSIFICATION OF HARRIS PHASE 1 ARRHYTHMIAS[11]

Current concepts describe the early post ligation arrhythmias as due to one mechanism, namely, reentry in the ischemic zone easily demonstrated by recording local activity with bipolar electrograms. In 41 consecutive animals, we have analyzed the relationship between the incidence and severity of early post ligation ventricular arrhythmias, and the extent to which local activation of the ischemic epicardium is delayed and fragmented. The latter was defined as the time interval between the onset of activation in the ischemic endocardium, and the last distinct activation spike in the ischemic epicardium.[11] This interrelationship was determined for the period of 30 minutes after ligation. The results are summarized in Figure 6-1. Immediately upon ligation, the activity of the ischemic epicardium becomes delayed and fragmented, reaching peak derangement at 5 to 6 minutes. As delay and fragmentation increase, arrhythmias appear. In the ensuing minutes, epicardial activation in the ischemic zone improves in the surviving animals and arrhythmias disappear. Following a period of quiescence, a second surge of arrhythmias is observed. These arrhythmias occur without any further deterioration in ischemic epicardial activation. As a matter of fact, epicardial activation continues to improve while arrhythmias reappear. Thus, the hallmark of the immediate ventricular arrhythmias (the first wave in Fig. 6-2) was the progressive delay and fragmentation of the activation of the ischemic epicardium preceding and sustaining the ectopic rhythms. In contrast, the delayed ventricular arrhythmias which occur 10 to 30 minutes after ligation were neither preceded nor sustained by such progressive delay in epicardial activation. The absence of delayed activity bridging the diastolic interval becomes the hallmark of the delayed ventricular arrhythmias.

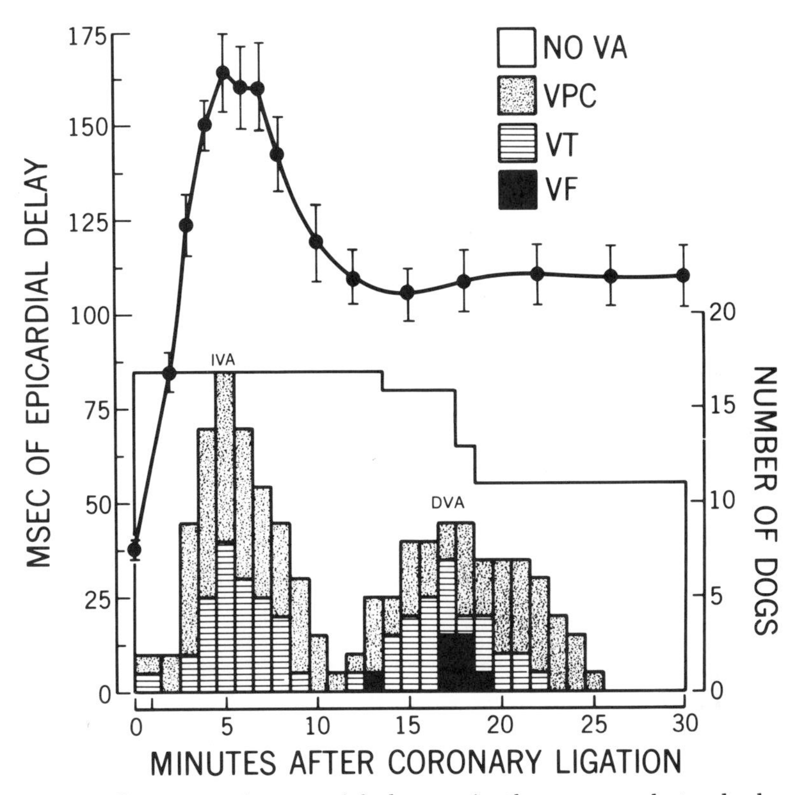

Figure 6–1. Summary of sequential changes in the mean and standard error of local subepicardial activation of the ischemic zone (indicated by the black dots), and the incidence and severity of ventricular arrhythmias (indicated by the lower vertical bars) in 41 dogs. The clear zone above the bars represents the number of dogs not showing arrhythmias at that particular time. VA = ventricular arrhythmias; VPC = ventricular premature complexes; VT = ventricular tachycardia; VF = ventricular fibrillation. The biphasic appearance of the ventricular arrhythmias during the first 30 minutes after ligation is clearly seen. The appearance and disappearance of the first wave of ectopic activity (the immediate ventricular arrhythmias, IVA) is closely associated with the rapid increase and subsequent decrease in local ischemic subepicardial delay of the normal sinus complexes. The second surge or the delayed ventricular arrhythmias (DVA), is clearly independent of further changes in local activation in the ischemic subepicardium. Note: Peak of subepicardial delay coincides with peak of ectopic activity. The stepwise decline in the total number of dogs represents the loss of animals due to ventricular fibrillation. (Used by permission of the American Heart Association, Inc.)

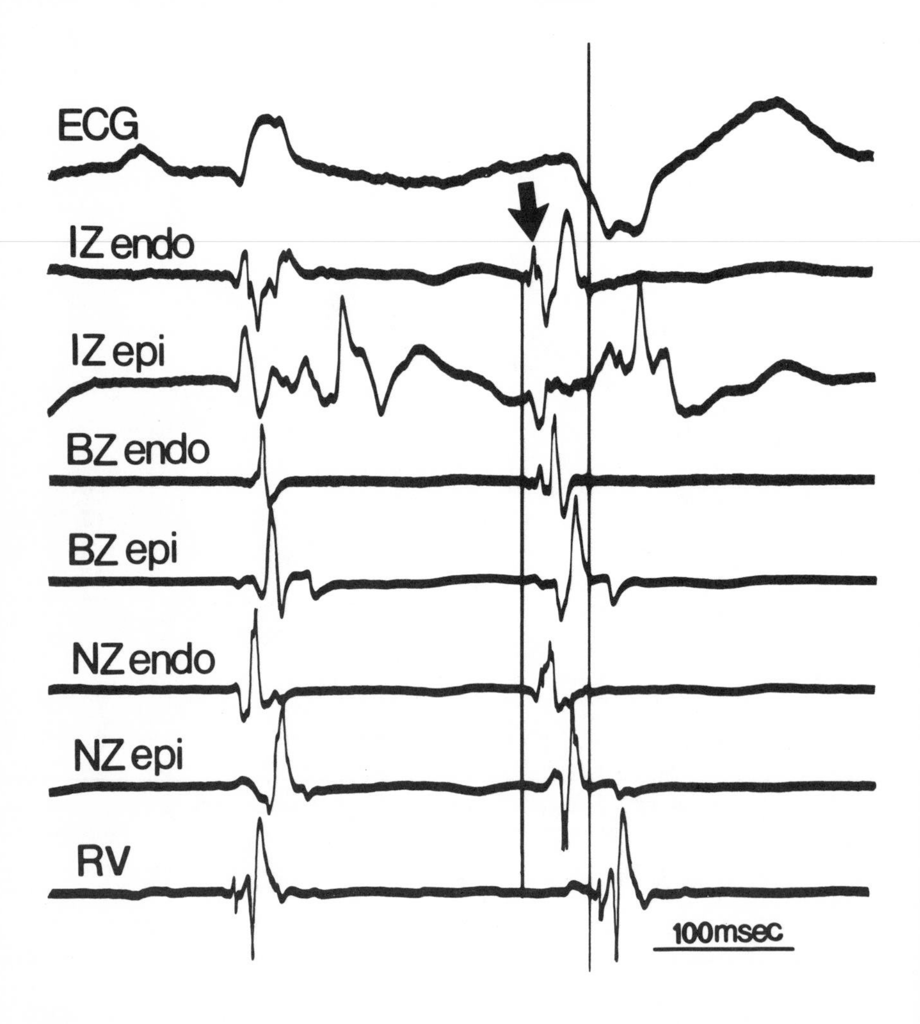

Figure 6–2. Lead 2 (ECG) of the electrocardiogram and seven composite electrograms recorded from a dog, 4 minutes after coronary artery ligation. IZ = ischemic zone; BZ = border zone, NZ = normal zone; RV = right ventricle; endo = endocardial; epi = epicardial. All electrograms were recorded through composites of several bipolar electrodes. The first complex is of sinus origin. Following it, the activation of the ischemic zone epicardium (IZepi) is markedly delayed and fragmented. This is associated with the appearance of an ectopic ventricular complex. The earliest activation is now noted in the IZendo (arrow). In all composites, endocardial activation precedes the corresponding epicardial. First vertical line—onset of IZendo activation—as part of the premature complex. Second verticle line is a time line. Paper speed is noted as part of the premature complex. Second verticle line is a time line. Paper speed is noted on the lower portion of the figure.

We therefore feel that the experimental arrhythmias which follow coronary artery occlusion have to be reclassified. The Phase 1 of Harris actually consists of two distinct periods of arrhythmias, the *immediate* and the *delayed* ventricular arrhythmias, all belonging to the hyperacute phase and both being extremely malignant with a high incidence of ventricular fibrillation.

PATTERNS OF ACTIVATION DURING THE EARLY POST LIGATION ARRHYTHMIAS[12]

Although the basic mechanisms of the ventricular arrhythmias associated with hyperacute ischemias began to unfold, the pathways linking the sites of the reentrant activity to the remaining normal portions of the heart were yet to be identified. Further studies utilizing multiple endocardial and epicardial composite electrodes were performed in 15 dogs.[12] The electrode arrangement permitted identification of the endocardial or epicardial spread of activation. All recorded episodes of the immediate and delayed ventricular arrhythmias (Phase 1 of Harris) were analyzed and the initial site of activation during arrhythmias was determined. In more than 99 percent of the ectopic complexes occurring during both periods of the early arrhythmias, the *endocardial* surface of the ischemic zone was the site of initial activation. Spread continued via the endocardium surface to the normal regions of the heart[12] (Fig. 6-2).

These studies suggested that (a) the efferent pathway of reentrant ventricular arrhythmias in acute ischemia is within the endocardial surface of the ischemic zone; (b) the Purkinje network may thus be a critical link in the genesis of the malignant arrhythmias during the acute phase of myocardial infarction.[12]

SIGNIFICANCE OF "RIGHT" VERSUS "LEFT" VENTRICULAR ARRHYTHMIAS[13]

The clinical significance of the ventricular origin of ventricular arrhythmias has been a controversial issue for many years. While some studies suggest that benign ventricular ectopic activity occurring in the young and healthy individual originates mainly in the right ventricle, other have shown that patients with coronary artery disease display ventricular arrhythmias originating from both ventricles.[14–20]

We have analyzed the ventricular ectopic activity in 32 dogs where bipolar electrodes were positioned in both ventricles.[13] The results clearly indicated that in the canine model of acute occlusion of the left anterior descending coronary artery, ventricular arrhythmias may appear from both the right and the left ventricles. It was of interest to note that during the immediate ventricular arrhythmias, similar delayed and fragmented activity of the ischemic epicardium was associated with both right and left ventricular exits (Fig. 6-3). Furthermore, ectopic activity exiting from either ventricle could be observed leading to ventricular fibrillation.[13]

These results are not surprising as the acutely ischemic zone extends into the right ventricle. It seems, therefore, that in the presence of coronary artery disease in general, and acute myocardial infarction in particular, the exact identification of the ventricle of "origin" in ventricular ectopic activity may not be of clinical significance.

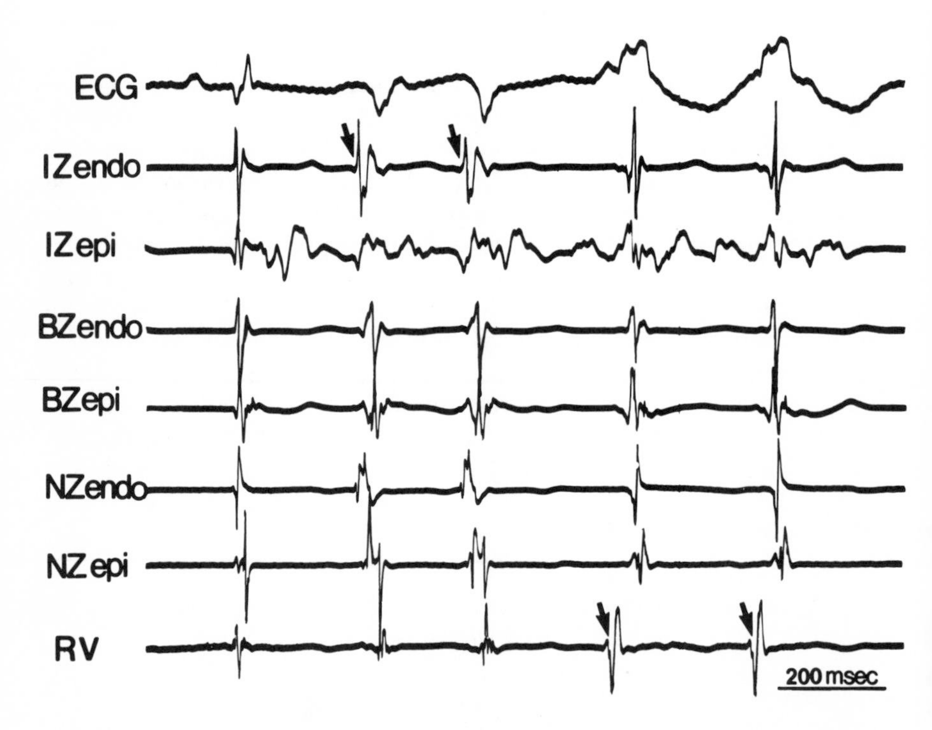

Figure 6-3. Lead 2 (ECG) of the electrocardiogram and seven composite electrograms from a dog 6 minute after coronary artery ligation. For abbreviations, see legend to Fig. 6-2. A multiform ventricular tachycardia is observed to follow the first QRS complex which is of normal sinus origin. The tachycardia is preceded by delayed and fragmented activation in IZepi. Note also that the activation of IZepi is further delayed and fragmented during the ventricular tachycardia. Earliest activation in the first two ectopic complexes is in the IZendo of the left ventricle while earliest activation in the last two complexes is in the right ventricle.

REPERFUSION ARRHYTHMIAS[21]

The intriguing phenomenon of the sudden and rapid onset of ventricular tachycardia and fibrillation following release of an occluded coronary artery has been known for more than a century.[1,22–28] The interest in reperfusion arrhythmias has come into sharp focus as more and more evidence has been accumulated to suggest the importance of spasm and release of spasm in the natural history of coronary artery disease.

Several investigators have suggested that the mechanism of reperfusion arrhythmias may differ from that of early post ligation arrhythmias. The onset of ventricular ectopy occurs within seconds after release of occlusion, compared to minutes after coronary ligation. The reperfusion arrhythmias are also more malignant and appear less responsive to antiarrhythmic intervention.[22–31]

We further observed that the severe and instantaneous reperfusion arrhythmias occurred only in the animals that displayed ventricular ectopic activity in the post ligation period.[21] In addition, a different and delayed onset variety of arrhythmia appeared within 2 to 5 minutes of reperfusion. This delayed ventricular arrhythmia was slower, more prolonged, and rarely was observed to deteriorate into ventricular fibrillation. While the instantaneous and more malignant arrhythmias showed an obvious similarity and correlation with post ligation arrhythmias, the delayed reperfusion arrhythmias were unrelated to any prior arrhythmia events.

The instantaneous reperfusion arrhythmias differed from the delayed variety not only in their malignancy but also in the characteristic electrophysiological changes noted in the ischemic zone prior to, and during, the arrhythmia.

Following a 20 to 30 minute ligation period the electrical activity in the ischemic epicardium became severely depressed.[6–9,11] However, upon release of the occlusion there is an immediate increase in the amplitude of local electrograms, and a majority of the dogs who developed instantaneous ventricular fibrillation, the "growth" of local activity resulted in the appearance of rapidly rising delayed and fragmented activity extending into diastole (Fig. 6-4).[21] No such activity was detected in the dogs that did not develop instantaneous reperfusion arrhythmias. Rapid recovery of activation within the ischemic zone was observed within 1 to 2 minutes after reperfusion. In contrast to the instantaneous arrhythmias, the activation of the ischemic zone remained intact with no delayed or fragmented activity.[21]

It seems that two mechanisms operate to produce reperfusion arrhythmias. The instantaneous rhythm disorders are associated with delayed and fragmented activation of the ischemic zone, very similar to the

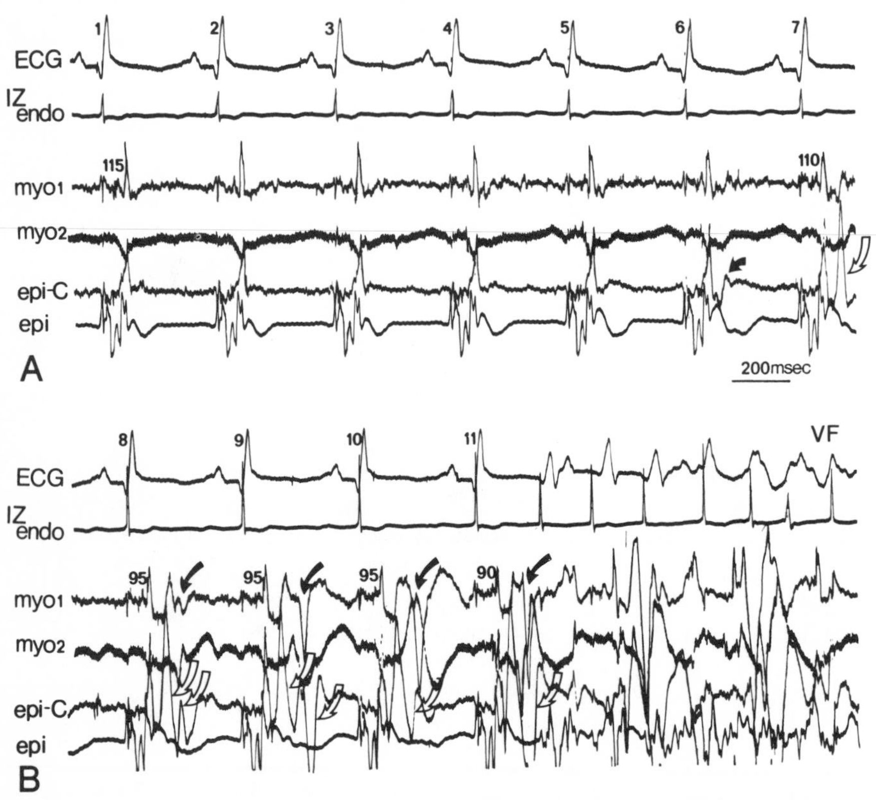

Figure 6–4. Continuous record of lead 2 (ECG) of the electrogram and five electrograms from various areas of the ischemic reperfused zone beginning 1.5 seconds after reperfusion. IZ = ischemic zone; endo = endocardial; myo_1 = myocardial, 7 mm below epicardial surface; myo_2 = myocardial, 5 mm below epicardial surface; epiC = a composite of four bipolar epicardial electrodes located at the central portions of the ischemic zone; epi = a single epicardial electrode in the ischemic zone; VF = ventricular fibrillation. The two tracings are continuous and the successive QRS complexes are indicated by numbers. *A*, Six seconds after reperfusion, the first ectopic ventricular complex was observed following complex 11. However, during the preceding normal sinus complexes (complexes 1 to 11, Fig. 6-4), marked changes were recorded in the local electrograms. Endocardial activity (see Fig. 6-4, IZendo) remained synchronous, but its amplitude was unstable and continued to increase. Extremely high gains, 75 mm/mv, were required to detect any periodic activity in myo_1, myo_2, and epiC. No significant changes were observed in the local activities of complexes 1 to 4. In complex 6, a small deflection of new activity immediately following the major deflection was noted (small curved black arrow). This change became more manifest in epiC of complex 7 as the new activity attained relatively enormous proportions *(white arrow)*, and the local electrical activity was now further fragmented.

activity observed during the immediate ventricular arrhythmias, and strongly suggest reentry as the basic mechanism. However, the delayed ventricular mechanisms display features suggesting increased automaticity, namely, slow frequency of discharge, gradual onset and offset, with frequent fusion complexes. Further support for a delayed transient rise in ventricular automaticity was obtained from studies incorporating vagal stimulation. Suppression of the sinus rhythm revealed a transient rise in the rate of the ventricular escape rhythm. A similar post reperfusion enhancement of automaticity was also described in cats.[32]

The results of these studies can be summarized as follows:

1. The Harris classification of post ligation ventricular arrhythmias in the dog must be modified. During the early, hyperacute phase of arrhythmia, two types of rhythm disturbances can occur. The Phase 1 of Harris consists of an immediate period clearly associated with delay and fragmentation of the activity of the ischemic zone, and a delayed period independent of it.
2. Efferent pathways from the ischemic zone to the normal portion of the heart involve the ischemic endocardial surface suggesting a critical role of the subendocardial Purkinje network as a link in the genesis of these ischemia-induced arrhythmias.
3. Both right and left ventricular arrhythmias occur in abundance in the canine model of acute anteroseptal ischemia.
4. Reperfusion arrhythmias are associated with two mechanisms: (a) an early instantaneous variety associated with the appearance of delayed and fragmented activity in the ischemic zone, and an extremely high incidence of ventricular fibrillation, and (b) a delayed, essentially benign, ectopic rhythm which is due to transient increase in ventricular automaticity.

Figure 6-4 *(Continued) B*, in complexes 8 to 11 the amplitude and further fragmentation (*white arrows* in epiC) became increasingly pronounced. A similar chain of events was noted in myo_1 beginning in complex 7 and attaining significant proportions in complexes 8 to 11 *(black arrows)*. Simultaneously, with the development of the new activity and its rapid increase in amplitude noted in myo_1, a decrease was observed in the delay of the main activation of myo_1, which was present initially from 115 msec in complex 1, to 90 msec in complex 11. Similar changes, although unmarked, were observed in myo_2, and to a lesser degree in epi. Only a moderate increase in amplitude with no delay and fragmentation was seen in IZendo.

REFERENCES

1. Cohnheim, J., von Schulthess, Rechberg, A.: Über die Folgen der Kranzarterienverschliessung für das Herz. *Virch. Arch. Pathol. Anat.* 85: 503–537, 1881.
2. Porter, W.T.: On the results of ligation of the coronary arteries. *J. Exp. Med.* **1**:46–70, 1896.
3. Johnson, F.D., Hill, I.G.W., and Wilson, F.N.: The form of the electrocardiogram in experimental myocardial infarction: The early effects produced by ligation of the anterior descending branch of the left coronary artery. *Am. Heart J.* **10**:889–902, 1935.
4. Harris, A.S., and Rojas, A.G.: The initiation of ventricular fibrillation due to coronary occlusion. *Exp. Med. Surg.* **1**:105–122, 1943.
5. Harris, A.S.: Delayed development of ventricular ectopic rhythms following experimental coronary occlusion. *Circulation* **1**:1318–1329, 1950.
6. Scherlag, B.J., Helfant, R.H., Haft, J.J., and Damato, A.N.: Electrophysiology underlying ventricular arrhythmias due to coronary ligation. *Am. J. Physiol.* **219**:1665–1671, 1970.
7. Boineau, J.P., and Cox, J.L.: Slow ventricular activation in acute myocardial infarction: A source of reentrant premature ventricular contraction. *Circulation* **48**:702–713, 1973.
8. Waldo, A.L., and Kaiser, G.A.: A study of ventricular arrhythmias associated with acute myocardial infarction in the canine heart. *Circulation* **47**:1222–1228, 1973.
9. Scherlag, B.J., El-Sherif, N., Hope, R., and Lazzara, R.: Characterization and localization of ventricular arrhythmias resulting from myocardial ischmia and infarction. *Circ. Res.* **35**:372–383, 1974.
10. El-Sherif, N., Scherlag, B.J., and Lazzara, R.: Electrode catheter recording during malignant ventricular arrhythmias following experimental acute myocardial ischemia: Evidence for reentry due to conduction and block in ischemic myocardium. *Circulation* **51**:1003–1014, 1975.
11. Kaplinsky, E., Ogawa, S., Balke, C.W., and Dreifus, L.S.: Two periods of early ventricular arrhythmias in the canine acute myocardial infarction model. *Circulation,* in press.
12. Kaplinsky, E., Ogawa, S., Balke, C.W., and Dreifus, L.S.: Endocardial pathways in malignant ventricular arrhythmias associated with acute ischemia. *J. Electrocardiol.*, in press.
13. Kaplinsky, E., Ogawa, S., Kmetzo, J., and Dreifus, L.S.: Origin of so-called right and left ventricular arrhythmias in acute myocardial ischemia. *Am. J. Cardiol.* **42**:774–780, 1978.
14. Hiss, R.G., Averill, K.H., and Lamb, L.E.: Electrocardiographic finding in 67,375 asymptomatic subjects. II. Ventricular rhythms. *Am. J. Cardiol.* **7**, 96–107, 1960.
15. Rosenbaum, M.B.: Classification of ventricular extrasystoles according to form. *J. Electrocardiol.* **2**:289–298, 1969.
16. Lown, B., Calvert, A.F., Armington, R., and Ryan, M.: Monitoring for serious arrhythmias and high risk of sudden death. *Circulation* **52 (Suppl. III)**:189–198, 1975.

17. Kennedy, H.L., and Underhill, S.J.: Frequent or complex ventricular ectopy in apparently healthy subjects: A clinical study of 25 cases. *Am. J. Cardiol.* **38**:141–148, 1976.
18. Pietras, R.J., Mautner, R., Denes, P., et al.: Chronic recurrent right and left ventricular tachycardia: Comparison of clinical, hemodynamic and angiographic findings. *Am. J. Cardiol.* **40**:32–37, 1977.
19. Bodenheimer, M.M., Banka, V.S. and Helfant, R.H.: Relationship between the site of origin of ventricular premature complexes and the presence and severity of coronary artery disease. *Am. J. Cardiol.* **40**:865–869, 1977.
20. Cohen, H.C., Gozo, E.G., Jr., Langendorf, R., et al.: Response of resistant ventricular tachycardia to bretylium: Relation to site of ectopic focus and location of myocardial disease. *Circulation* **47**:331–340, 1973.
21. Kaplinsky, E., Balke, C.W., Ogawa, S., and Dreifus, L.S.: Reperfusion arrhythmias: Evidence for early reentry and delayed increased automaticity. *Am. J. Cardiol.*, in press (abstract).
22. Tennant, R., and Wiggers, C.J.: The effect of coronary occlusion on myocardial contraction. *Am. J. Physiol.* **112**:351–361, 1935.
23. Harris, A.S., Estandia, A., and Tillotson, R.F.: Ventricular ectopic rhythms and ventricular fibrillation following cardiac sympathectomy and coronary occlusion. *Am. J. Physiol.* **165**:505–512, 1951.
24. Sewell, W.H., Koth, D.R., and Huggins, C.E.: Ventricular fibrillation in dogs after sudden return of flow to the coronary artery. *Surgery* **38**:1050–1053, 1955.
25. Petropoulos, P.C., and Jaijne, N.G.: Cardiac function during perfusion of the circumflex coronary artery with venous blood, low molecular weight dextran or Tyrode's solution. *Am. Heart J.* **68**:370–373, 1964.
26. Battle, W.E., Naimi, S., Avitall, B., et al.: Distinctive time course of ventricular vulnerability to fibrillation during and after release of coronary ligation. *Am. J. Cardiol.* **34**:42–47, 1974.
27. Levites, R., Banka, V.S., and Helfant, R.H.: Electrophysiologic effects of coronary occlusion and reperfusion: Observations of dispersion of refractoriness and ventricular automaticity. *Circulation* **52**:760–765, 1975.
28. Corhblan, R., Verrier, R.L., and Lown, B.: Differing mechanisms for ventricular vulnerability during coronary artery occlusion and release. *Am. Heart J.* **92**:223–230, 1976.
29. Bigger, J.T., Jr., Dresdale, R.J., Heissenbuttel, R.H., et al.: Ventricular arrhythmias in ischemic heart disease: Mechanism, prevalence, significance and management. *Prog. Cardiovasc. Dis.* **19**:255–300, 1977.
30. Stephenson, J.E., Jr., Cole, R.K., Parrish, T.F., et al.: Ventricular fibrillation during and after coronary artery occlusion: Incidence and protection afforded by various drugs. *Am. J. Cardiol.* **5**:77–87, 1960.
31. Axelrod, P.J., Verrier, R.L., and Lown, B.: Vulnerability to ventricular fibrillation during acute coronary occlusion and release. *Am. J. Cardiol.* **36**:776–782, 1975.
32. Penkoske, P.A., Sobel, B.E., and Corr, P.B.: Disparate electrophysiological alterations accompanying dysrhythmia due to coronary occlusion and reperfusion in the cat. *Circulation* **58**:1003–1035, 1978.

7

Electrophysiological Studies in Patients With Ventricular Tachycardia

Jerónimo Farre, M.D.
Isaac Wiener, M.D.,
David Ross, M.B., B.S., F.R.A.C.P.,
Frits W. Bär, M.D., and
Hein J.J. Wellens, M.D.

The technique of programmed electrical stimulation of the heart for the study of ventricular tachycardia in man has been in use since 1972.[1] In this article the purpose and results of these electrophysiological investigations in patients with ventricular tachycardia (VT) will be reviewed.

THE METHOD

In patients with VT, five external electrocardiographic leads (I,II, III,V_1 and V_6) are simultaneously recorded with up to six intracardiac electrograms by a 16 channel ink-jet direct recorder (Mingograf, Siemens-Elema, Sweden). Routine intracardiac recordings in these patients currently include bipolar electrograms from the high right atrium (HRA), coronary sinus (CS), His bundle region (HB) and right ventricular outflow tract (RVOT). All signals are stored on tape by a 14 channel tape-recorder (Ampex PR-2200). Stimulation is performed with a programmable stimulator (Janssen Pharmaceutica, Belgium) which can deliver up to four consecutive premature stimuli following a paced or spontaneous rhythm. Electrical impulses are delivered which are 2 ms

Dr. Farré has been supported by the Fundacion Conchita Rabago de Jiminez Diaz, Spain.
Dr. Ross is supported by the National Heart Foundation of Australia.

wide and have a stimulus strength of twice diastolic threshold. The protocol of stimulation is shown in Table 7-1. If tachycardia is initiated during the stimulation study or if the patient enters the investigation in tachycardia, single and multiple atrial and ventricular test stimuli are delivered by synchronizing the stimulator to either an intracardiac or surface electrocardiographic signal. If a ventricular tachyarrhythmia which is poorly tolerated by the patient is induced during the study, immediate DC shock cardioversion is performed.

Table 7-1. Protocol of Stimulation in Patients with Ventricular Tachycardia

A. Basic Procedure
1. HRA extra-stimulus technique*
2. CS extra-stimulus technique
3. HRA pacing at increasing rates†
4. CS pacing at increasing rates
5. RV apex extra-stimulus technique
6. RV outflow tract extra-stimulus technique
7. RV apex pacing at increasing rates
8. RV outflow tract pacing at increasing rates

B. During Tachycardia
1. Single and multiple atrial premature stimuli
2. Single and multiple ventricular premature stimuli

**Extra-stimulus technique*: performed at three different BCL
†*Pacing at increasing rates*: performed up to the rate in which (1) tachycardia develops, (2) hemodynamic intolerance is observed, (3) A-V block results (during atrial pacing).

CS atrial stimulation is optional; occasionally CS left ventricular stimulation is performed.

Abbreviations: HRA=high right atrium; CS=coronary sinus; RV=right ventricle; BCL=basic cycle length

AIMS OF ELECTROPHYSIOLOGICAL STUDIES IN VENTRICULAR TACHYCARDIA

The purposes of these studies are: (1) to confirm the diagnosis of VT, (2) to study the mechanism of the arrhythmia, (3) to select antiarrhythmic drug prophylaxis, (4) to study the potential benefits of specially designed pacemakers in patients refractory to conventional drug treatment, (5) to help in the selection of patients for surgical treatment. Most of these goals cannot be accomplished unless VT is reproducibly initiated and terminated during the stimulation study.

MODES OF INITIATION AND TERMINATION OF VENTRICULAR TACHYCARDIA

As shown in Table 7-2, neither short-lasting episodes of ventricular tachycardia nor ventricular tachyarrhythmias in patients with QT prolongation can be reproducibly induced and/or terminated by pro-

Table 7-2. Results of Programmed Electrical Stimulation in a Series of 110 Patients with Ventricular Tachycardia

Group of Patients	No. of Patients	Initiation	Termination
Short-lasting VT	21	1 (5%)	1 (5%)
VT and long QT	8	0	0
Sustained VT	81	56 (69%)	63 (78%)
MI < 24 hrs	7	0	2 (28%)
MI 24 hrs to 5 weeks	3	0	2 (66%)
MI > 5 weeks	42	36 (85%)	40 (95%)
Idiopathic VT	20	17 (85%)	17 (85%)
Others	9	3 (33%)	2 (22%)

Abbreviations: VT=ventricular tachycardia; MI=myocardial infarction

grammed electrical stimulation of the heart. In patients with sustained VT, there are two subsets in which initiation and termination of the arrhythmia is particularly frequent: (1) patients with so-called idiopathic VT in whom no cardiac abnormality can be identified, and (2) patients with sustained VT and an old myocardial infarction. These observations probably indicate that the underlying pathophysiology in human VT is complex and that the mechanisms involved in the different types of VT are diverse.

Factors Influencing Initiation of VT

Initiation of VT during the stimulation study depends on (1) the basic cycle length (BCL) of the regular ventricular paced rhythm, (2) the site of stimulation in the ventricle, (3) the number of ventricular premature stimuli delivered.[2] In our laboratory, three different BCL are employed during the extra-stimulus testing. The slowest BCL is just above the mean rate of the basic rhythm of the patient. The other two BCL are 600 and 500 ms, respectively.

As previously reported,[2] when a single ventricular premature stimulus can initiate the tachycardia, the zone of premature beat intervals resulting in tachycardia (tachycardia zone) is widest at the slowest possible basic pacing rate in 85 percent of the instances. Most of the time, initiation of VT is easier during right ventricular apical stimulation. In a few patients, however, the tachycardia zone is widest or its initiation is accomplished only during pacing of the outflow tract of the right ventricle.[2] Other investigators have more systematically employed left ventricular as well as right ventricular stimulation.[3] However, left ventricular stimulation is not routinely required since in most patients in whom VT can be induced from the left ventricle it can also be initiated from the right.[3]

Initiation of VT is frequently accomplished with a single ventricular premature stimulus. In our series of 56 sustained ventricular tachycardias induced during the stimulation study, 42 (75%) could be initiated by single ventricular premature stimuli during a ventricular paced rhythm.[4]

Two ventricular premature stimuli were required in 11 patients (20%), three stimuli in two patients and in one instance four consecutive ventricular premature stimuli were needed to initiate VT.

In seven out of 56 patients (12%) VT could also be initiated by timed atrial stimuli during atrial pacing. As reported elsewhere, these patients usually had wide tachycardia-zones and relatively slow tachycardia rates.[5]

Factors Influencing Termination of VT

Termination of VT during the stimulation study depends on: (1) the ventricular rate during tachycardia, (2) the site of stimulation in the ventricles, (3) the number of ventricular premature beats delivered.

In general, the faster the rate of the ventricular tachycardia, the more difficult it is to terminate by means of ventricular premature stimuli.[4] Very fast rates during VT (above 220 per minute) frequently result in rapid hemodynamic deterioration. Termination of these tachycardias by pacing is extremely difficult and DC shock cardioversion should be utilized instead.

The site of stimulation plays an important role in the termination of tachycardia. Most of the times, termination is facilitated by pacing from the apex of the right ventricle as compared to the right ventricular outflow tract. In the occasional patient, however, interruption of VT can only be accomplished by stimulating from the outflow tract of the right ventricle.[2] We have been able to terminate sustained attacks of VT during the stimulation study in 63 patients.[4] In 38 patients (60%) a single ventricular premature beat was able to terminate VT. In 21 patients (33%) two ventricular premature stimuli were required. Three ventricular premature beats were needed in three patients and four consecutive ventricular stimuli in only one patient. There is no relationship between the number of ventricular premature beats required to initiate and terminate VT in a given patient.[4]

CONFIRMATION OF THE DIAGNOSIS OF VT

The electrocardiographic diagnosis of VT can only be made with confidence when all the following features are observed during a tachycardia: (1) wide QRS complex (more than 0.12 secs.), (2) atrioventricular (A-V) dissociation, and (3) capture beats showing normal intraventricular conduction.

Our group has recently reviewed the electrocardiogram in 70 episodes of sustained VT.[6] A-V dissociation was present in 32 instances (45%) but capture beats were only observed in four patients. In this study we reported on some electrocardiographic criteria which are of help in making the diagnosis of VT. The most important of these criteria were: (1) QRS complex during tachycardia showing left axis deviation, (2) QRS width of more than 0.14 seconds, and (3) certain configurational characteristics of the QRS complex in leads V_1 and V_6.[6]

There are instances, however, in which the electrocardiographic diagnosis of VT may be difficult, such as: (1) presence of 1:1 V-A conduction during a wide QRS complex tachycardia, (2) tachycardia with left bundle branch block (BBB) configuration showing an intermediate or right axis in the frontal plane, (3) presence of previous organic BBB, (4) previous administration of drugs which prolong the duration of the QRS complex, and (5) identification of uncommon configurations for VT or configurations that can be seen both in ventricular and supraventricular tachycardias with aberrant conduction.

As differentiation between supraventricular and ventricular tachycardia has important therapeutic and prognostic implications, the correct diagnosis should be established. Figure 7-1 illustrates an example of a questionable VT in a patient with an old inferior wall myocardial infarction.

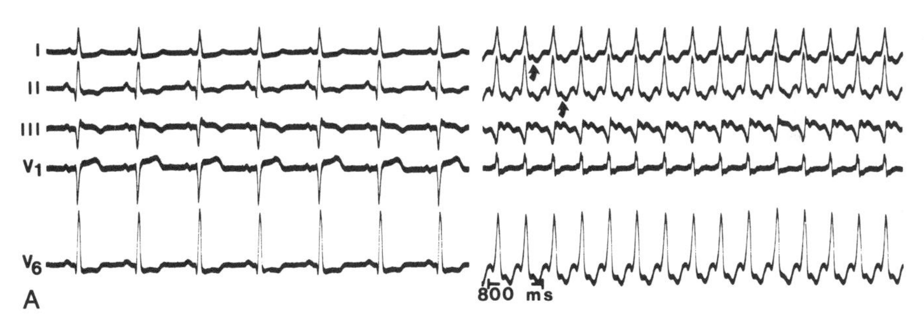

Figure 7-1. Example of recurrent sustained ventricular tachycardia in a patient with an old inferior wall infarction who had a posteroinferior left ventricular aneurysm. Panel *A* show five simultaneously recorded electrocardiographic leads at 25 mm/sec paper speed during sinus rhythm (left upper panel) and during tachycardia (right upper panel). The arrows point to retrograde P waves during tachycardia. The patient was referred to our hospital with the presumptive diagnosis of supraventricular tachycardias. During the stimulation study the tachycardia was reproducibly initiated with three consecutive ventricular premature stimuli.

Electrophysiological Diagnosis of VT

The electrophysiological diagnosis of VT is based on the demonstration

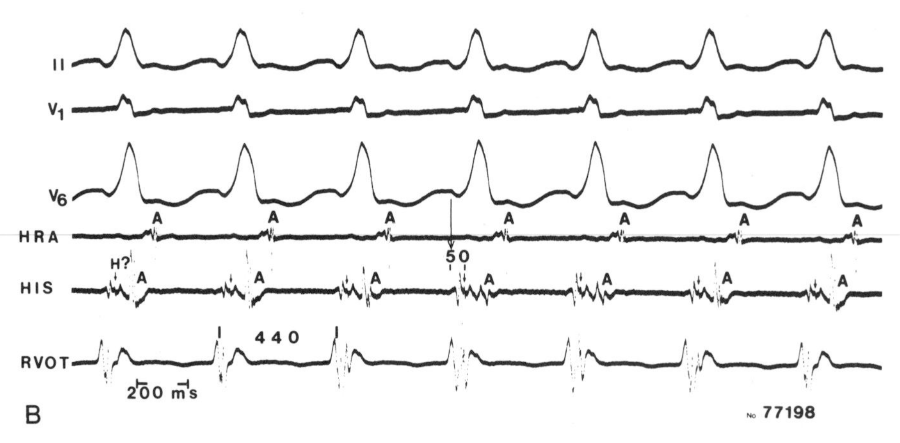

Figure 7-1 *(Continued).* As shown in *B* the QRS complex during tachycardia was not preceded by a His bundle potential. A questionable His potential was identified within the QRS complex (small arrows). During the study spontaneous and pacing induced A-V dissociation was observed without affecting the tachycardia. For abbreviations see text.

that only ventricular structures are required to sustain the tachycardia. Therefore, the following two criteria should be fulfilled: (1) spontaneous or pacing induced A-V dissociation, and (2) identification of a His bundle potential which either (a) is dissociated from the QRS complex, (b) follows the beginning of the QRS, or (c) precedes the ventricular activity by an H-V interval which is shorter than that observed during a supraventricular rhythm.

In patients with a wide QRS complex tachycardia not preceded by a His potential and with 1:1 V-A conduction, pacing induced A-V dissociation needs to be provoked to discard an A-V junctional mechanism utilizing an accessory pathway in the antegrade direction. Single or multiple atrial premature stimuli during tachycardia will demonstrate that the atria are not required to sustain the arrhythmia (Fig. 7-2).

In an earlier report from this laboratory, deflections compatible with a His potential were identified in 54 percent of the patients during VT.[2] Most of the time the His potential is localized in the middle of the QRS complex. The timing of the His potential relative to the beginning of the QRS complex has a limited value as indicator of the site of origin of the VT. As shown in Figure 7-3, during the same VT without change in rate or QRS configuration, the His bundle can be invaded more or less prematurely. As discussed elsewhere, we believe that an early appearance of the His potential indicates a close relation between the tachycardia exit point and the His-Purkinje system. The absence of this feature has no value at all in determining the relationship between site of origin of VT and His-Purkinje system.[4]

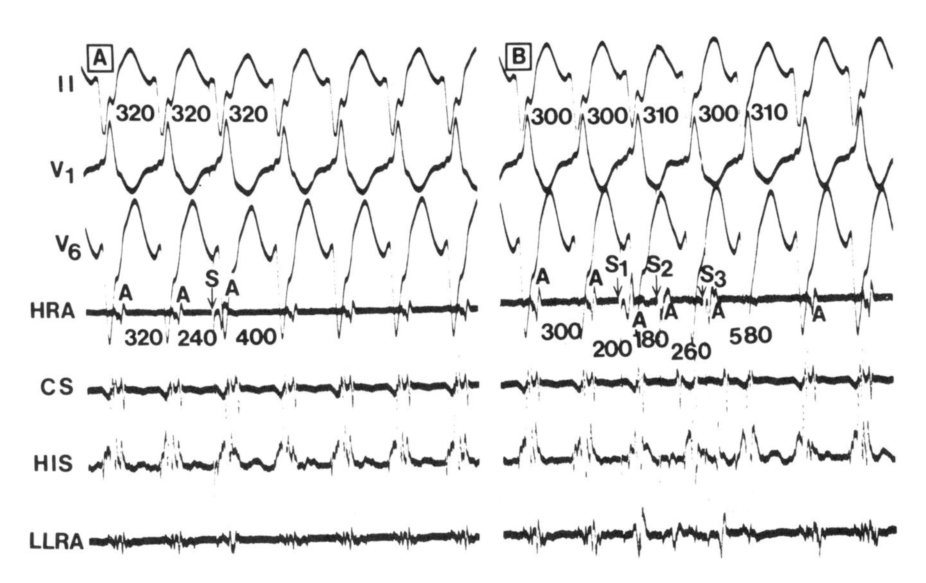

Figure 7–2. Demonstration of pacing-induced dissociation in a patient with 1:1 V-A conduction during ventricular tachycardia. Panel A shows that a single atrial premature stimulus (S) does not affect the tachycardia. In panel B after three consecutive atrial premature stimuli (S_1, S_2, S_3) a ventricular complex of the tachycardia is not followed by retrograde atrial activity. Despite this, tachycardia continues at the same rate.

MECHANISM OF HUMAN VENTRICULAR TACHYCARDIA

Until recently initiation and termination of VT during the stimulation study was considered as evidence for reentry.[2] Several investigators have demonstrated, however, that under certain experimental conditions focal arrhythmias can be triggered and terminated by appropriate modes of stimulation.[7] The relevance of triggered focal activity as an underlying mechanism of ventricular tachycardia in man is unknown. The differentiation between triggered focal activity and reentry cannot be made with certainty at this time by stimulation techniques. Josephson et al. have recently shown that in some patients with recurrent sustained VT, the initiation of the arrhythmia depended on the development of a critical degree of fragmentation and delay in local left ventricular electrograms.[8] Sustainment of VT in these patients was associated with the recording of a continuous local electrical activity. The identification of diastolic and systolic continuous activity during VT is probably the strongest available argument to support an underlying reentrant mechanism.

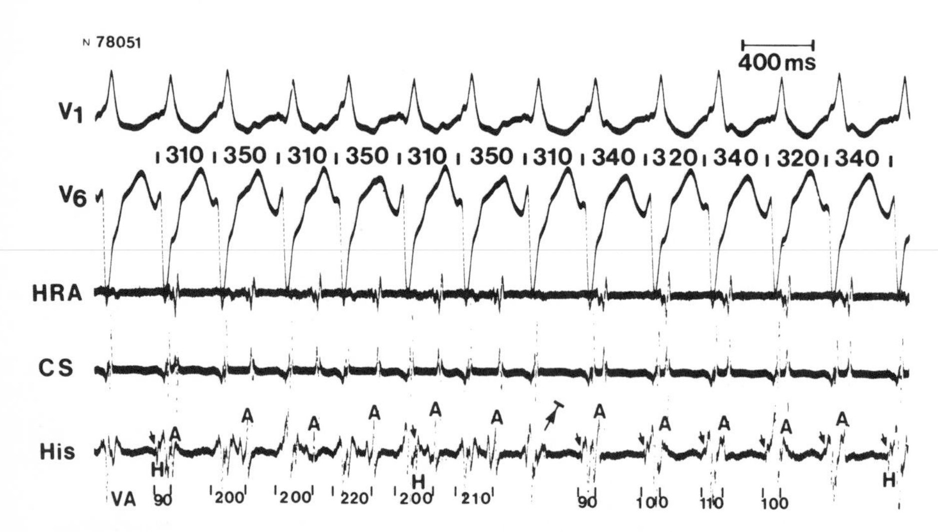

Figure 7-3. This figure belongs to the same patient as Figure 7-2. During tachycardia spontaneous variation of the relationship between the His potential and the beginning of ventricular activation is illustrated. Alternating cycle lengths during tachycardia are observed. At the beginning of the tracing the His potential is identified early after the onset of the QRS complex, the V-A time being 90 ms (from the earliest ventricular forces in the surface leads to the beginning of the atrial electrogram in the His lead). A sudden change in V-A time occurs in the next beat and the timing of the His potential also changes. In the middle of the tracing V-A block occurs when the His potential is again invaded early after the onset of ventricular activation so that this impulse find the A-V node refractory. For abbreviations, see text.

The characterization of the components of the reentrant circuit in patients in whom this mechanism is thought to be responsible for the VT, is difficult. Fascicular reentry was not found to be a plausible explanation in most cases of sustained VT studied in our laboratory.[2,4] As mentioned above, activation of the His-Purkinje system seemed to be a secondary phenomenon. Josephson et al. have recently demonstrated that in many of these patients, ventricular capture by either ventricular or supraventricular impulses during tachycardia frequently does not affect the arrhythmia, thus suggesting that the reentrant circuit is small in size.[9]

DRUG STUDIES IN VT

Stimulation studies can be a valuable tool helping in the selection of more adequate modes of therapy in some patients with VT. This obviously applies to the forms of VT that can be reproducibly induced and terminated during the stimulation study. Therefore, these investigations should in practice be restricted to patients with sustained VT and either an old myocardial infarction or an otherwise normal heart.

In conducting drug studies in patients with sustained VT, the following data should be analyzed: (1) ability of the drug to terminate VT, (2) modification of the tachycardia cycle length after the drug, (3) number of ventricular premature stimuli required to terminate the tachycardia following the drug as compared with before drug administration, (4) modification of the tachycardia-zone both during atrial and ventricular extra-stimulus testing, and (5) presence of spontaneous terminations of the VT induced following the administration of the drug.

Procainamide was studied in 12 patients with sustained VT in whom the arrhythmia was reproducibly inducible prior to drug administration.[10] In ten out of twelve patients (83%), procainamide terminated the arrhythmia. In four patients (33%), VT could no longer be induced following procainamide administration. In all patients the tachycardia cycle length was prolonged after the drug. No relationship was found between the tachycardia cycle length before and after the administration of procainamide. The slowing in heart rate after procainamide made it possible to terminate tachycardia with fewer premature ventricular stimuli than before drug administration. Chronic drug studies in patients with chronic recurrent VT have recently been reported by others.[11]

STIMULATION TECHNIQUES IN THE TREATMENT OF VT

As recently reviewed, information derived from the stimulation studies has resulted in the application of different modalities of pacing in the treatment of certain patients with VT.[12] Conventional antiarrhythmic medication sometimes fails to prevent the development of sustained recurrent attacks of VT. Frequently in these patients, a single ventricular premature stimulus is capable of terminating the arrhythmia when before drug administration more ventricular premature stimuli were required to stop the tachycardia. These patients can be successfully controlled by combining the administration of drugs that slow the ventricular rate during tachycardia (amiodarone, quinidine etc.) and the so-called underdrive pacing, as discussed elsewhere.[4,12]

More recently, "burst" pacemakers have been introduced in the management of drug-resistant recurrent sustained VT.[12] Burst pacemakers should probably be considered only in patients with idiopathic recurrent sustained VT (Fig. 7-4). However, this mode of pacing in patients with severely diseased hearts (cardiomyopathy, severe ischemic heart disease, etc.) may be potentially very harmful.

Sophisticated implantable units capable of recognizing the onset and termination of the tachycardia and able to scan the cardiac cycle with

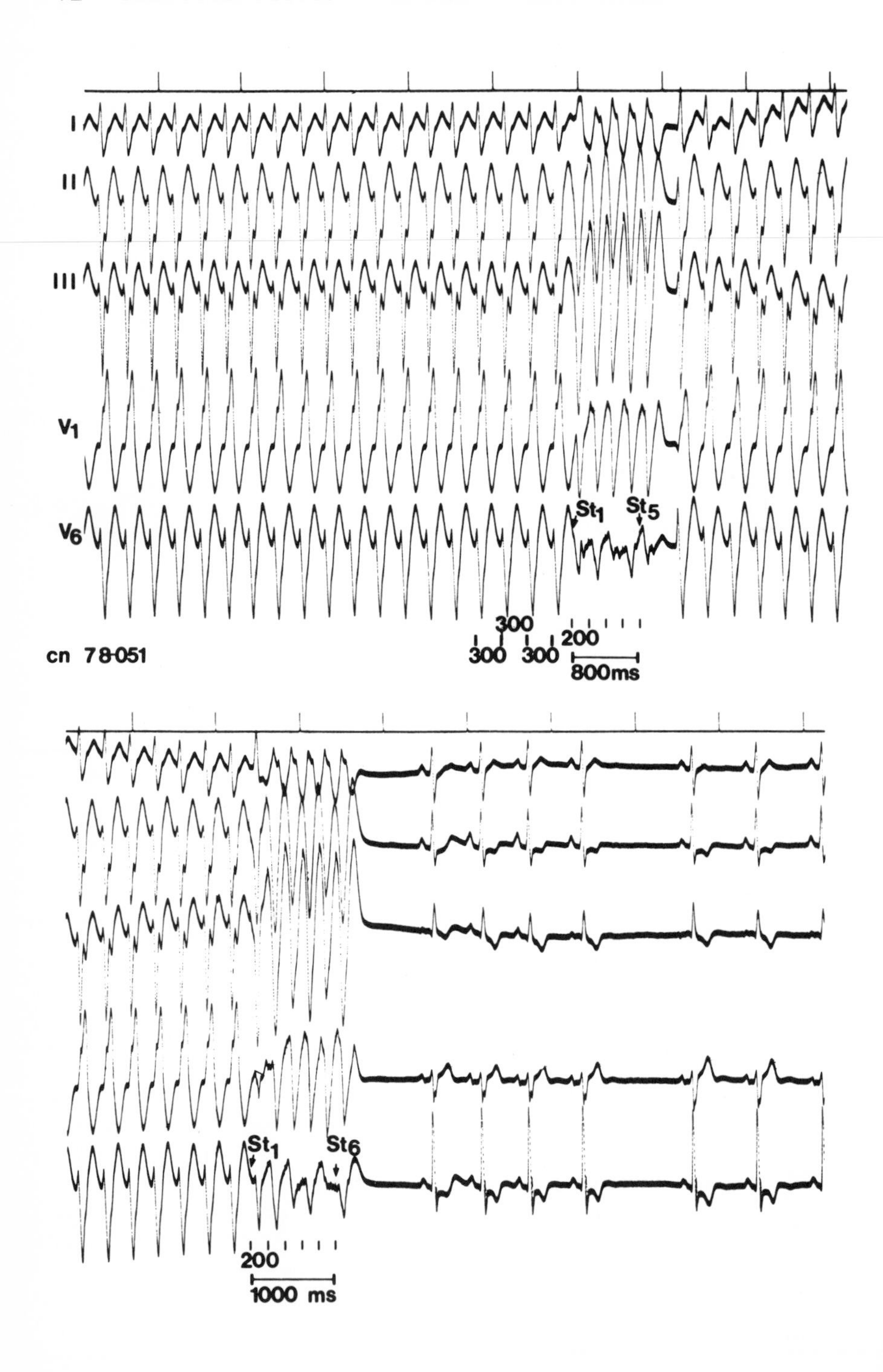
I
II
III
V1
V6
St1
St5
cn 78-051
300
300
300
300
200
800ms
St1
St6
200
1000 ms

single and multiple premature stimuli are needed. These units will represent an useful therapeutic tool to improve the quality of life in some young and healthy patients who otherwise are crippled by both the arrhythmia and the antiarrhythmic medication.

RELEVANCE OF STIMULATION STUDIES IN THE SELECTION OF SURGICAL CANDIDATES

The success of surgical techniques in preventing further development of medically refractory recurrent ventricular tachycardia has been variable. Electrophysiological investigations may provide some useful data helping in the selection of better surgical candidates. Fontaine has shown that success of surgical therapy for VT is higher in those patients in whom the arrhythmia was thought to be based on reentry because of its reproducible initiation and termination by premature stimulation.[13] Recently, Josephson et al.[14] have reported on their findings with the technique of endocardial mapping from both ventricles in patients with recurrent sustained VT. This technique may have potential practical applications in the selection of better surgical candidates and as a complement of epicardial mapping during the operation.

REFERENCES

1. Wellens, H.J.J., Schuilenburg, R.M., and Durrer, D.: Electrical stimulation of the heart in patients with ventricular tachycardia. *Circulation* **46**: 216, 1972.
2. Wellens, H.J.J., Düren, D.R., and Lie, K.I.: Observations on mechanisms of ventricular tachycardia in man. *Circulation* **54**: 237, 1976.
3. Josephson, M.E., Horowitz, L.N., Farshidi, A., and Kastor, J.A.: Recurrent sustained ventricular tachycardia. 1. Mechanisms. *Circulation* **57**: 431, 1978.

Figure 7–4. This figure belongs to the same patient illustrated in Figures 7-2 and 7-3. Because of the recurrent nature of the tachycardia despite intensive drug therapy, a "burst" pacemaker was indicated in this patient since during the stimulation study four consecutive ventricular premature stimuli were required to terminate the arrhythmia. We have observed that in some patients a critical number of extra-stimuli are needed in order to terminate successfully the episode of VT. For example in this patient, as mentioned above, four ventricular premature impulses could terminate the tachycardia, whereas as illustrated in the upper panel of this figure, a burst consisting of 5 stimuli at a rate of 300 per minute did not terminate the arrhythmia despite capturing the ventricles. In the lower panel a burst of 6 stimuli terminates the episode of ventricular tachycardia. The possible explanations for this phenomenon have been discussed elsewhere.[4]

4. Wellens, H.J.J., Farré, J. and Bär, F.W.: Value and liminations of stimulation studies in patients with ventricular tachycardia. In Narula, O. (ed.): Clinical Electrophysiology. Philadelphia, F.A. Davis, 1979 (in press).
5. Wellens, H.J.J., Bär, F.W., Farré, J., and Gorgels, A.P.: Characteristics of patients with ventricular tachycardia initiated by supraventricular stimuli. *Circulation* **58**: II-154, 1978.
6. Wellens, H.J.J., Bär, F.W., and Lie, K.I.: The value of the electrocardiogram in the differential diagnosis of a tachycardia with a widened QRS complex. *Am. J. Med.* **64**: 27, 1978.
7. Ferrier, G.F.: Digitalis arrhythmias:Role of oscillatory afterpotentials. *Prog. Cardiovasc. Dis.* **20**: 459, 1977.
8. Josephson, M.E., Horowitz, L.N., and Farshidi, A.: Continuous local electrical activity; A mechanism of recurrent ventricular tachycardia. *Circulation* **57**: 659, 1978.
9. Josephson, M.E., Horowitz, L.N., Farshidi, A., et al.: Sustained ventricular tachycardia: Evidence for protected localyzed reentry. *Am. J. Cardiol.* **42**: 416, 1978.
10. Wellens, H.J.J., Bär, F.W., Lie, K.I., et al.: Effect of procainamide, propanolol and verapamil on mechanism of tachycardia in patients with chronic recurrent ventricular tachycardia. *Am. J. Cardiol.* **40**: 579, 1977.
11. Denes, P., Wu, D., Wyndham, C., et al.: Chronic electrophysiological study of paroxysmal ventricular tachycardia. *Circulation* **58**: II-155, 1978.
12. Wellens, H.J.J., Bär, F.W., Gorgels, A.P., and Farré, J.: Electrical management of arrhythmias with emphasis on the tachycardias. *Am. J. Cardiol.* **41**: 1025, 1978.
13. Fontaine, G., Guiraudon, G., Frank, R., et al.: Stimulation studies and epicardial mapping in ventricular tachycardia: Study of mechanisms and selection for surgery. In Kulbertus, H.E. (ed.): Re-entrant Arrhythmias, Mechanism and Treatment Lancaster, MTP Press, 1977.
14. Josephson, M.E., Horowitz, L.N., Farshidi, A., et al.: Recurrent sustained ventricular tachycardia. 2. Endocardial mapping. *Circulation* **57**: 440, 1978.

8

Acute and Chronic Aspects of Conduction Disturbances in Acute Myocardial Infarction

K.I. Lie, M.D.,
and D. Durrer, M.D.

PATHOPHYSIOLOGICAL BASIS

The mechanism, clinical course, and prognosis of conduction disturbances following acute myocardial infarction are closely related to the blood supply of the specific conduction system and the site of infarction.[1–3] Conduction disturbances in the A-V node are usually the consequence of an occlusion proximal to the origin of the A-V nodal artery, which in 90 percent of the cases originates from the right coronary artery.[3] Therefore, conduction disturbances in the A-V node are associated with acute inferior wall myocardial infarction.[4] On the other hand, the right bundle branch and the anterior division of the left bundle branch, receive their blood supply from the septal perforating branches of the left anterior descending artery.[3] Therefore, right bundle branch block, with or without concomitant left anterior hemiblock, is usually associated with extensive anteroseptal infarction, due to an occlusion proximal to the origin of the septal perforating branches of the left anterior descending artery. The posterior division of the left bundle has a dual blood supply from both the posterior descending branch of the right coronary artery and the anterior descending branch of the left coronary artery. This implies that an involvement of the posterior division of the left bundle branch is usually associated with two vessel disease in both the right coronary artery and the proximal part of the left anterior descending artery. Therefore, the development of left posterior hemiblock is always associated with massive myocardial damage.

Clinicopathologic studies also indicate the relationship between the site of infarction and involvement of the conduction system.[1,5-7] It is of interest to note that in many of the cases, no actual necrosis was found in either the A-V node or bundle branches. Moreover, in those cases in which necrosis was present, it was frequently not extensive and was present only within or adjacent to the specific conducting system.[5,6] It is still unclear whether the focal necrosis, when found, is sufficient to cause the interruption of impulse conduction. A recent clinicopathologic study has revealed that hydropic cell swelling (with infiltration of polymorphonuclear leukocytes in some cases) was present in those exhibiting conduction disorders, whereas it was absent in a control group without conduction disturbances but with the same site of infraction.[7] These data correlate very well with the transient nature of the conduction disorders associated with acute myocardial infarction.

A-V NODAL CONDUCTION DISORDERS

Intranodal conduction disorders occur almost exclusively with acute inferior myocardial infarction. In this clinical setting, their occurrence shows a bimodal pattern. During the first hour of myocardial infarction, intranodal conduction disorders occur very frequently. Observations from the mobile coronary care units have revealed that second and third degree A-V blocks occur in approximately 11 percent of the patients with inferior myocardial infarction examined within one hour after onset of symptoms.[8] In contrast, this incidence was extremely low in those seen during the second hour after onset of symptoms. The very short duration, and its immediate response to atropine, suggest that vasovagal mechanisms probably play a very important role in the genesis of these conduction disorders.[8] Intranodal conduction disturbances occur in approximately 20 percent of hospitalized patients with inferior myocardial infarction, which are usually manifested several hours after onset of symptoms.[9] In the majority of these patients, block first appeared between two and 72 hours after onset of symptoms. In our experience, the latest time of onset of intranodal conduction disturbances was on the fifth day of infarction.

First degree A-V block has been reported to occur in 7 to 13 percent of patients admitted with acute myocardial infarction, and is usually observed in those with an inferior myocardial infarction.[9] Norris has reported that of the 64 patients with first degree A-V block and acute inferior infarction, 75 percent subsequently developed second degree A-V block.[10] Second degree A-V block, in association with acute inferior myocardial infarction, usually manifests as a progressive lengthening of the P-R interval until a successive P wave is blocked (Wenkebach Type

I). In the minority on cases, 2:1 A-V block occurs in association with inferior myocardial infarction.

During inferior myocardial infarction and second degree A-V block, we have frequently observed that following a blocked P wave the next conducted sinus impulse shows a left bundle branch block pattern (Fig. 8-1). This pattern of bradycardia-related left bundle branch block was noted in approximately one-third of our patients with second degree A-V block. Of interest in these patients is the fact that bradycardia-dependent left bundle branch block occurred only during second degree A-V block and did not occur during sinus bradycardia despite comparatively slower rates.

In 91 of our cases with second degree A-V block as a complication of inferior myocardial infarction, approximately half progressed to a high degree A-V block or third degree A-V block (Table 8-1). It has been

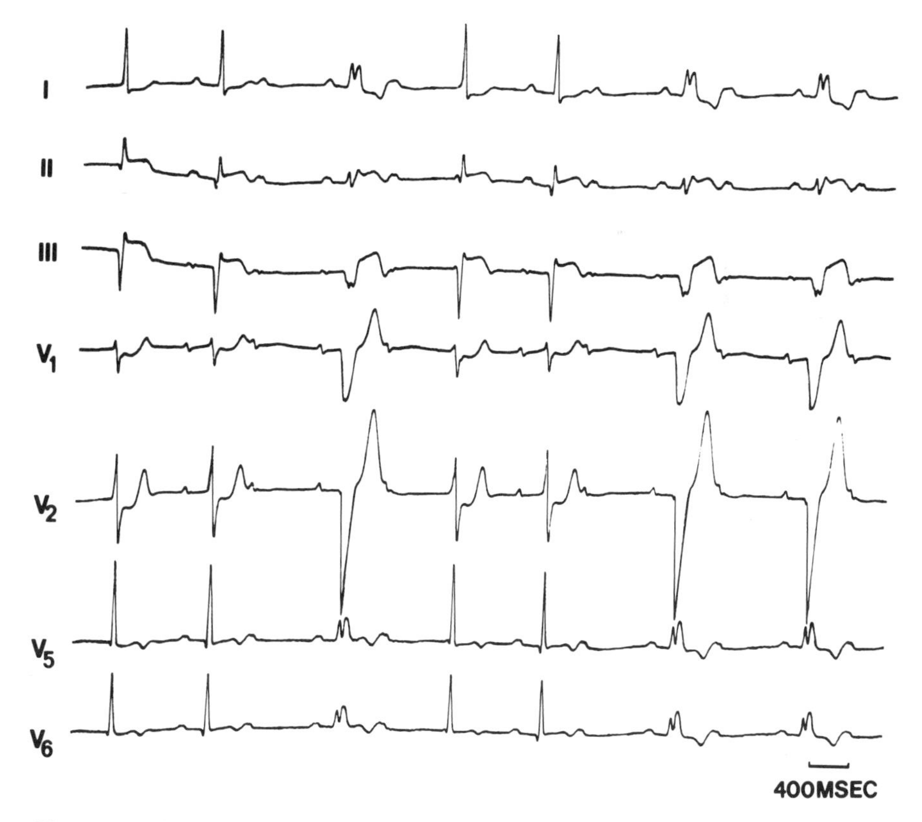

Figure 8-1. Second degree A-V block with bradycardia-dependent left bundle branch block in a patient with acute inferior myocardial infarction.

TABLE 8-1. ECG Prior to and Following Second Degree AV-Block

	No.	No.		No.
1 → 2	59	91	→ 3	41
normal PR → 2	7		→ 1	43
on admission 2	25		→ †	7

1= first degree AV-block.
2= second degree AV-block.
3= third degree AV-block.
†= death during second degree AV-block.
PR= PR interval.

TABLE 8.2. Escape Frequency During Third Degree AV-Block

Beats/min.	No.		Mortality No.		P.M.* No.	
<30	8	74	4	14	7	60
31 - 40	34		6		26	
41 - 50	32		4		27	
51 - 60	15	20	5	6	9	11
61 - 70	3		1		1	
>70	2		0		1	

*P.M.= temporary pacemaker therapy.

generally believed that under these circumstances, the escape pacemaker during complete A-V block or dissociation produces an acceptable and dependable heart rate.[2,5] However, in our 94 patients with complete A-V block or dissociation, only 20 (21%) had a ventricular rate of more than 50 beats per minute and 42 (44%) actually had a ventricular rate of less than 40 beats per minute (Table 8-2). Previously, it has also been supposed that the escape pacemaker, during intranodal block complicating acute inferior infarction, usually produces narrow QRS complexes as it originates from a site just below the A-V node. However, an escape rhythm with wide QRS complexes (0.12 sec) was seen in 35 of our 94 patients (37%) with intranodal block as a complication of inferior myocardial infarction.

The above data suggests that intranodal conduction disturbances following acute inferior infarction are frequently associated with escape mechanisms showing either slow ventricular rates or wide QRS complexes.

Another interesting phenomenon was that in some cases the escape beats showed right bundle branch block and in others, left bundle branch block pattern. The escape pacemakers with left bundle branch block pattern had higher ventricular rates as compared to those with a right bundle branch block configuration. His bundle studies in these patients showed that all escape beats were preceded by a His bundle potential at a normal H-V interval, revealing an escape pacemaker site located in the A-V junction with a relatively higher rate. In some of the latter patients, His bundle pacing normalized the QRS duration and abolished left bundle branch block by an increase in frequency. These findings indicate that bradycardia-dependent left bundle branch block was the underlying mechanism responsible for the wide QRS complexes.

On the other hand, the escape beats with a right bundle branch block pattern either showed no His bundle potential or had a His bundle potential just at the onset of the QRS complex. In addition, His bundle deflections were absent after each atrial depolarization. These findings indicate that these beats were either of ventricular or fascicular origin and also explain the relatively slow frequency of the escape mechanism. The escape rhythms with a right bundle branch configuration sometimes alternated with an escape A-V junctional mechanism which had a much slower rate (Fig. 8.2).

In our series of 144 patients with second or third degree A-V block and inferior myocardial infarction, the duration of block varied from several minutes to 16 days. The conduction defect lasted for less than 24 hours in 37 percent, from one to three days in 30 percent, and for more than three days in 33 percent of the cases. All patients with high degree A-V block who survived resumed 1:1 A-V conduction.

Prognosis

The presence of high degree A-V block affected the immediate prognosis of patients with inferior myocardial infarction. The hospital mortality was more than two times higher in those with A-V block as compared to those without intranodal block (Table 8-3). The size of infarction was also significantly larger in patients with high degree A-V block.

TABLE 8-3. Incidence, Age, Sex, Mean Peak SGOT and Mortality

	All Patients with IMI	Patients Without High Degree AV-block	Patients With High Degree AV-Block
Number	843	699	144
Mean age (yr)	63	62	65
Sex: male	627	517	110
Sex: female	216	182	34
Mean peak SGOT (I.U.)	100	92	140
Mortality (%)	12	9	22

In our series neither degree, duration, time of onset of block and QRS width, nor frequency of the escape pacemaker affected immediate prognosis. However, most patients with complete A-V block of longer duration, or an escape pacemaker with a low ventricular rate, were usually paced. Therefore, the fact that pacemaker intervention might have influenced the immediate prognosis cannot be excluded. The reason why

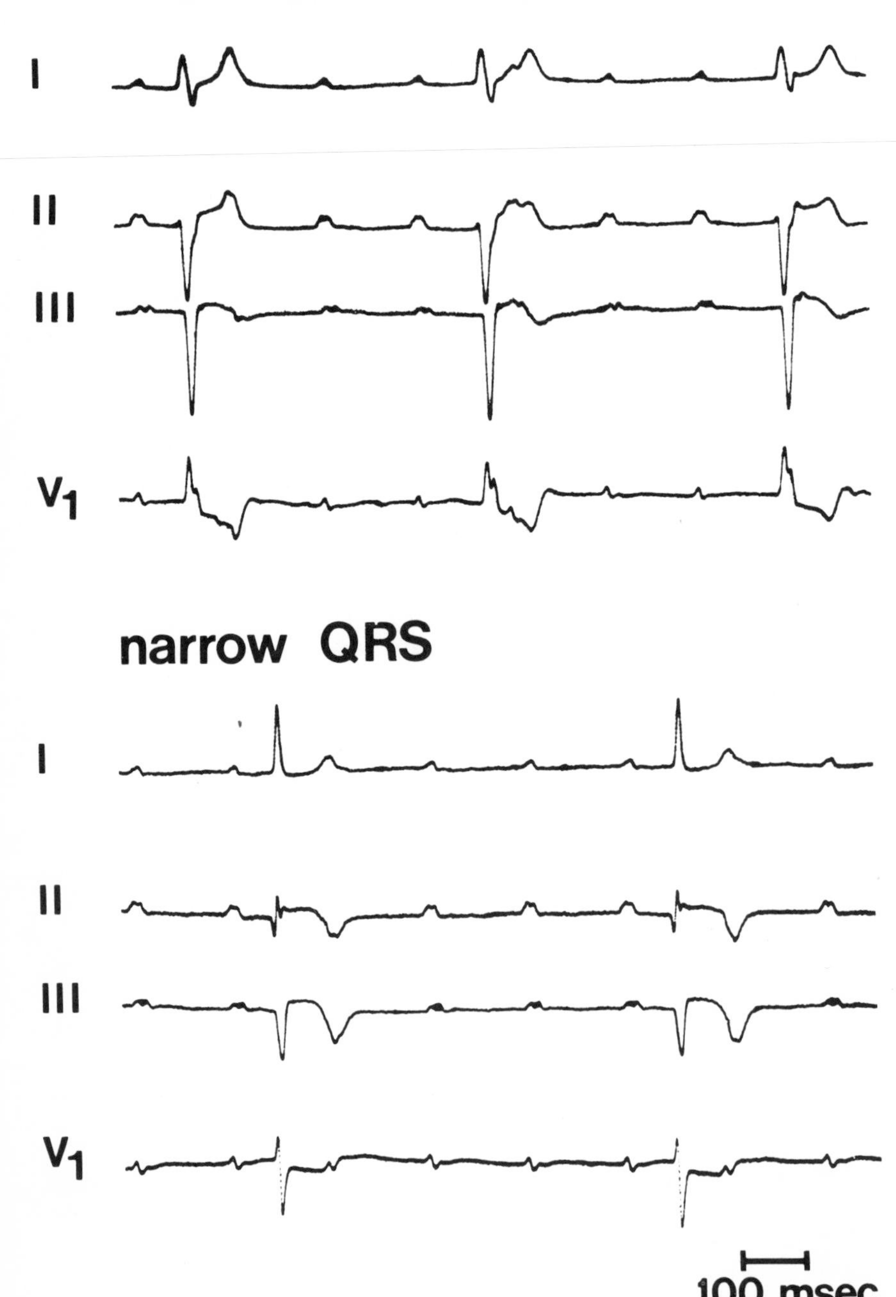
wide QRS RBBB
I
II
III
V1
narrow QRS
I
II
III
V1
100 msec

patients with wide QRS complexes did not have a higher mortality rate, as compared to those with narrow QRS complexes during intranodal block in inferior infarction, is related to the fact that the site of block is still located in the A-V junction.

INTRAVENTRICULAR CONDUCTION DISORDERS

Incidence

Following acute myocardial infarction, intraventricular conduction disturbances are usually located in the bundle branches and are associated with an anteroseptal site of infarction.[5] Bundle branch block has been reported to occur in 6 to 10 percent of patients with acute myocardial infarction.[5] However, the diagnosis of bundle branch block as a consequence of acute myocardial infarction is often difficult, as in 40 to 83 percent of reported cases the conduction defect was already present on admission and may have reflected a preexistent conduction disorder.[11]

In an attempt to determine the true incidence of acquired and preexistent bundle branch block in acute myocardial infarction, we tried to obtain previous ECGs of those patients who on admission presented with a bundle branch block pattern. Bundle branch block was considered to be a consequence of infarction if it developed after admission, or if the conduction disorder was not present on an ECG taken within six months of admission. Of the 1200 consecutive admissions for an acute myocardial infarction, 106 (9.6%) had an acquired bundle branch block, and 42 (3.8%) had a preexistent bundle branch block. Thirty (2.5%) others in whom the acquired or preexistent nature of the bundle branch block could not be determined, were excluded from this study.

Our data revealed that especially patients with *acquired* right bundle branch block and anteroseptal infarction are at risk of developing complete infranodal block. However, only 50 percent of our patients with acquired right bundle branch block actually developed the conduction disturbance after admission. In the other 50 percent a previous electrocardiogram was usually not readily available. Moreover, 28 percent of the patients with bundle branch block on admission had not had an ECG recorded in the preceding six months. These considerations stress the importance of evaluating those factors which may help in the early

---

Figure 8–2. Escape beats showing a right bundle branch block configuration *(top)* alternating with an A-V junctional escape mechanism (*bottom*). Note that the frequency of the right bundle branch block escape rhythm is higher than that of the A-V junctional escape rhythm.

identification of patients with an acquired bundle branch block, from those with a preexistent bundle branch block.

The QRS configuration in V_1 is helpful in differentiating acquired from preexistent right bundle branch block. Ninety percent of patients with acquired right bundle branch block and acute anteroseptal infarction showed a QR complex in V_1 during the first 24 hours of admission, whereas 90 percent of the patients with pre-existent right bundle branch block showed either a qR or a trifasic QRS pattern in V_1. Two patients with a preexistent right bundle branch block also showed a QRS pattern in V_1 and each had had a previous anteroseptal infarction. Therefore, the QRS configuration in V_1 is probably more valuable in patients with a first attack than in those with a recurrent infarct.

Diagnosis of Fascicular Block

During acute myocardial infarction, the diagnosis of fascicular block may be hampered by two factors which influence the frontal plane QRS axis: (1) In transmural myocardial infarction the frontal QRS axis may change to a direction away from the leads showing QS complexes, i.e., away from the site of infarction. (2) In nonintramural myocardial infarction, the frontal QRS axis may shift toward the site of infarction due to intramural conduction block near the site of infarction with delayed activation of this area forming QR complexes. In an attempt to evaluate the nature of true fascicular block complicating acute myocardial infarction, we observed the pattern and degree of changes in frontal QRS axis in 12 patients with acute anteroseptal infarction who on admission had nonaberrant conduction and subsequent to a phase of bifascicular block developed complete infranodal block. During these observations, the shift in axis occurred gradually over a period of hours, in contrast to the usual sudden development of right bundle branch block.

All patients developed right bundle branch block with left anterior fascicular block, had left axis deviation of at least $-60°$, and a change of frontal QRS axis of $60°$ or more prior to the development of complete infranodal block. Patients who developed right bundle branch block with left posterior fascicular block, showed an axis of $+90°$ or more and a rightward shift of frontal QRS axis of $60°$ or more, before they progressed to complete infranodal block. These data suggest that the classical criteria for diagnosis of fascicular block in acute anteroseptal infarction, as far as deviation of frontal QRS axis is concerned, should probably be corrected by a factor of 30 to the left. A possible explanation is that in acute anteroseptal infarction, the frontal QRS axis has usually already shifted to a horizontal position, presumably due to loss of forces in the apical area.

We also observed that the classical initial QRS patterns of fascicular block are often not present if fascicular block complicates acute anteroseptal infarction. This could possibly be attributed to the fact that the areas activated early by the anterior or posterior fascicle of the left bundle are involved by the interaction with the resultant absence of an initial r wave if the fascicular block occurs contralaterally to the infarcted area. Since our results indicate that in acute anteroseptal infarction the classical criteria of fascicular block are often not present, the following new characteristics may be diagnostically helpful: (1) a left or rightward shift of 60° or more in frontal QRS plane, and (2) a frontal QRS axis of $\geqq -60°$ or $\geqq +90°$ when a hemiblock pattern is already present on admission.

Evolution of Right Bundle Branch Block

The evolution of right bundle branch block was registered in ten patients during continuous tape recordings. Five patients developed incomplete right bundle branch block over periods ranging from several minutes to two hours. This was followed by the occurrence of sudden onset (within one beat) of complete right bundle branch block without a change in the preceding RR intervals (Fig.8-3). The other five patients abruptly (within one beat) developed complete right bundle branch block without either passing through a phase of incomplete right bundle branch block or a change in the preceding cycle length. In nine of these ten patients, the onset of complete right bundle branch block was associated with a concomitant shift of the frontal QRS axis to the left (10 to 30 degrees). Concomitant right axis deviation was observed in only one patient (Fig. 8-3). In the patients with a transient right bundle branch block, the pattern disappeared within one beat. These observations suggest that the conduction disorder is located in the proximal right bundle. His bundle recordings and stimulation studies further favor this concept and are discussed later.

The duration of complete infranodal block varied from several hours to ten days. Onset of complete infranodal block was usually noted during the first three days after infarction. However, we have observed two cases in which complete infranodal block occurred during the second week of infarction. In all cases with infranodal block, the escape pacemaker showed a wide QRS complex. In a surprisingly high percentage (50%) of cases, the escape pacemaker had an acceptable heart rate. In the other 50 percent, escape mechanism was unreliable and showed either a very slow ventricular rate or complete ventricular asystole (Fig. 8-4).

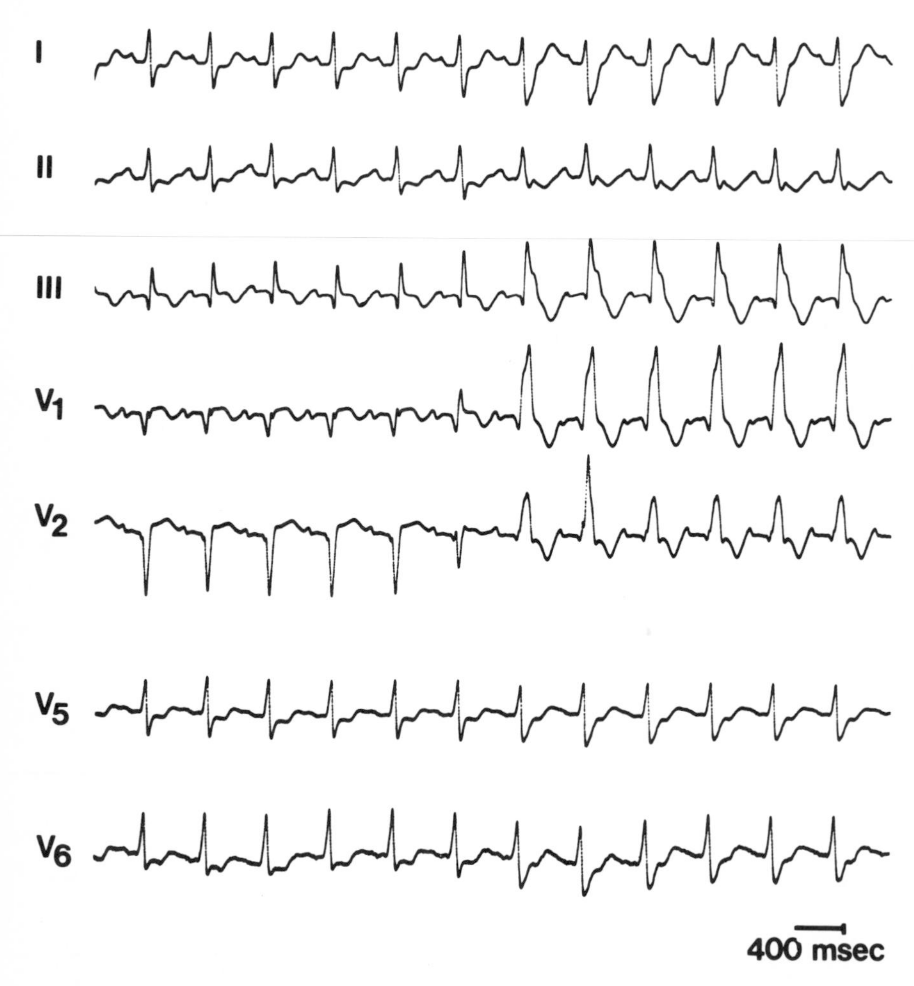

Figure 8-3. Acute anteroseptal infarction complicated by right bundle branch block. Note the sudden onset of right bundle branch block without change of the preceding RR interval. There is a concomitant rightward shift of the QRS axis.

Prognosis

In 434 patients with acute anteroseptal infarction (collected through 1978) the incidence of acquired right bundle branch block (with or without hemiblock) was 25 percent (Table 8-4). In patients with acquired right bundle branch block, the mortality rate was more than three times higher than that of patients with acquired left bundle branch block. This difference could be attributed to the site of infarction associated with the

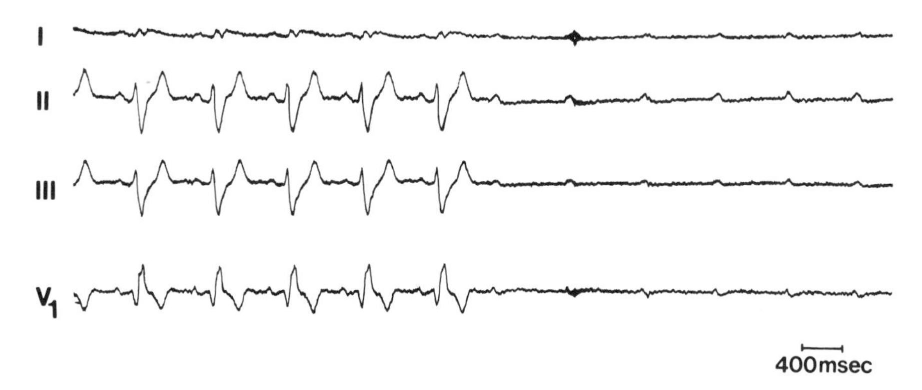

Figure 8-4. Sudden onset of complete infranodal block in a patient right bundle branch block and left anterior fascicular block.

Note that no subsidiary escape pacemaker occurs after onset of complete infranodal block. The mechanism of induction of complete infranodal block may be caused by paroxysmal A-V block, since the complete block starts with a sinus impulse occurring at a shorter PP interval than the previous ones.

TABLE 8-4. Incidence of RBBB in Anteroseptal Infarction and Its Relation to Mortality.

	Incidence		Mean	Mortality	
	No.	%	age	No.	%
All patients with AS infarct	434	100	63.3	151	35
Patients with RBBB	108	25	63.4	80	74
Patients without RBBB	326	75	63.2	71	22

type of bundle branch block. In addition, anteroseptal infarction complicated by right bundle branch block has a higher mortality rate than that without right bundle branch block, as it requires a more proximal occlusion of the left anterior descending artery. The various types of conduction disturbances observed in acute anteroseptal infarction are presented in Table 8-5. Although patients with right bundle branch block and left posterior hemiblock had a higher mortality than the other subgroups, and a higher incidence of progression to complete infranodal block than those with right bundle branch block and left anterior hemiblock, these differences were statistically not significant. Prior to complete infranodal block, all patients showed bifascicular block. Patients with right bundle branch block of short duration (6 hours) or of delayed onset after infarction) had a better prognosis and tended not to progress to complete infranodal block (Tables 8-6 and 8-7).

Table 8-5. Incidence of Type of RBBB and Relation to Mortality and Complete Infranodal Block.

	Incidence		Mortality		Complete Block	Infranodal
	No.	%	No.	%	Number	Percent
RBBB	35	32	24	69	0	0
RBBB + LAH	47	44	33	70	15	32
RBBB + LPH	26	24	23	90	10	38

Table 8-6. Duration of RBBB in Relation to Mortality and Complete Infranodal Block

	No.	Mortality	Complete Infranodal Block
1 to 6 hours	16	2	0
6 to 24 hours	9	3	2
1 to 6 days	6	6	3
pers until discharge	9	0	1
pers until death	69	69	19

Table 8-7. Onset of RBBB in Relation to Mortality and Complete Infranodal Block

Onset of RBBB		Mortality		Complete Infranodal Block	
	No.	No.	%	No.	%
Within 24 hours of infarction	78	66	84	22	29
After 24 hours of infarction	30	14	47	3	10

The prognosis of patients with acquired left bundle branch block was not influenced if the left bundle branch block was due to a rate-dependent mechanism. The latter was especially observed in those with an inferior infarction who developed bradycardia-dependent left bundle branch block during high degree intranodal block (Fig. 8-1). In contrast, acquired non-rate dependent left bundle branch block was associated with a poor prognosis, if the site of infarction was anteroseptal; and the mortality rate was twice as high as compared to those with anteroseptal infarction unassociated with conduction disturbances.

It was initially believed that the dismal prognosis of those with anteroseptal infarction bundle branch block was primarily due to the massive myocardial damage.[11] However, recent observations have revealed that a considerable number of these patients die from late in-hospital ventricular fibrillation.[12,13] During a prospective study, more than one-third of CCU survivors with bundle branch block and an anteroseptal infarction developed late in-hospital ventricular fibrillation one to six weeks after onset of infarction.[13] As a result, it is our current practice to keep all CCU survivors with acquired bundle branch block and anteroseptal infarction in the monitoring area for six weeks. With this policy, the immediate prognosis of these patients might well be improved due to early institution of cardiopulmonary resuscitation, when lethal late arrhythmias supervene. Since the mortality rate of patients with preexistent bundle branch block could be influenced by differences in age, the clinical data of these patients were compared to that of patients without bundle branch block who were matched for age and sex. It then appeared that a preexistent bundle branch block was not associated with a significantly higher mortality rate.

The prognosis of patients with a peripheral intramural block is difficult to establish as the latter diagnosis cannot always be established with certainty. Our observations indicate that a peripheral intramural block can only be considered if other causes for intraventricular conduction disorders are unlikely. On this basis, our data indicate that the presence or development of peripheral intramural block does not affect immediate prognosis.

The prognosis of acquired fascicular block is dependent upon its type. As mentioned earlier, acquired isolated fascicular block is difficult to recognize if frequent 12-lead ECGs are not recorded. Based on those cases in whom the diagnosis of fascicular block could be established with some certainty it appeared that the isolated left anterior fascicular block was not associated with a poor prognosis, whereas all of our few cases with isolated left posterior fascicular block died in the hospital mainly due to pump failure.

The prognosis of patients with complete infranodal block following acute anteroseptal infarction is very poor.[11,14] It is generally accepted that the dismal prognosis of these patients is mainly due to the extensive myocardial damage rather than to the conduction disturbance itself, as temporary pacing does not seem to affect the immediate prognosis significantly. Our data in 35 patients with complete infranodal block are in accordance with previous reports, as 32 of these died in the hospital due to either pump failure or cardiac rupture.[11,14] Of the three survivors, in two temporary pacing might have influenced the immediate prognosis. These two patients may have benefited from cardiac pacing as they had either a slow ventricular rate or complete ventricular asystole.

We have also utilized His bundle recordings in patients with acute anteroseptal infarction complicated by bifascicular block, to determine the value of H-V interval in identifying a subset of patients who are at high risk for subsequent development of complete infranodal block. We have previously reported that the H-V interval in these patients proved to be a predictor of high risk for development of complete block. Our observations in 34 patients with anteroseptal infarction and bifascicular block reconfirm these previous conclusions (Table 8-8). The P-R interval is of limited value in identifying this high risk group as eight of the 21 patients with a normal P-R interval had a prolonged H-V interval (Table 8-9); and three of these eight developed complete heart block. In these patients, the discrepancy between the P-R and the H-V intervals is caused by a short A-H interval. The latter is probably short due to an increased sympathetic tone, which usually accompanies large infarcts.

Table 8-8. H-V Interval in Patients With Bifascicular Block and Relation to Complete A-V Block.

H-V Interval	No. of Patients	Progression into Complete A-V Block
Normal	18	1
Prolonged	16	12

Table 8-9. P-R Interval in Relation to H-V Interval in Patients With Bifascicular Block and ASMI.

		P-R Interval	
		Normal	Prolonged
H-V interval	normal	18	1
	prolonged	8	8

INDICATIONS FOR PACING

Controversy still exists as to the indications for cardiac pacing in conduction disturbances following acute myocardial infarction.[15-17] These controversies are primarily due to a lack of data on the natural history of conduction disturbances, as most patients who manifested these conduction disturbances were treated either medically or with a pacemaker. In this subset of patients, no controlled studies have been performed to determine the value of these interventions.

Temporary Pacing

It was initially believed that in acute inferior wall myocardial infarction with A-V block temporary pacing was usually not necessary as the escape pacemaker emerges just below the A-V node with an acceptable and dependable rate. However, our observations in 94 patients with complete A-V block or A-V dissociation reveal that 74 (78%) of these had ventricular rates of less than 50 beats per minute (Table 8-2). The slow ventricular rates were often caused by unstable escape mechanisms either fascicular or ventricular in origin.[18]

Patients with acute inferior wall myocardial infarction complicated by high degree A-V block, had a high incidence of severe power failure, especially when high degree A-V block was first manifested in the coronary care unit (Table 8-10). These findings may be explained by the following two possibilities: (1) The high degree of A-V block was only a manifestation of an inferior infarction with more extensive myocardial damage, as suggested by a higher mean peak SGOT (Table 8-3). (2) The conduction disturbance itself may have contributed to the development of power failure and extension of infarction with a higher mortality.

Table 8-10. Hemodynamic Condition and Ventricular Rate During High Degree A-V Block in Inferior Infarction.

	HEMODYNAMIC DETERIORATION						NORMAL CLINICAL CONDITION		
	V.R. < 50/min.			V.R. ≥ 50/min.					
		Mortality			Mortality			Mortality	
Management	No.	No.	%	No.	No.	%	No.	No.	%
P.M.	29	6	21	6	4	67	50	8	16
None or Atropine	2	0	0	5	5	100	52	9	17
Total	31	6	19*	11	9	82*	102	17	17

* p < (2 =13.80)
V.R.=ventricular rate.
P.M.=temporary pacemaker therapy.

Forty-two of the 144 patients with inferior infarction and conduction disturbances had hemodynamic deterioration coincident with a high degree of A-V block (Table 8-10). Of these 42 patients, 31 had ventricular rates of less than 50 beats per minute. Although 11 of these 31 patients were initially treated with atropine, only one benefited from atropine. In 29 of the 31 patients, treatment with a temporary pacemaker was instituted. After pacing was started, the clinical condition improved in 24, and of these only one patient died later. The remaining five patients did not respond to pacemaker therapy and died of true cardiogenic shock. Eleven other patients with a ventricular rate more than 50 beats per minute had hemodynamic deterioration. Of these 11 patients, six were paced, and five despite the presence of second degree A-V block were not paced due to a ventricular rate ≧ 80 beats per minute. Three of the six patients who were paced initially showed an improvement in hemodynamic status, although one of these three died later of cardiogenic shock. The other three who did not respond to pacemaker therapy and the three who were not paced died of true cardiogenic shock. Of the remaining 102 patients who were not in shock at the time of the onset of high degree A-V block, 17 died.

Our data indicate that even without severe power failure, patients with high degree A-V block had a higher mortality (17%) than those without high degree A-V block (9%; $p < 0.05$). In the subgroup with high degree A-V block but without severe power failure, there was no difference in mortality between those who were paced (16%) and those who did not require a temporary pacemaker (17%) because of an acceptable ventricular rate. We believe that in this group of patients without severe power failure the higher mortality is mainly due to more extensive myocardial damage and not to the A-V block itself.

On the other hand, in patients with severe power failure at the time of onset of the high degree A-V block and a slow ventricular rate, pacemaker therapy may have been beneficial. Most of these patients were paced and it was found that in the majority, the shock was reversible soon after pacing was started. In addition, the 19 percent mortality in this group is not significantly different from the 17 percent morality in the group without severe power failure. However, when the ventricular rate was more than 50 per minute, most of the patients in shock did not respond to treatment and died in cardiogenic shock. These data correspond very well with the above-described effects of pacing on cardiac index in patients with slow heart rates and complete A-V block.

In these patients, another serious complication secondary to the bradyarrhythmia may be the occurrence of bradycardia-dependent ventricular tachycardia or ventricular fibrillation. Under these circumstances, cardiac pacing may be the only successful means of managing these arrhythmias. In our experience, these arrhythmias are relatively rare but are very resistant to anti-arrhythmic interventions.

From the above discussion it can be concluded that certainly there are some indications for temporary pacing in conduction disturbances during acute inferior wall myocardial infarction. These are: (1) a slow ventricular rate associated with hemodynamic deterioration or Stokes Adams attacks, (2) unstable escape mechanisms especially when the escape beats show a right bundle branch block configuration, (3) bradycardia-dependent ventricular arrhythmias.

The indications for temporary pacing in conduction disturbances following acute anteroseptal infarction are also controversial. One report has suggested that in patients with anteroseptal infarction complicated by complete infranodal block, temporary pacing did not affect the immediate prognosis and was associated with a high incidence of catheter-induced ventricular tachycardia or fibrillation. These authors found that, despite temporary pacing, most deaths occurred from complications of the massive myocardial damage. Others have suggested that temporary pacing should be instituted in these patients.[11,19] The rationale for this policy is based on two considerations: (1) the obvious prevention and/or treatment of Stokes Adams attacks and (2) the possibility that temporary pacing may be a life-saving procedure in some individual cases.

We generally agree with the former policy as, in our opinion, it is unethical to withhold treatment if Stokes Adams attacks supervene. However, we feel that to prevent Stokes Adams attacks, prophylactic temporary pacing should be instituted in those with intact A-V conduction at high risk for the subsequent development of complete infranodal block, i.e., right bundle branch block with either anterior or left posterior fascicular block acquired as a consequence of infarction. These high risk patients have been discussed in detail above (Table 8-5).

If facilities to record the His bundle electrogram are available, the H-V interval may be of help in identifying those with trifascicular block, since 75 percent of the cases with a prolonged H-V interval will develop complete A-V block (Table 8-8). However, if facilities for His bundle recordings are not available, we recommend institution of temporary pacing in every patient suspected of bifascicular block as a complication of anteroseptal infarction. These patients should be paced for five days as the development of complete block usually occurs within this period. In these patients, the P-R interval is not helpful in predicting those at high risk for complete A-V block (Table 8-9).

Temporary pacing is probably not necessary in those with a bifascicular block of delayed onset (later than 24 hours) or of short duration (less than 6 hours) since the latter subgroups are at a very low risk for progression to complete block (Tables 8-6 and 8-7). The indications for temporary pacing in both inferior and anteroseptal infarction are summarized in Table 8-11.

Table 8-11. Indications for Temporary Pacing in Ischemic Conduction Disturbances

A. Inferior infarction:	1. Ventricular rate under 50 beats per minute with power failure or Stokes Adams attacks.
	2. Unstable escape mechanisms (right bundle branch block configuration).
	3. Bradycardia dependent ventricular arrhythmias.
B. Anteroseptal infarction:	Right bundle branch block and left anterior or posterior hemiblock.
	Note: 1. Prophylactic temporary pacing is especially indicated when the H-V interval is prolonged; the the P-R interval is of limited value in identifying those at high risk for development of complete block.
	2. Prophylactic pacing is not indicated when the conduction disturbance is of delayed onset (> 24 hours) or of short duration(< 6 hours).

Permanent Pacing

There is little controversy on the indications for permanent pacing in conduction defects associated with inferior infarction, as these are always transient and do not tend to recur. In our view, permanent pacing is generally not necessary in this setting. However, the indications for permanent pacing in patients with conduction disturbances in association with anteroseptal infarction are very controversial.

Atkins et al. suggested that patients with right bundle branch block and left anterior hemiblock who develop transient complete heart block are at a particularly high risk for sudden death after discharge from the hospital.[19] After combining their cases with those of Scanlon et al.[20] and Godman et al.,[17] they noted that of the 21 patients with right bundle branch block and left anterior hemiblock who had transient complete heart block during acute myocardial infarction, eight of eight with permanent pacemakers were alive at an unspecified period post discharge; whereas 11 of the 13 without permanent pacemakers had died suddenly.

Similarly, Waugh et al. reported that seven of the ten patients with transient infranodal block who were discharged without a permanent pacemaker developed syncope (2 patients) or sudden death (5 patients) within one year, compared to six of seven patients discharged with pacemakers.[21] Of the 16 patients with right bundle branch block and left anterior hemiblock with or without a prolonged P-R interval, or alternating right and left bundle branch block but without a progression to complete heart block, five died suddenly within the first year after myocardial infarction. On the other hand, sudden death may also occur in these patients even after pacemaker implantation.[19] Contrary to these reports, Waters and Mizgala did not notice sudden death in 15 patients with incomplete bilateral bundle branch block, as a complication of acute myocardial infarction, who were followed up for five to 35 months.[22]

Although some of these observations suggest that certain patients with fascicular block and an acute myocardial infarction are at a high risk for sudden death, these are based on uncontrolled studies. In addition, as shown in a recent study, sudden death may also result from ventricular fibrillation and may not necessarily be due to complete A-V block.[13] Therefore, more data on the long-term prognosis of bundle branch block as a complication of anteroseptal infarction are needed, since the actual incidence and the precise mechanism of sudden death in these patients after hospital discharge remain unknown.

REFERENCES

1. Sutton, R., and Davies, M.: The conduction system in acute myocardial infarction complicated by heart block. *Circulation* **38**: 987–992, 1968.
2. Norris, R.M.: Heart block in posterior and inferior infarction. *Br. Heart J.* **31**: 352–356, 1969.
3. James, T.N., and Burch, G.E.: Blood supply of the human interventricular septum. *Circulation* **17**: 391–396, 1958.

4. Kostuk, W.J., and Beanlands, D.S.: Complete heart block associated with acute myocardial infarction. *Am. J. Cardiol.* **26**: 380–384, 1970.
5. Rotman, M., Wagner, G.S., and Wallace, A.G.: Bradyarrhythmias in acute myocardial infarction. *Circulation* **45**: 703–722, 1972.
6. Blondeau, M., Rizzon, P., Lenègre, J.: Les troubles de la conduction auriculo-ventriculaire dans l'infarctus du myocarde récent. *Arch. Mal. Coeur* **54**: 1104–1117, 1961.
7. Becker, A.E., Anderson, B., and Lie, K.I.: Bundle branch block and antero-septal infarction. Clinicopathologic correlations. *Br. Heart J.* **40**: 773, 1978.
8. Adgey, A.A., and Pantridge, J.F.: Acute phase of myocardial infarction. *Lancet* **2**, 501–504, 1971.
9. Meltzer, L.E., and Cohen, H.E.: The incidence of arrhythmias associated with acute myocardial infarction. In Meltzer, L.E., and Dunning, A.J. (eds.): *Textbook of Coronary Care.* Amsterdam, Excerpta Medica, 1972.
10. Norris, R.M.: Arrhythmias in acute myocardial infarction. In Sandoe, E., Flensted-Jensen, E., and Olesen, K. (eds.): *Symposium on Cardiac Arrhythmias.* Sweden, Astra AB, 1970, p. 734.
11. Lie, K.I., Wellens, H.J., Schuilenburg, R., et al.: Factors influencing prognosis of bundle branch block complicating acute anteroseptal infarction. *Circulation* **50**: 935–941, 1974.
12. Lichstein, E., Gupta, P.K., and Chadda, K.D.: Long-term survival of patients with incomplete bundle branch block complicating acute myocardial infarction. *Br. Heart J.* **37**: 294–930, 1975.
13. Lie, K.I., Schuilenburg, R.M., David, G.K., and Durrer, D.: A 5½-year retro- and prospective study on early identification of candidates developing late in-hospital ventricular fibrillation. *Am. J. Cardiol.* **41**: 674–677, 1978.
14. Godman, M.J., Alpert, B.A., and Julia, D.G.: Bilateral bundle branch block complicating acute myocardial infarction. *Lancet* **2**: 345–347, 1971.
15. Bruce, R.A., Blackmon, J.R., Cobb, L.A., et al.: Treatment of asystole or heart block during acute myocardial infarction with electrode catheter pacing. *Am. Heart J.* **69**: 460–469, 1965.
16. Chatterjee, K., Harris, A., and Leatham, A.: The risk of pacing after infarction, and current recommendations. *Lancet* **2**: 1061–1063, 1969.
17. Godman, M.J., Lassers, B.W., and Julian, D.G.: Complete bundle-branch block complicating acute myocardial infarction. *N. Eng. J. Med.* **282**: 237–240, 1970.
18. Lie, K.I., Wellens, H.J., Schuilenburg, R.M., et al.: Mechanism and significance of widened QRS complexes during complete atrioventricular block in acute inferior myocardial infarction. *Am. J. Cardiol.* **33**: 933–939, 1974.
19. Atkins, J.M., Leshin, S.J., Blomqvist, G., et al.: Ventricular conduction blocks and sudden death in acute myocardial infarction. *N. Eng. J. Med.* **288**: 281–284, 1973.
20. Scanlon, P.J., Pryor, R., and Blount, S.G.: Right bundle branch block associated with left superior or inferior intraventricular block associated with acute myocardial infarction. *Circulation* **42**: 1135–1142, 1970.
21. Waugh, R.A., Wagner, G.S., Haney, T.L., et al.: Immediate and remote prognostic significance of fascicular block during acute myocardial infarction. *Circulation* **47**: 765–775, 1973.

9

Recent Concepts in Electrophysiology of Antiarrhythmic Drugs in Man

Paul Touboul, M.D.

Electrophysiological changes induced by antiarrhythmic agents can be studied in isolated cardiac tissues using microelectrodes and voltage clamp techniques. Such methods have provided some possible explanations for the antiarrhythmic action. Further advances have resulted from the development of electrophysiological studies in man and their extension to clinical pharmacology. The aim of this chapter is to give details of clinical electrophysiological methods, to stress their value and limitations and to report the results. A new classification of antiarrhythmic drugs is proposed.

METHODS

The studies are performed in patients in the nonsedated, postabsorptive state who are not taking any cardioactive drugs. Syncope or dizziness are the main clinical disorders leading to the indication of electrophysiological study. Patients presenting with a patent, atrioventricular (A-V) block or conduction disturbances detected by intracardiac recording were not included. Cases of Wolff-Parkinson-White (WPW) syndrome provide study material for the pharmacological effects on accessory pathways.

Four 6 or 7F electrode catheters were introduced percutaneously via the right and left femoral veins using Seldinger technique. A tripolar catheter was used for recording the His bundle activity. Another was used to obtain a bipolar electrogram in the upper lateral part of the right atrium. The remaining two catheters are used to pace the right atrium at the upper third of the septum and the right ventricle respectively. Recordings were made using an eight-channel direct ink-jet recorder. Paper speeds were 100 or 200 mm per second. Five external leads I, II, III, V1, and V6 were always recorded in addition to the intracardiac electrograms. The signals from the His bundle area were transmitted through pre-amplifiers and filtered (recording frequencies:50 to 700 Hz). All data were stored on magnetic tape.

A programmable modular stimulator was used. The electrical impulses have a duration of 1.5 msec and are delivered at a twice diastolic threshold intensity. Stimulation provides a constant cycle length. Moreover, after every eighth beat, premature depolarizations can be induced and the coupling interval is shortened by 10 msec each time. The delivery of atrial extrastimuli provides a method for studying the behavior of the A-V conducting system and of the right atrium.

The electrophysiological measurements were repeated 5 to 30 minutes after intravenous administration of antiarrhythmic drugs. Blood samples were drawn at the same time to assess the plasma levels of drug. The electrophysiological changes were statistically analyzed using the Student t test for paired data.

TERMINOLOGY

S represents the electrical impulse. H is the His bundle deflection, A and V the atrial and ventricular electrograms recorded in the His bundle lead. In the case of paired stimulation, the same symbols are used with the Figure 9-1 for the basic beat and the Figure 9-2 for the premature beat.

Spontaneous cardiac cycle length is taken as the average of at least five consecutive sinus beats.

A-V nodal conduction time (A-H interval) is measured from the first rapid deflection of the low atrial electrogram (A) to the onset of the His bundle activity.

His-Purkinje conduction time (H-V interval) is taken from the initial deflection of the His potential to the earliest point of ventricular depolarization from either the ECG leads or the intracardiac electrogram. Changes in conduction time after drug administration were assessed at identical rates. QRS duration and QT interval are recorded as a measure of intraventricular conduction and repolarization respectively. These data are determined during stimulation and comparisons are made at similar paced cycles. Effective refractory period (ERP) of the atrium is the longest S1S2 interval at which the premature impulse S2 does not result in atrial response. ERP of the AV node is the longest A1A2 interval at which A2 is not conducted to the His bundle.

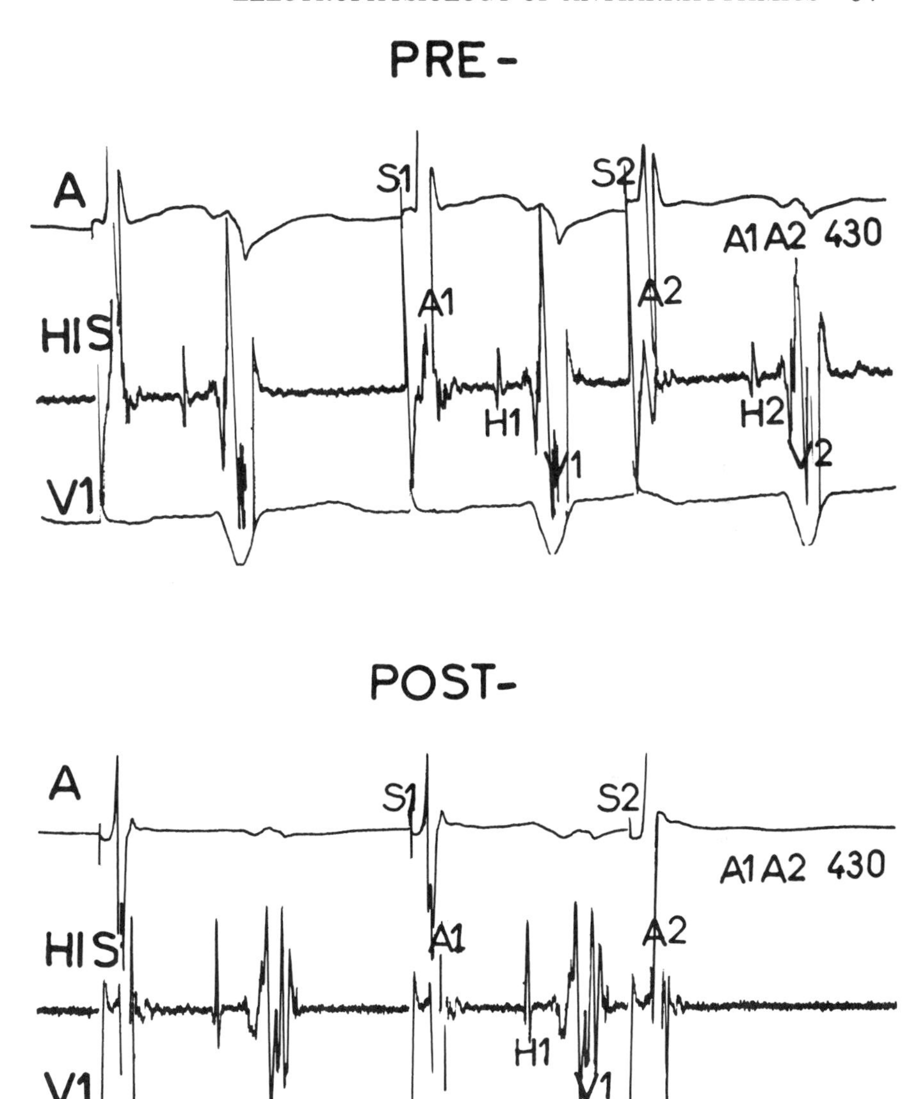

Figure 9–1. Effect of acebutolol, a beta-blocking agent, on the effective refractory period of the A-V node. Extrastimulus method. In the upper panel, before acebutolol (*Pre* -), an atrial premature depolarization A2 induced at a coupling interval of 430 msec is transmitted to the ventricles. After acebutolol administration (*Post* -), at the same coupling interval, the A2 response is blocked within the A-V node. Abbreviations: A = right atrial electrogram; HIS = His bundle lead; S = electrical impulse.

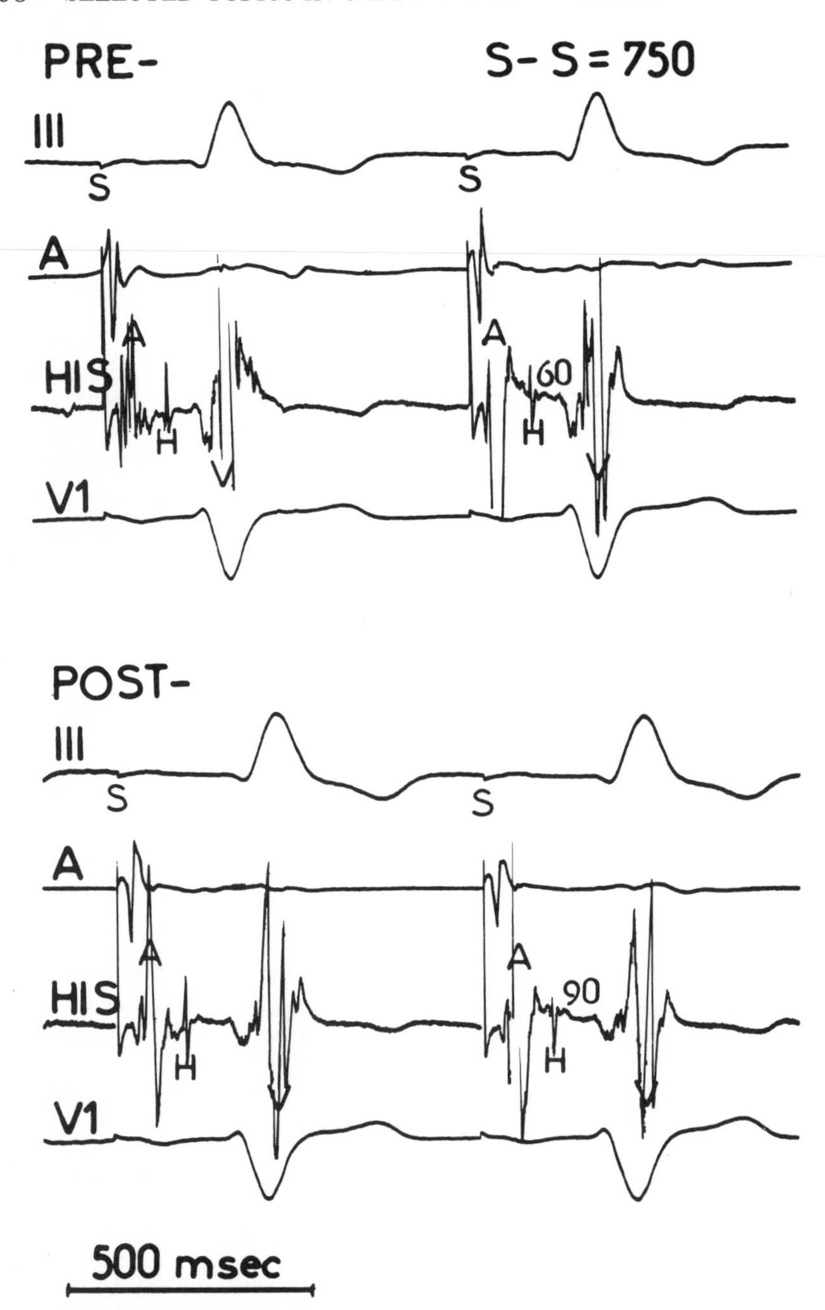

Figure 9–2. Effect of a new quinidine-like compound on the A-V conduction intervals. H-V interval is increased from 60 to 90 msec. The QRS duration is also prolonged.

Functional refractory period (FRP) of the AV node is defined as the shortest H1H2 interval that results from any A1A2.

ERP of the His-Purkinje system is defined as the longest H1H2 interval at which the H2 response fails to propagate to the ventricles.

Relative refractory period of the His-Purkinje system corresponds to the longest H1H2 interval at which the premature His bundle depolarization H2 is followed by a QRS of aberrant configuration or by a longer H-V time than that of the basic drive beat.

ERP of the right ventricle can be determined during ventricular pacing. It is the longest S1S2 interval at which S2 fails to depolarize the ventricle.

In the WPW syndrome, the S-delta interval represents the conduction time through the accessory pathway. ERP of the bypass is defined as the longest A1A2 interval at which the A2 response results in AV block or is conducted to the ventricles along the normal pathway only. The changes observed during reciprocating tachycardia provide an opportunity for assessing the action of drugs on the antegrade and retrograde part of the circuit.

The electrophysiological properties of the human heart have been shown to remain stable for a long time in the basal state, except for a reduction in A-V nodal FRP during the hour following the beginning of the study. The reproducibility of the measurements mean that the electrophysiological changes can be attributed to the action of the antiarrhythmic drugs.

RESULTS

The following classification is based on several years experience of electrophysiological effects induced by antiarrhythmic drugs in man. Three classes can be distinguished in relation to the site of action of these substances within the A-V specialized tissue.

Class I : Drugs depressing the A-V nodal function

A-V nodal conduction, represented by the A-H interval, is slowed. ERP and FRP of the A-V node are increased (Fig. 9-1). On the other hand, the properties of the His-Purkinje system are unchanged. Three types of drugs belong to this group : digitalis,[8] beta-blocking agents,[11] and verapamil.[2]

Class II : Drugs acting on the His-Purkinje system

This class includes two subdivisions based on the presence or absence of depressed His-Purkinje conduction.

IIa : H-V interval is increased (Fig. 9-2)

Conduction is depressed within the Purkinje fibers. Of these drugs, some (quinidine,[6], procainamide,[5] disopyramide[4]) lengthen the refractory periods of the His-Purkinje system, others (ajmaline,[10] chloro-acetyl-ajmaline,[16]) shorten them. Moreover, an increase in ERP of the atrium and of the accessory pathways is also usually observed.[17,18]

IIb : Electrophysiological changes do not involve the H-V interval

Only the refractory periods of the His-Purkinje system are altered: decreased (lidocaine,[3] mexiletine,[7] diphenylhydantoin[1]) or increased (bretylium[15]) (Fig. 9-3 and 9-4).

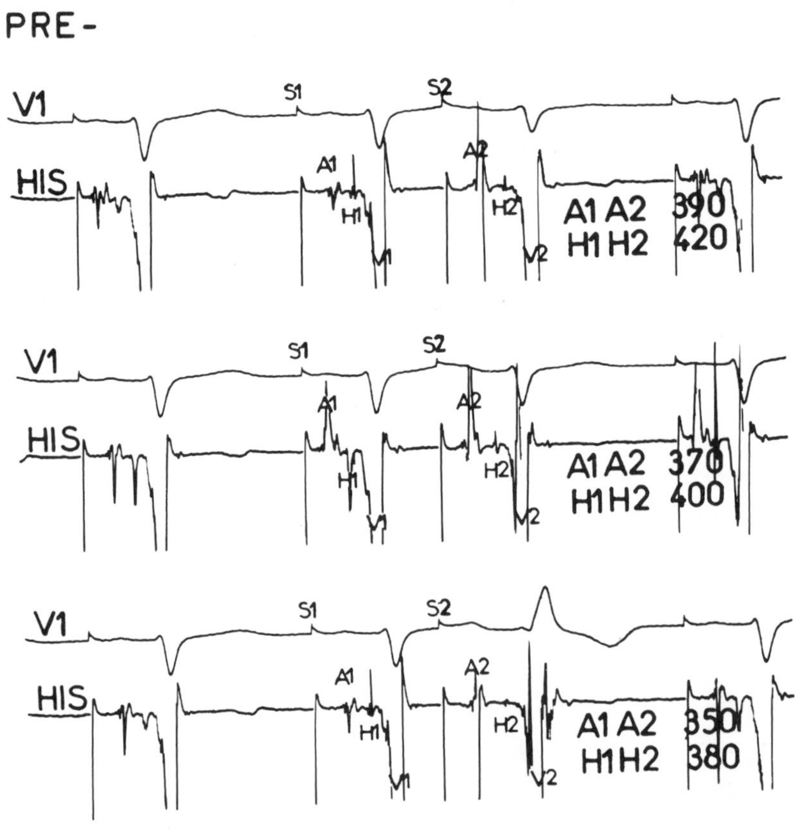

Figure 9-3. Effect of bretylium tosylate on the His-Purkinje system in man. Before drug (*Pre -*), a right bundle branch block appears during atrial premature stimulation at a H1H2 interval of 380 msec.

Class III : drugs changing the properties of both A-V nodal and His-Purkinje tissues (amiodarone, aprindine)

In all cases, there is A-V nodal depression : slowed A-H conduction and increased refractory periods of the A-V node. The effect on the distal conducting fibers varies according to drugs : aprindine prolongs His-Purkinje conduction,[12] whereas amiodarone has no effect on the H-V interval but increases the refractory periods of the His-Purkinje system.[13] Amiodarone also delays recovery of atrial and ventricular tissues. Finally both drugs lengthen ERP of the accessory pathways.[9,14]

DISCUSSION

Electrophysiological studies of drugs in man provide the opportunity of assessing changes within the tissues involved by antiarrhythmic treatments. The site of drug action can thus be located. The present clas-

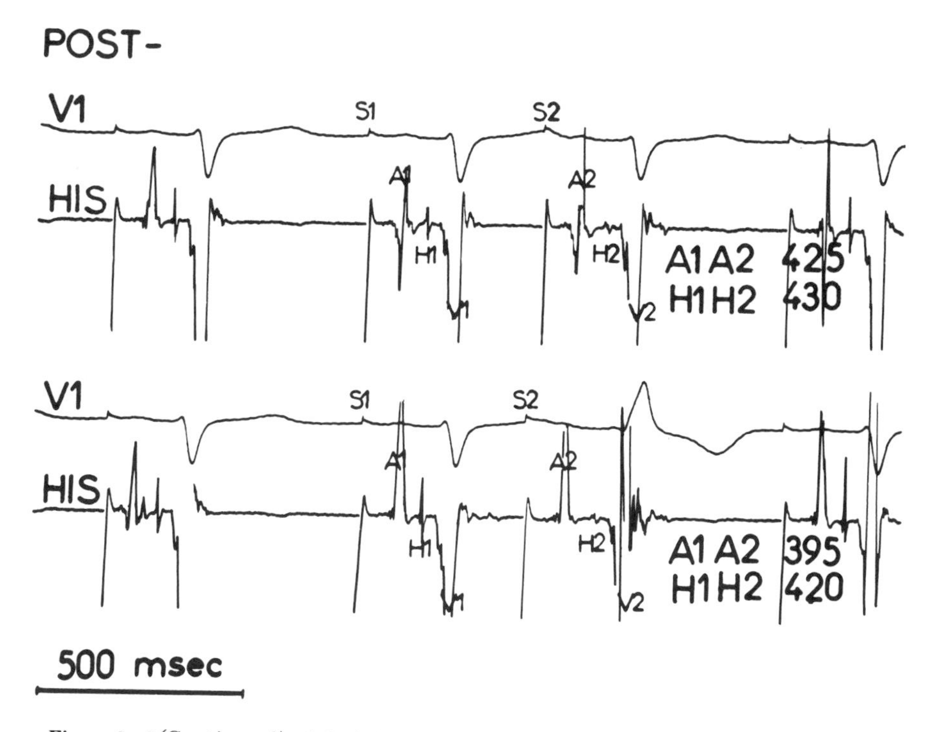

Figure 9-3 *(Continued).* Administration of bretylium results in increased relative refractory period of the His-Purkinje system, the right bundle branch block appearing at a H1H2 interval of 420 msec. On the other hand, His-Purkinje conduction time is not altered following drug.

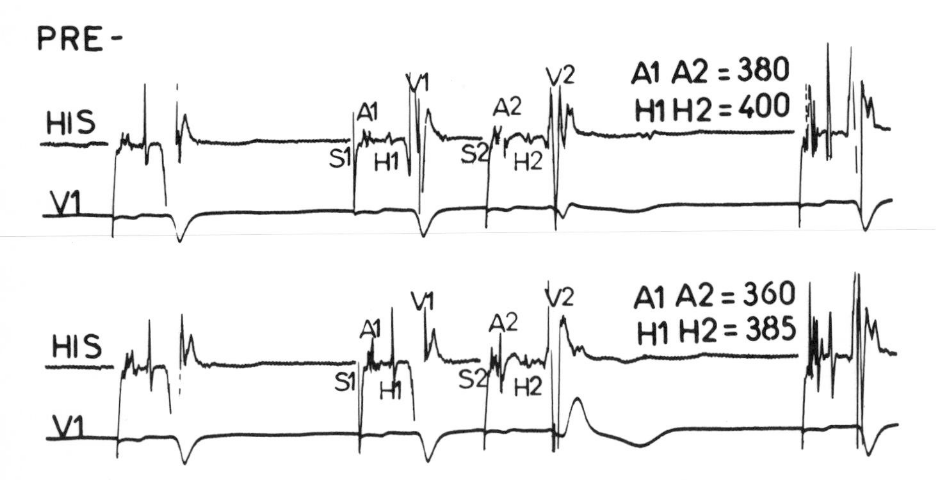

Figure 9–4. Action of mexiletine on the relative refractory period of the His-Purkinje system. Before drug (*Pre* -), an atrial premature depolarization induced at a coupling interval of 380 msec is followed by an aberrant QRS complex. The relevant H1H2 interval measures 400 msec. At a shorter coupling interval, a right bundle branch block becomes apparent.

sification utilizes the effects on the A-V conducting tissue. As a matter of fact, such effects are commonly seen after drug administration. Moreover, on this basis a clear separation can be made between substances acting either on supraventricular or ventricular arrhythmias. Thus depression of the A-V node contributes to the slowing of heart rate during rapid atrial rhythms and to the control of reciprocating tachycardias. Electrophysiological changes within the His-Purkinje system support the possible effectiveness of drugs on ventricular arrhythmias. These changes may involve conduction velocity or refractory periods. Two subdivisions have been distinguished in class II in relation to the presence or absence of H-V prolongation. Lengthening of the H-V interval indicates slowed conduction in the His-Purkinje tissue suggestive of membrane depressant effect. On the other hand, drugs which have no action on conduction velocity may increase or decrease the refractory periods. These data are well correlated with the observations made in isolated cardiac fibers.

However appraisal of drugs must also take into account other possible effects on atrial tissue or A-V accessory pathways. Changes induced within accessory pathways are of special interest due to the common occurrence of supraventricular tachyarrhythmias associated with preexcitation syndromes. Such properties may then increase significantly the spectrum of antiarrhythmic action.

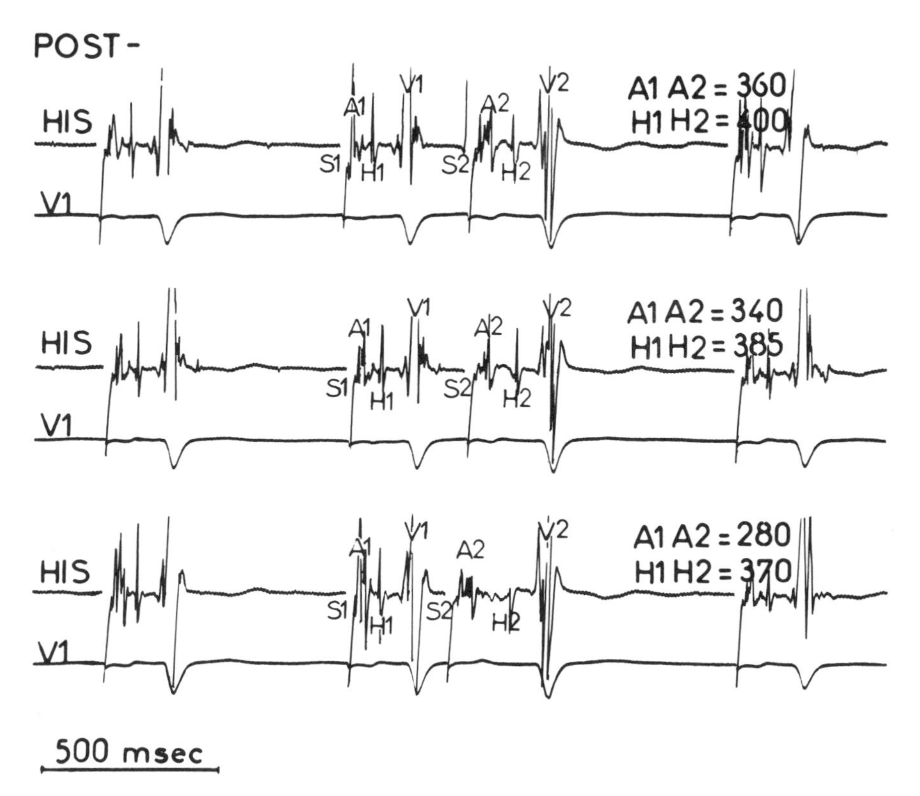

Figure 9–4 *(Continued).* After mexiletine administration (*Post* -), the premature beats exhibit normal intraventricular conduction despite H1H2 intervals similar to control values or even shorter.

There are several criticisms of this kind of study:

1. The relative inaccuracy of the measurements makes it difficult to estimate variations in conduction times of less than 5 msec. Minimal changes in the H-V interval may then pass unnoticed.
2. Drugs are usually given intravenously, and the changes observed are not necessarily the same as those resulting from prolonged, oral administration of the same drug.
3. A single dose is generally used. It is not impossible that other effects might occur with different doses.
4. The action of drugs is complex. Some changes in autonomic tone may combine with the direct cardiac action or even mask its effect. Such phenomena are noted in particular when drugs with vagolytic properties are used. Studies after atropine pretreatment could be useful.

5. Patients selected for study have no A-V conduction disturbances. The mode of action of drugs may change in the presence of damaged tissues providing a different basis for antiarrhythmic effectiveness.

More recently electrophysiological assessment of drugs has been extended to the sinus node. The data studied are the sinus node recovery time, as determined by overdrive atrial pacing, and the sinoatrial conduction time estimated by premature atrial stimulation. The results are related to possible side-effects of therapy.

Finally the knowledge of electrical properties of drugs in the human heart has obvious clinical implications. The classification herein reported aims at giving a basis for proper selection of drugs in clinical practice, allowing a more rational approach to the use of antiarrhythmic therapy.

REFERENCES

1. Caracta, A.R., Damato, A.N., Josephson, M.E., et al.: Electrophysiologic properties of diphenylhydantoin. *Circulation* **47**: 1234, 1973.
2. Husaini, M.H., Kvasnick, A.J., Ryden, L., and Holmberg, S.: Action of verapamil on sinus node, atrioventricular and intraventricular conduction. *Br. Heart J.* **35**: 734, 1973.
3. Josephson, M.E., Caracta, A.R., Lau, S.H., et al.: Effects of lidocaine on refractory periods in man. *Am. Heart J.* **84**: 778, 1972.
4. Josephson, M.E., Caracta, A.R., Lau, S.H., et al.: Electrophysiological evaluation of disopyramide in man. *Am. Heart J.* **86**: 771, 1973.
5. Josephson, M.E., Caracta, A.R., Ricciutti, M.A., et al.: Electrophysiologic properties of procainamide in man. *Am. J. Cardiol.* **33**: 596, 1974.
6. Josephson, M.E., Seides, S.F., Batsford, W.P., et al.: The electrophysiological effects of intramuscular quinidine on the atrioventricular conducting system in man. *Am. Heart J.* **87**: 55, 1974.
7. McComish, M., Crook, B., Kitson, D., and Jewitt, D.: Clinical electrophysiological effects of mexiletine and its mechanism of antidysrhythmic action. *Br. Heart J.* **38**: 311, 1976.
8. Przybyla, A.C., Faulay, K.L., Stein, E., and Damato, A.N.: Effects of digoxin on atrioventricular conduction patterns in man. *Am. J. Cardiol.* **33**: 344, 1974.
9. Reid, P.R., Greene, H.L., Schaeffer, A.H., and Varghese, P.J.: Effects of aprindine in refractory Wolff-Parkinson-White syndrome. *Circulation* **54** **(Suppl. II)**: 18, 1976.
10. Schlepper M., and Neuss, H.: Changes of refractory periods in the A-V conduction system induced by antiarrhythmic drugs. A study using His bundle recordings. *Acta Cardiol.* **Suppl. XVIII**: 269, 1974.
11. Seides, S.F., Josephson, M.E., Batsford, W.P., et al.: The electrophysiology of propranolol in man. *Am. Heart J.* **88**: 733, 1974.
12. Seipel, L., Both, A., Breithardt, G., et al.: Action of antiarrhythmic drugs on His bundle electrogram and sinus node function. *Acta Cardiol.* **Suppl. XVIII**: 251, 1974.

13. Touboul P., Porte J., Huerta, F., and Delahaye, J.P.: Electrophysiological effects of amiodarone in man. *Am. J. Cardiol.* **35**: 173, 1975.
14. Touboul, P., Porte, J., Huerta, F., and Delahaye, J.P.: Effects of amiodarone hydrochloride given intra-atrially in patients with the Wolff-Parkinson-White syndrome. *Circulation* **52** (**Suppl. 1**): 252, 1975.
15. Touboul, P., Porte, J., Huerta, F., and Delahaye, J.P.: Etude des propriétés électrophysiologiques du tosylate de bretylium chez l'homme. *Arch. Mal. Coeur* **69**: 503, 1976.
16. Touboul, P., Jandot, V., Thizy, J.F., et al.: Action de la chloro-acetyl-ajmaline sur les propriétés électriques du coeur humain. *Arch. Mal. Coeur* **70**: 973, 1977.
17. Touboul, P., Gressard, A., Atallah, G., et al.: Action de la chloro-acétyl-ajmaline dans le syndrome de Wolff-Parkinson-White. *Arch. Mal. Coeur* **71**: 808, 1978.
18. Wellens, H.J.J., and Durrer, D.: Effects of procainamide, quinidine, and ajmaline in the Wolff-Parkinson-White syndrome. *Circulation* **50**: 114, 1974.

10

Newer Antiarrhythmic Agents

Henri E. Kulbertus, M.D.

The renewed interest in sudden death and its protection accounts for the recent developments which have taken place in the field of antiarrhythmic agents. Although clinicians are very satisifed with the use of lidocaine in acute conditions, it seems generally agreed that there is still a need for an antiarrhythmic drug, active in the management of ventricular dysrythmias and which could be administered intravenously for example in the acute phase of a myocardial infarction and orally later during the long-term treatment of this condition.

The purpose of this presentation is to summarize the results obtained in our hospital with some of the newer antiarrhythmic agents.

DRUGS TESTED

Disopyramide

Disopyramide (Rythmodan, Norpace) is a class I antiarrhythmic drug with a half-life of 5 to 8 hours. Its oral form has been available for almost 10 years in Europe; the intravenous form is more recent. Carlier and his co-workers[1] were the first to use it. They injected 1.5 mg of disopyramide per kg of body weight, thus obtaining drug plasma levels ranging from 1.7 to 3.0 μg/ml. They studied 146 patients of whom 102 had an acute myocardial infarction. Altogether, disopyramide showed a clearcut beneficial effect in 68.6 percent of the patients with myocardial infarction and in 36.4 percent of those with other etiologies. Table 10-1 presents in greater details the results obtained in the series with myocardial infarction.

Table 10-1. Results of Disopyramide Use in Patients with Myocardial Infarction

Type of Arrhythmia	No. of Cases	No. of Successes*
Supraventricular ectopic beats	21	16
Atrial fibrillation	19	11
Atrial flutter	5	2
Supraventricular tachycardia	9	3
Ventricular ectopic beats	36	30
Ventricular parasystole	5	4
Ventricular tachycardia	7	4
	102	70 (68.6%)

*Return to normal regular sinus rhythm.

A drop of blood pressure greater than 20 mmHg was observed in eight cases, a PR lengthening ($\geq$ 0.24 sec) in two, and a short-lasting atrioventricular dissociation in one. The QRS significantly widened in three subjects. In eight patients who had an atrial fibrillation or flutter, the injection of disopyramide was followed by an increase of ventricular rate by facilitation of atrioventricular conduction. Another two subjects suffered from gastrointestinal symptoms.

Other studies[2] have indicated that disopyramide is a good antiarrhythmic which is reasonably well tolerated in long-term administration. Its side-effects are well known: 10 to 40 percent of the patients taking this substance complain of dry mouth or urinary hesitancy; 3 to 9 percent report urinary retention, constipation, blurred vision, dry mouth, eyes or throat and finally, some 5 to 6 percent suffer from gastrointestinal discomfort.[2]

Mexiletine

Mexiletine is another class 1 antiarrhythmic agent with a half-life of 10 hours. It has been used widely in England and Germany for a few years. In our study,[3] 12 patients with refractory ventricular arrhythmias were treated with one single dose of 250 mg of mexiletine injected intravenously over a 15-minute period. The mean peak drug plasma concentration was 1.61 μg/ml. Some therapeutic effect was obtained in each case. Total suppression of the ectopic beats was accomplished in nine out of the 12 patients. A direct relationship between plasma level and therapeutic effect was disclosed. Three patients reported side-effects: one vomited, one had tremor, the third developed a short-lasting phase of sinus arrest with slow junctional escape.

During long-term oral administration, side-effects occur when the plasma level is higher than 2.0 μg/ml.[2] They may consist of neurological signs (tremor, nystagmus, diplopia, dizziness, dysarthria, paresthesia, ataxia, confusion) or, more frequently, of gastrointestinal distress (vomiting, nausea, dyspepsia).

Tocainide

Tocainide, a lidocaine congener, is a class I antiarrhythmic agent with a half-life of 10 to 17 hours. We used it intravenously at a dose of 0.75 mg/kg producing a mean peak plasma concentration of 6 μg/ml in three patients with intranodal reentrant tachycardia, five patients suffering from circus movement tachycardia incorporating an accessory pathway and two patients with ventricular tachycardia.[4] The drug was found to have no effect on AH time and refractory periods of the AV node. It produced a 20 msec. increase of the HV time in three subjects. It did not influence the refractory periods of the atrial or ventricular muscle but lengthened the refractory periods of the bypasses at least when they were initially fairly long. Injected during six episodes of tachycardia, tocainide interrupted the rhythm disorder in one out of two patients with intranodal tachycardia, three patients with circus movement tachycardia involving an accessory pathway and one patient with ventricular tachycardia. No side-effects were noted. Others have demonstrated that tocainide is an effective antiarrhythmic agent which is well tolerated in long-term administration.[2] It also has possible side-effects which, as with mexiletine, may be classified into neurological and gastrointestinal disorders.

Aprindine

Aprindine is one of the most powerful class I antiarrhythmic agent that we ever had to study. It has a half-life of 22 to 30 hours and, as opposed to the previously discussed drugs, deeply affects the His-Purkinje system and significantly lengthens the conduction times in all structures.[5]

With this drug, the toxic to therapeutic ratio is very low. Neurological side-effects are very frequent if the plasma levels reach 1 μg/ml or higher. They consist of tremor, dizziness, ataxia, hallucinations and even seizures. Gastrointestinal disorders are rare. Unfortunately, sporadic cases of cholestatic jaundice and agranulocytosis have been reported.

New molecules derived from aprindine and hopefully devoid of its side-effects are now being tested. We are presently investigating moxaprindine and believe that it is extremely promising.

Lorcainide

Lorcainide is another class I antiarrhythmic agent. We studied[6] its electrophysiologic effects in nine patients using a dose of 150 mg injected over a 5-minute period. No significant effects on the A-H time was noted whereas the HV time increased (15 to 50 msec.) in all patients. The refractory period of the atrial and ventricular muscle consistently increased. It is apparent that the doses we used and the mode of administration that we followed were not suitable: toxic effects were observed. Two patients developed left bundle branch block during the injection. In addition, lorcainide injected during an episode of supraventricular tachycardia interrupted the rhythm disorder but the return to sinus rhythm was followed by QRS widening and ventricular fibrillation. Kesteloot[7] using a more cautious regimen reports excellent results. Van Durme also describes favorable data with this drug used orally on a long-term basis.[8]

Amiodarone

Amiodarone is another type of antiarrhythmic agent which possesses class III properties. Its half-life still remains unknown but is surely extremely long. Initially used as an antianginal substance, it has been reported by Rosenbaum to be an excellent antiarrhythmic which can produce total suppression and control of supraventricular (98 out of 106 patients: 92.4%) as well as ventricular (119 out of 145 patients: 82%) arrhythmias.[9,10]

We have used it[11] intravenously at a dose of 300 mg in 12 patients with paroxysmal supraventricular tachycardia. Four subjects had, at least intermittently, electrocardiographic evidence of the Wolff-Parkinson-White syndrome. In four patients, a concealed accessory pathway was present. In the remaining four cases, the circuit was confined to the AV node. Amiodarone lengthened the effective and refractory periods of the AV node, the AV nodal conduction time and the refractory period of the atrial muscle. Administrated intravenously during tachycardia, amiodarone terminated the rhythm disorder in five out of six patients. It also slowed the heart rate during the tachycardic episodes. In two of the four subjects with intranodal tachycardia, no arrhythmia could be initiated after amiodarone administration.

Most authors agree that amiodarone is one of the best drugs for the treatment of arrhythmias related to the Wolff-Parkinson-White syndrome.[10] It may have significant side-effects[2] (corneal deposits, skin pigmentation, thyroid dysfunction, severe bradycardia) but surely deserves a place among the modern antiarrhythmic substances.

CONCLUSION

With Jewitt[12] we believe that "an ideal antiarrhythmic drug should demonstrate selective efficacy against a specific type of arrhythmia in a manner unassociated with general side-effects, particularly cardiovascular side-effects. It should be effective and safe following intravenous administration and when given orally should have a long therapeutic half-life."

In spite of the efforts of the industry, we do not as yet have such a drug at our disposal.

REFERENCES

1. Carlier, J., Andriange, M., Lisin, N., and Vandenbosch, R.: A clinical trial of intravenously administered disopyramide in man. Second International Symposium on Disopyramide, 1972, pp. 9–10.
2. Zipes, D.P., and Troup, P.J.: New antiarrhythmic agents. *Am. J. Cardiol.* **41**: 1005, 1978.
3. Waleffe, A., and Kulbertus, H.: The efficacy of intravenous mexiletine on ventricular ectopic activity. *Acta Cardiol.* **4**: 269, 1977.
4. Waleffe, A., Mary-Rabine, L., Bruninx, P., and Kulbertus, H.E.: Effects of tocainide studied by programmed electrical stimulation of the heart in patients with reentrant arrhythmias. *Am. J. Cardiol.* (in press).
5. Bordalo, A., and Kulbertus, H.: Electrophysiological effects of aprindine in the anesthetized dog. In Seipel, L. Breithardt, G., and Loogen, F. (eds.): *Experience with Aprindine. New Aspects of Antiarrhythmic Therapy.* Aulendorf, Germany, Editio Cantor, 1976, p. 45.
6. Waleffe, A., Mary-Rabine, L., Bruninx, P., and Kulbertus, H.E.: Electrophysiological effects of lorcainide studied by programmed electrical stimulation of the heart in man. (In preparation).
7. Kesteloot, H., and Stroobandt, R.: Clinical experience with lorcainide, a new antiarrhythmic drug. *Arch. Int. Pharmac. Ther.* **230**: 225, 1977.
8. Van Durme, J.P., Bogaert, M., Weyne, A., and Pannier, R. Comparative study of lorcainide, mexiletine and placebo in patients with chronic ventricular dysrhythmias. (In press)
9. Rosenbaum, M.B., Chiale, P.A., Halpern, M.S., et al.: Clinical efficacy of amiodarone as an antiarrhythmic agent. *Am. J. Cardiol.* **38**: 934, 1976.
10. Rosenbaum, M.B., Chiale, P.A., Ryba, D., and Elizari, M.V.: Control of tachyarrhythmias associated with Wolff-Parkinson-White syndrome by amiodarone hydrochloride. *Am. J. Cardiol.* **34**: 215, 1974.
11. Waleffe, A., Bruninx, P., and Kulbertus, H.E.: Effects of amiodarone studied by programmed stimulation of the heart in patients with paroxysmal reentrant supraventricular tachycardia. *J. Electrocardiol.* **11**: 253, 1978.
12. Jewitt, D.J.: Limitations of present drug therapy of cardiac arrhythmias: a review. *Postgrad. Med. J.*, **53 (Suppl. 1)**: 12, 1977.

11

The Arrhythmogenic Effects of Antiarrhythmic Agents

Henri E. Kulbertus, M.D.

Every clinician is aware that most antiarrhythmic drugs may develop an arrythmogenic effect when they are administered in high doses or in particular clinical conditions.

The purpose of this presentation is to describe three possible mechanisms by which antiarrhythmic agents may produce rhythm disturbances.

"TORSADES DE POINTE"

Torsades de pointe consist of an unusual form of reentrant ventricular tachycardia (Fig. 11-1). Its electrocardiographic features are very characteristic and may be described as follows[1–3]:

1. The episodes are generally initiated by a ventricular ectopic beat falling late after the preceding sinus complex;
2. The successive QRS complexes during tachycardia show an "undulating series of rotations"[4] of the electrical axis; and
3. The episodes most frequently cease spontaneously.

Torsades de pointe may remain asymptomatic, produce syncope or Adams-Stokes attacks, or seldom degenerate into ventricular fibrillation.

This clinical entity has long been recognized in Europe. Different causes (bradycardia, electrolytes deficits, variant angina, hereditary prolongation of QT interval) may be responsible for torsades de pointe, but one of the most frequent is the administration of medications which prolong ventricular repolarization. It is now generally agreed that quinidine syn-

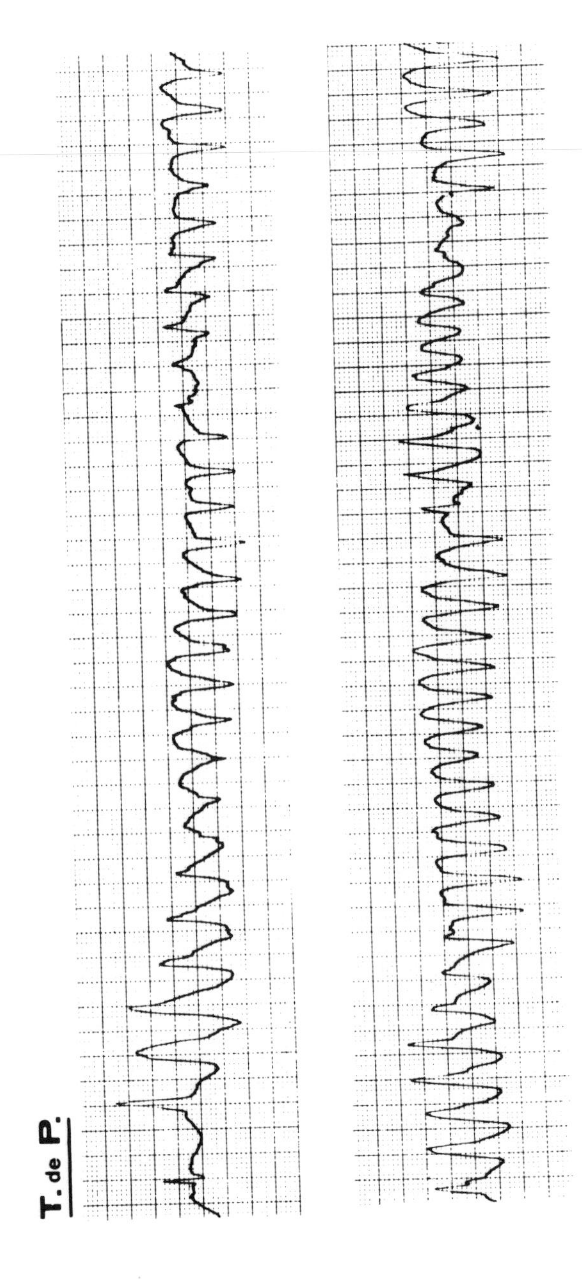

Figure 11-1. Typical of torsades de pointe.

cope reflects a torsades de pointe phenomenon. It is less well known that the same complications can occur especially in the elderly with other drugs producing QT prolongation. This is, for example, the case for amiodarone and prenylamine and also for some phenothiazines and tricyclic antidepressants. Admittedly, most patients with iatrogenic torsades de pointe receive several drugs simultaneously and it may appear hazardous to blame one rather than another. Nonetheless, the reports describing cases in which torsades de pointe were associated with the administration of the above-mentioned drugs are sufficiently frequent to have a reasonable suspicion.

FACILITATION OF CIRCUS MOVEMENT TACHYCARDIA

Any clinician dealing with patients suffering from rhythm disorders knows that, in some instances, the administration of an antiarrhythmic agent may actually increase the frequency and/or the duration of episodes of circus movement tachycardia involving the A-V node and an overt or concealed accessory pathway. This paradoxical effect has received a satisfactory explanation from investigations using intracardiac recordings and programmed electrical stimulation of the heart. It is frequently observed with drugs slowing A-V nodal conduction without significantly affecting the bypass. In those circumstances, an atrial ectopic beat, for example, which would normally have initiated no tachycardia may, after drug administration, be sufficiently delayed within the node to reach the distal end of the bypass after the end of its refractory period, thus starting a sustained circus movement tachycardia.

This phenomenon has been observed with digitalis,[4] verapamil[5] and beta-blockers[6]. We reported it in patients treated by amiodarone[7] and one of its congeners benzoyl-indolizine.[8] It can also be encountered with drugs acting not on the A-V node, but on the intraventricular conduction system. This is, for example, the case for tocainide.[9] With the latter drug, we have even observed a patient with a concealed bypass who, after intravenous administration of the drug, developed the "incessant" form of supraventricular tachycardia in which the episodes were almost continuous and were repeatedly initiated by trivial shortenings of the sinus cycle length without precipitating extrasystole.

ENHANCEMENT BY ANTIARRHYTHMIC AGENTS OF VENTRICULAR ARRHYTHMIAS INDUCED BY ACUTE CORONARY OCCLUSION IN THE DOG

Delayed activation of the ischemic myocardium has been observed by many investigators and recently correlated with the incidence of ventricular tachyarrhythmias occurring at the time of the coronary occlusion.[10] Aprindine, a drug which increases the degree of ischemia-induced conduction delay, was demonstrated to increase the incidence of the ventricular tachycardia and fibrillation developing after experimental myocardial infarction.[11] We undertook a study[12] to evaluate whether other antiarrhythmic agents might also lengthen the conduction delay produced by myocardial ischemia and thus favor the development of ventricular tachycardia and fibrillation, when they were administered intravenously prior to occlusion of the left anterior descending artery in the dog.

The study was carried out on 81 open-chest German shepherd dogs. The experimental protocol was similar to that described by Zipes' group[10] and was based upon the repetition of the same sequence three consecutive times. During the basic sequence, the atrium was continuously paced at 120/min, the sinus node being crushed. Pacing was raised to 150/min for 30 seconds and to 200/min for another 30 seconds and then set back to 120/min for 1 minute. The left anterior descending artery was then ligated for 6 minutes. During the first 5 minutes, the rate remained set at 120/min. It was then raised to 150/min and 200/min for consecutive periods of 30 seconds. Ligation was then released and the heart was paced at the basic rate of 120/min. A 30-minute recovery period was allowed between successive occlusions. The basic sequence was performed three times. The responses were first assessed in the control state. After 30 minutes, the antiarrhythmic agent (or saline in the controls) was administered as follows: the total dose prepared as a 0.1 percent injectable solution was divided into eight equal doses injected intravenously over a 30-second period and 2 minutes apart. Drug administration therefore took 14.5 minutes. The basic experimental sequence was repeated 9 minutes after the last injection. Left anterior descending artery ligation thus occurred 11 minutes after the last injection at a time when the myocardial content of the antiarrhythmic agent was presumably high. After 30 minutes, the basic sequence was repeated once more so that the third left anterior descending artery occlusion took place 48 minutes after the last injection at a time when the myocardial content of the antiarrhythmic agent was presumably lower. It was thus possible to investigate separately the effects of (a) increased heart rate alone; (b) ischemia alone; (c) both factors together.

Repetition of the sequence three times allowed study of these effects in the control state (first sequence) in the presence of a high serum level and myocardial content of an antiarrhythmic agent (second sequence) and in the presence of a lower serum level and myocardial content of the antiarrhythmic agent (third sequence). If an animal developed ventricular fibrillation during the first sequence, no attempt was made to defibrillate the heart. So all dogs submitted to the whole protocol were free of arrhythmia during the initial control occlusion. Fourteen dogs were excluded for this reason. At the end of the third occlusion, the left anterior descending artery was severed downstream from the occlusion site. If a significant backflow was observed, the animal was disregarded for the study (10 instances). Altogether, 57 dogs were retained for analysis. The various categories are indicated in Table 11-1.

Table 11-1. Distribution of Antiarrhythmic Agents in Experimental Animals

Groups	No. of Animals
Saline	11
Quinidine (16 mg/kg)	7
Quinidine (8 mg/kg)	9
Aprindine (2.86 mg/kg)	8
Mexiletine (15 mg/kg)	9
Drobuline (2.86 mg/kg)	6
Lorcainide (2.86 mg/kg)	7

All drugs studied, at the doses used, produced a lengthening of the resting QRS duration. The extent of the conduction delay recorded in the subepicardial electrogram of the ischaemic zone after coronary occlusion was significantly increased by all drugs. All agents studied increased the incidence of ventricular tachycardia and fibrillation observed after left anterior descending artery occlusion. This effect was particularly obvious 11 minutes after drug administration (Table 11-2).

Table 11-2. Analysis of Post-infarction Arrhythmias

	Before Drug		11 Minutes After		48 Minutes After	
Group	QRS Duration (msec)	VF-VT*	QRS Duration (msec)	VF-VT	QRS Duration (msec)	VF-VT
Control	50.1 ± 1.1	—	51.9 ± 1.0	1/11	51.3 ± 1.3	0/10
Quinidine (8 mg/kg)	50.9 ± 1.7	—	58.4 ± 1.3	5/9	55.0 ± 1.6	0/5
Quinidine (16 mg/kg)	49.9 ± 1.4	—	67.4 ± 2.4	6/7	66.3 ± 2.4	1/3
Aprindine	49.8 ± 1.0	—	62.8 ± 1.6	7/8	56.5 ± 1.6	1/3
Mexiletine	49.8 ± 0.6	—	60.0 ± 2.3	9/9	59.0 ±	1/1
Drobuline	47.5 ± 1.1	—	56.4 ± 1.8	4/6	50.5 ± 1.2	0/2
Lorcainide	47.6 ± 1.5	—	59.6 ± 2.5	7/7	—	—

*VT = ventricular tachycardia defined as bursts of 25 consecutive ventricular beats or more.

These results which will be described in details elsewhere further illustrate the fact that there is a relationship between the extent of ischemia-induced conduction delay and the incidence of ventricular arrhythmias developing early after coronary occlusion. Any drug which significantly increases the ischemia-induced conduction delay may increase the incidence of these arrhythmias. The results described by Zipes' group are therefore not applicable to aprindine only. The experimental model used in this study is characterized by three major features. The post LAD ligation arrhythmias which are observed develop (1) when the myocardial content of the antiarrhythmic agent is very high as we have demonstrated for the aprindine and quinidine-treated dogs (unpublished data); (2) when heart rate is high; (3) when left anterior descending artery occlusion is performed in the presence of an otherwise normal coronary circulation. Clinically, such a situation may be encountered at times, but it is likely to be rare. The model is therefore better for the understanding of the mechanisms of post-infarction arrhythmias than for the appraisal of the safety of antiarrhythmic substances.

REFERENCES

1. Dessertenne, F.: La tachycardie ventriculaire à deux foyers opposés variables. *Arch. Mal. Coeur* **59**: 263, 1966.
2. Krikler, D.M., and Curry, P.V.L.: Torsade de pointes: An atypical ventricular tachycardia. *Br. Heart J.* **38**, 117, 1976.
3. Kulbertus, H.: La torsade de pointes. *Rev. Med. Liège* **33**: 63, 1978.
4. Wellens, H.J.J., Duren, D.R., Liem, K., and Lie, K.I.: Effect of digitalis in patients with paroxysmal atrioventricular nodal tachycardia. *Circulation* **52**: 779, 1975.
5. Wellens, H.J.J., Tan, S.L., Bar, F.W.H., et al.: Effects of verapamil studied by programmed electrical stimulation of the heart in patients with paroxysmal re-entrant supraventricular tachycardia. *Br. Heart J.* **39**: 1058, 1977.
6. Wu, D., Denes, P., Dinghra, R., et al.: The effects of propranolol on induction of AV nodal reentrant paroxysmal tachycardia. *Circulation* **52**: 201, 1975.
7. Waleffe, A., Bruninx, P., and Kulbertus, H.: Effects of amiodarone studied by programmed electrical stimulation of the heart in patients with paroxysmal reentrant supraventricular tachycardia. *J. Electrocard.* **11**: 253, 1978.
8. Waleffe, A., Bruninx, P., Bordalo, A., et al.: Electrophysiological effects of a derivative of amiodarone, benzoyl-indolicine. *Br. Heart J.* (in press).
9. Waleffe, A., Mary-Rabine, L., Bruninx, P., and Kulbertus, H.E.: Effects of tocainide studied by programmed electrical stimulation of the heart in patients with reentrant tachyarrhythmias. *Am. J. Cardiol.* (in press).
10. Boineau, J.P., and Cox, J.L.: (1973). Slow ventricular activation in myocardial infarction: a source of reentrant premature ventricular contraction. *Circulation* **48**: 702, 1973.
11. Zipes, D.P., Elharrar, V., Noble, R.J., et al.: Effects of various drugs on ventricular conduction delay and ventricular arrhythmias during myocardial ischaemia in the dog. In Kulbertus, H.E. (ed.): *Reentrant Arrhythmias : Mechanisms and Treatment*. Lancaster, MTP Press, 1976, p. 312.

12. Gerin, M.G., and Kulbertus, H.E.: Effects of various antiarrhythmic agents on conduction delay and incidence of ventricular arrhythmias induced by acute coronary occlusion in the dog. In Sandoe, E., Julian, D.G., and Bell, J.W. (eds.): *Management of Ventricular Tachycardia.* Amsterdam, Excerpta Medica, 1978, p. 299.

12

Sick Sinus Node Syndrome: Clinical Manifestations and Physiologic Assessment

Benjamin Befeler, M.D.

The sick sinus node syndrome is made up of a spectrum of abnormalities in the function of the sinoatrial node which manifest themselves clinically by two types of electrocardiographic patterns: bradycardias of various types and supraventricular tachycardias and their combination. The syndrome may present with a number of signs and symptoms resulting from the electrophysiologic derangements, but with some frequency patients present for initial evaluation with nonspecific sinus bradycardia[1] which can be classified as: (1) Disease of the atrial wall—this occurs in a group of patients who present themselves with clinical manifestations of bradycardia and normal sympathetic responses. (2) Patients with physiologic bradycardia but with abnormal or supernormal sympathetic responses to various stressful situations, which include: (a) patients with Stokes-Adams attacks with or without vasomotor instability, and (b) patients with hyperactive vagus. (3) Patients with combinations bradycardia and supraventricular tachycardia of various types.

The first description of the syndrome showing manifestations of brady-cardia-tachycardia was published by Short in 1954.[2] In 1957[3] a comprehensive description of this syndrome was published which characterized the clinical manifestations. Lown[4] subsequently identified an interesting subgroup of patients with abnormalities of sinoatrial function which became manifest after direct current cardioversion for atrial fibrillation. Figure 12-1 shows such a case from our own series. Ferrer[5] described the clinical aspects in 1968. Other authors have called this syndrome the sluggish sinus node syndrome[6] or simply sinoatrial syncope.[7] It is quite interesting to note that at the beginning of this century[8-10]

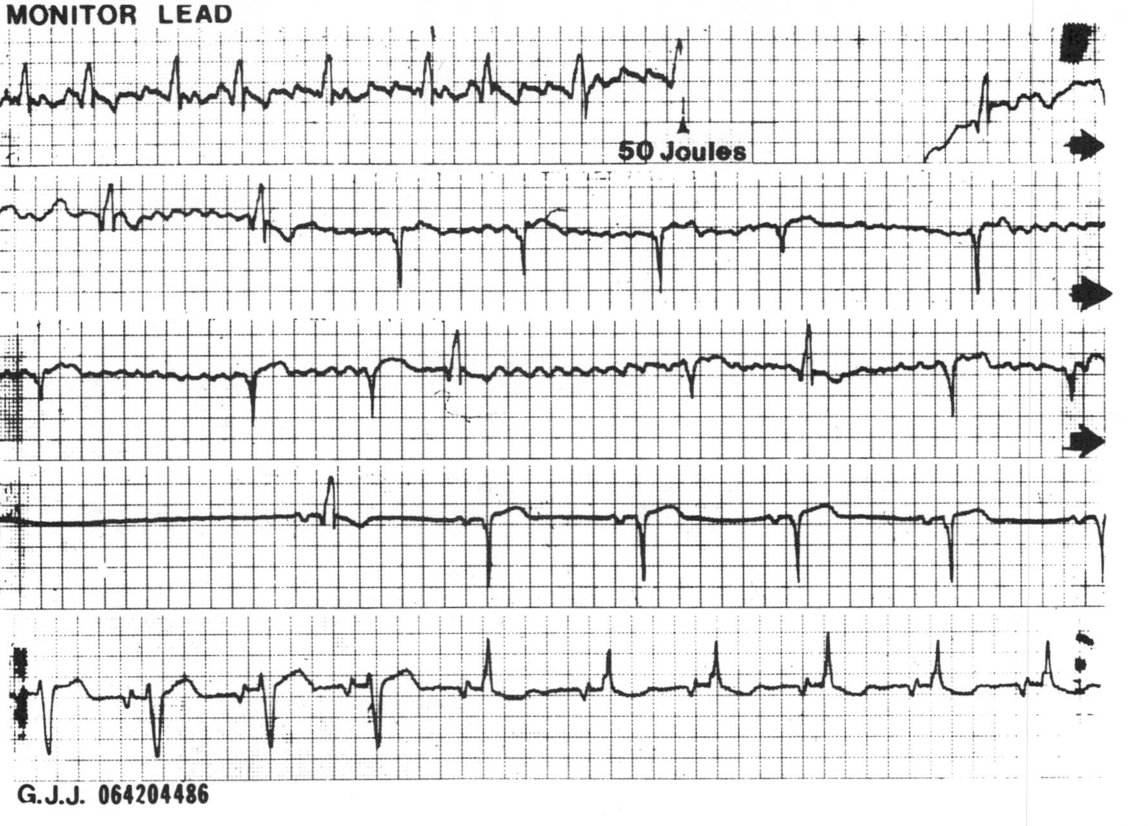

Figure 12–1. Continuous monitor lead of a patient who presented with atrial flutter. The patient was given DC cardioversion with 50 joules and converted to atrial fibrillation with slow ventricular rate, followed by sinus arrest and sinus bradycardia. Also note rate-related abnormalities of intraventricular conduction.

there were a number of publications which dealt with various manifestations of what we recognize today as this syndrome.

The symptomatology in these patients has to be differentiated from those alterations of heart rate and abnormalities of reflex blood pressure control due to carotid sinus dysfunction.[11]

CLINICAL PRESENTATION

As this syndrome complex is the result of abnormalities of the sinoatrial node, the atrial muscle, and alterations in the balance between these structures and sympathetic and parasympathetic control of heart rate, symptoms can be most varied.

The underlying pathophysiology of the main symptom, syncope, is sinus bradycardia or sinoatrial block, occurring spontaneously or at the cessation of a bout of overdrive suppression produced by a tachycardia and episodes of bradycardia combined with episodes of supraventricular tachycardia.

Syncope[6–10] is the most common symptom and is seen in 25 to 45 percent of the cases, depending on the series. This symptom is the most striking feature of the sick sinus node syndrome because it invariably leads the patient to the physician's attention. According to Easley and Goldstein,[7] syncope can be due to (I) severe sinoatrial block and (II) bradycardia-tachycardia. The number of patients who present type I or type II forms of syncope is about equal in their series.

Dizziness is the next most frequent complaint noted and it has been found in various series between 7 to 45 percent. Patients who eventually are diagnosed as having the sick sinus node syndrome, a number of them present with symptoms which in no way suggest the presence of a rhythm abnormality. The proportion of patients in this category varies from series to series. These symptoms include angina pectoris, dyspnea on exertion, and ill-defined motion disorders. A clinical feature which is quite characteristic of this group of patients is that they have a variable and unexpected response to various antiarrhythmic agents.

From the functional standpoint, the abnormalities in this syndrome are due to abnormalities of the automaticity of the sinus node, alterations of sinoatrial conduction, and abnormalities of the sympathetic control of heart rate. In a number of patients, the clinical symptomatology is the result of cerebrovascular disease in individuals in whom even minor changes of the rhythm and rate cause symptoms. It is important to note that in some patients the symptomatology takes place not during the periods of established bradycardia or tachycardia, but rather at the time of the asystole which occurs after a run of supraventricular tachycardia ceases. This situation is akin to the overdrive suppression which is employed in the laboratory to bring out abnormalities of the sinus node function. As mentioned before, clinically it is also important to differentiate the patients who have hypersensitivity of the carotid node from those who have sick sinus syndrome. Patients with hypersensitivity of the carotid node manifest clinically in two different ways: those patients who have marked bradycardia after stimulation of the carotid body and those patients who have changes of vasomotor control; that is, changes in blood pressure as a result of stimulation of the carotid body.

It has been known for a long time[12] that the recovery time of subsidiary pacemakers can be depressed when an idioventricular rhythm is interrupted by single or multiple premature beats, leading to Stokes-Adams attacks. Furthermore, recent experimental evidence[13] suggests that these attacks of complete heart block in the sick sinus node syndrome may be due to ventricular standstill following paroxysmal or atrial or ventricular tachycardia. It is also known that in normal individuals and dogs, there is a difference in response to overdrive pacing, depending on the location of the pacemaker within the conduction system. During atrial pacing, the escape pacemaker (sinoatrial) recovery time was 600 msec, maximum 540 msec ± 43 msec. in contrast to recovery time after ventricular pacing subsidiary pacemaker which was 2840 msec ± 83 msec. Post-recovery sinus node acceleration was consistently observed after atrial overdrive pacing, whereas subsidiary pacemaker "depression" was seen with overdrive ventricular pacing.[13-14]

ELECTROCARDIOGRAPHIC FINDINGS

The electrocardiogram in this syndrome may show sinus bradycardia usually of a severe degree. This bradycardia may be persistent, intermittent, or inappropriate; that is, the patient may not respond with an increase in rate to physiologic stress. One can also find sinus arrest and various degrees of sinoatrial block. Patients demonstrate episodes of tachycardia which can be atrial flutter, atrial fibrillation of paroxysmal atrial tachycardia alone or in combination with episodes of bradycardia.

PHYSIOLOGIC EVALUATION

This syndrome can be evaluated by invasive and noninvasive means. Holter monitoring, utilizing the single or two-lead electrocardiogram, provides useful information, particularly when the patient is allowed to continue to perform his usual activities. Invasive studies include the measurement of the sinus node recovery time after overdrive suppression (Table 12-1), and all other derived parameters, such as the recording of the ten first beats following overdrive suppression with atrial stimulation which has been useful in evaluating secondary pauses[15] (Table 12-2). The study of the sinoatrial conduction time, although cumbersome, may be of some usefulness and this is done with paired atrial stimulation during the "reset" period.[16] The study of overdrive suppression gives an indication of the state of automaticity of the sinus node and the measurement of the sinoatrial conduction time reflects conductivity. The administration of various drugs with performance of overdrive suppression before and after the drug may be useful; particularly when drugs can decrease the amount of entry block into the SA node and in that way the overdrive suppression creates a more definite effect on the sinus node. In some instances, abnormalities can only be demonstrated after the administration of drugs such as atropine, disopyramide, or quinidine. Not all patients show abnormalities during the physiologic testing,[17] and the diagnosis may have to be based either on a clinical history or on the information obtained from the longterm electrocardiographic monitoring with the Holter system.

Table 12-1. Sinus Node Dysfunction: Corrected Sinus Node Recovery Time*

Series	Number of Cases	Percent Prolonged	Normal†
Mandel et al.[14]	31	93.0	7.0
Gupta et al.[20]	17	35.5	64.7
Rosen et al.[18]	10	40.0	60.0
Narula et al.[19]	28	57.0	43.0

*Corrected sinus node recovery time = SNRT (basic heart rate)
†375 msec (210 msec ± 131)

Table 12.2. Sinus Node Dysfunction: Comparison Between the Occurrence of Abnormal Secondary Pauses (SP) and Prolonged CSRT in Patients with Sick Sinus Node Syndrome

Dysfunction	Percent
CSRT	56.3%
SP[15]	91.7%

Several studies have demonstrated that patients who have the sick sinus node syndrome also demonstrate abnormalities of atrioventricular conduction.[19-20] These consist of first degree AV block, prolonged AH interval, and various forms of second degree block. Patients also demonstrate abnormalities of His-Purkinje conduction manifested by the presence of bundle branch block. This may be of relevance when the treatment is undertaken utilizing pacemakers since atrial pacing, although the treatment of choice at first glance, may not be possible because of subsequent development of AV block or intra-Hisian abnormalities of conduction.

PATHOLOGIC ASPECTS

In general, tissues have a limited manner to respond to injury. When tissue becomes available at autopsy for morphologic studies, changes found may reflect more accurately the duration of disease than a specific process; hence when correlative studies of individuals with sick sinus node syndrome have been made with autopsy findings, no specific lesions (specific for certain arrhythmias) can be found.

Fibrosis is the main feature of sinoatrial disease.[21] Its etiology can only be associated to specific causes in a small number of cases, such as carcinomatosis, infectious pericarditis, and atrial infarction. Nonetheless, several conclusions can be made from such studies: (1) The number of nodal cells (pacemaker cells) in the sinoatrial node is inversely proportional to age, rather than underlying arrhythmias. (2) Normal sinus rhythm can be present in cases with severe fibrosis of the sinoatrial node. (3) Atrial fibrillation does not correlate well with fibrosis of the sinoatrial node, but rather with abnormalities of atrial tissue. (4) Sinoatrial block was associated with extensive lesions of the sinoatrial node and the approaches of the SA node and the AV node itself. (5) The tachycardia-bradycardia syndrome showed underlying disease of the sinoatrial node and atrial muscle. Once the injury occurs, nodal cells degenerate, become highly vacuolated and poorly stained and are replaced by fibrous and elastic tissue. The underlying fate of the coronary circulation does not appear to play a role on the etiology of these lesions.

James[22] has advocated the notion that certain supraventricular arrhythmias in myocardial infarction are due to interference with the blood supply to the SA node. This has not been corroborated by other workers.[21] The artery to the SA node may be patent even in individuals with very serious cerebrovascular difficulties in the presence of extreme bradycardia or significant tachycardia (Fig. 12-2 and 12-3).

TREATMENT

In the usual situation, it makes good clinical sense that the control of symptoms may improve survival and prevent catastrophic events. There is no longitudinal study demonstrating that the treatment in fact lengthens life. In a recent study[23] and as previously suggested,[24] there sounds a voice of warning on the widespread use of pacemakers in this syndrome. It has also been known for some time that symptoms improve when patients develop stable atrial flutter[27] or atrial fibrillation.[24–26] The overall survival of these patients appears to be more related to the presence or absence of myocardial disease and not to the cerebral symptoms or arrhythmias. The tremendous clinical importance of this syndrome is reflected by the numerous publications of the subject.[28–31]

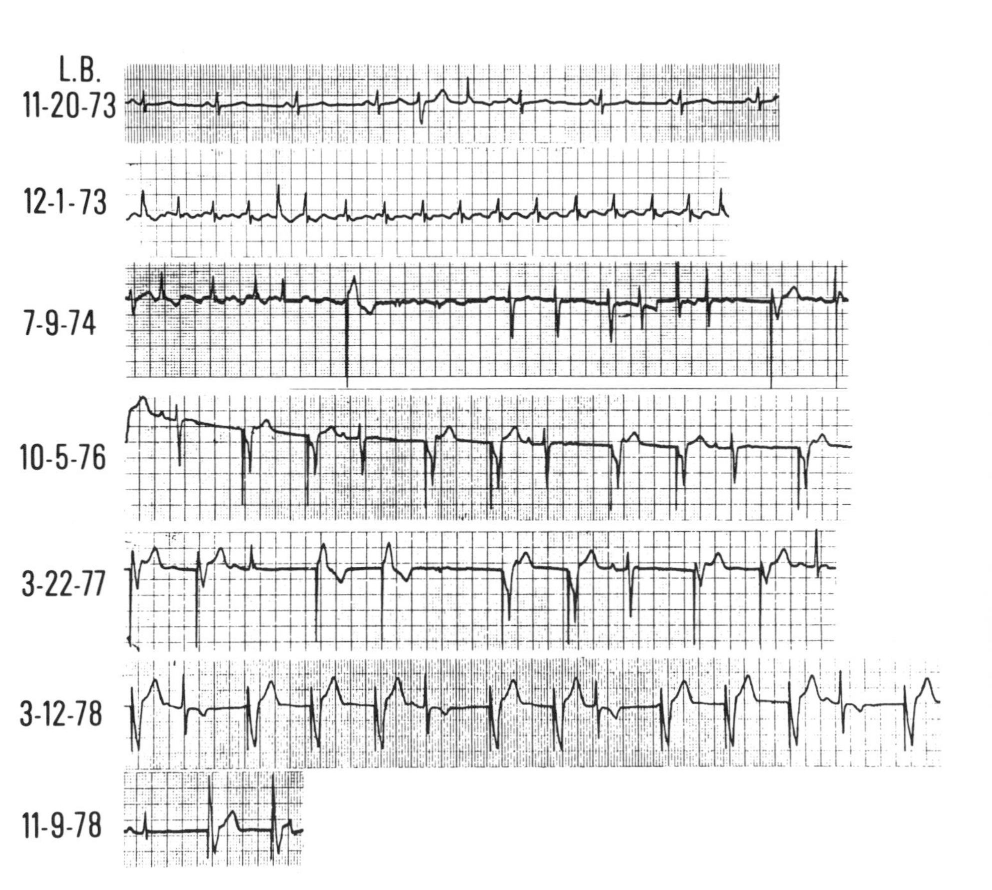

Figure 12–2. L.B., a patient followed for 5 years who presented with dizzy spells had underlying sinus bradycardia and premature beats, followed by atrial fibrillation and rapid ventricular response. Patient had a syncopal episode with documented sinus arrest, was given a ventricular demand pacemaker plus oral propranolol and has remained essentially asymptomatic with episodes of sinus arrest, sinus bradycardia, and periods of atrial fibrillation.

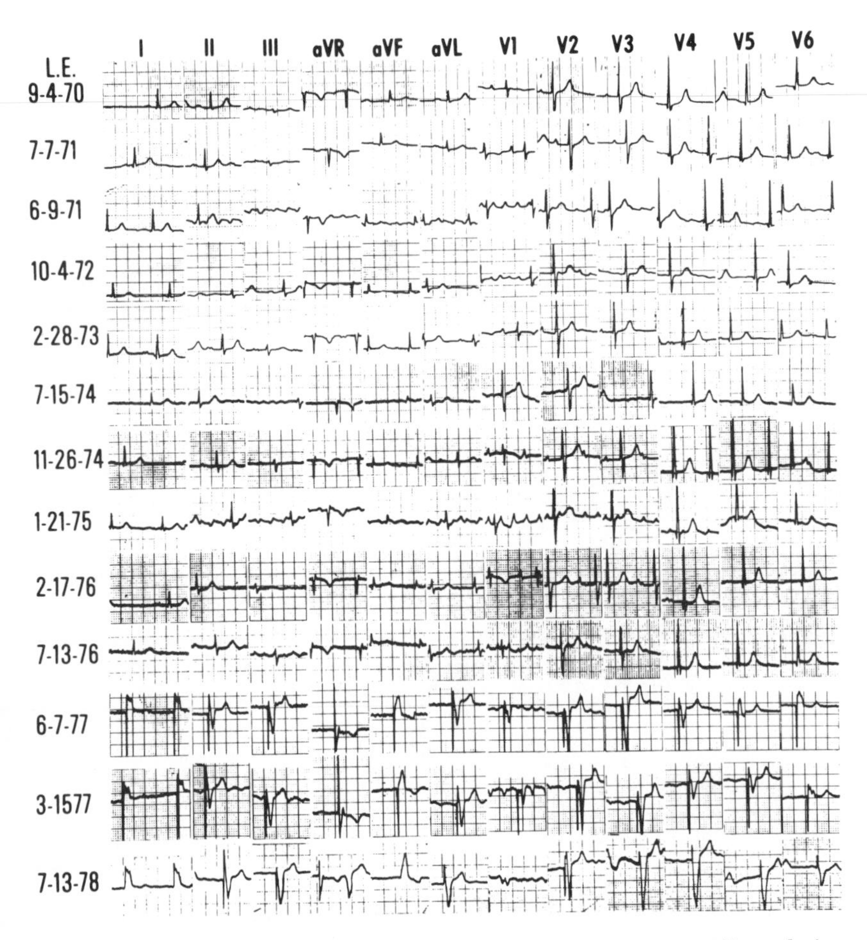

Figure 12-3. L.E., an elderly gentleman, presented with dizzy spells and sinus bradycardia in September of 1970. In the ensuing years, he showed transient atrial flutter and fibrillation without change in his symptoms. In June of 1976, six years later, he had a syncopal episode and a permanent demand pacemaker was implanted and he was given propranolol. He remained asymptomatic, with similar underlying arrhythmias.

REFERENCES

1. Dighton, D.H.: Sinus bradycardia. Autonomic influence and clinical assessment. *Br. Heart J.* **36**: 791–796, 1974.
2. Short, D.S.: The syndrome of alternating bradycardia and tachycardia. *Br. Heart J.* **16**: 208, 1954.
3. Birchfield, R.I., Menefee, E.E., and Bryant, G.D.N.: Disease of the sinoatrial node associated with bradycardia, asystole, syncope, and paroxysmal atrial fibrillation. *Circulation* **16**: 20, 1957.
4. Lown, B.: Electrical reversion of cardiac arrhythmias. *Br. Heart J.* **29**: 469–489, 1967.
5. Ferrer, M.I.: Sick sinus syndrome in atrial disease. *J.A.M.A.* **206**: 645–646, 1968.
6. Tabatznik, B., Mowrer, M.M., Samson, E.B., and Prempree, A.: Syncope in the "sluggish sinus node syndrome". *Circulation* **40 (Suppl. III)**: 200, 1969.
7. Easley, R.M., and Goldstein, S.: Sino-atrial syncope. *Am. J. Cardiol.* **50**: 166–177, 1971.
8. Laslett, E.E.: Syncopal attacks, associated with prolonged arrest of the whole heart. *Quart. J. Med.* **2**: 347, 1908–1909.
9. Eyster, J.A.E., and Evans, J.S.: Sino-auricular heart block. *Arch. Intern. Med.* **16**: 832, 1915.
10. Levine, S.A.: Obsevations on sino-auricular heart block. *Arch. Intern. Med.,* **17**: 153, 1916.
11. Sigler, L.H.: The cardio-inhibitory carotid sinus reflex. *Am. J. Cardiol.* **12**: 175, 1963.
12. Pick, A., Langendorf, F., and Katz, L.N.: Depression of cardiac pacemakers by premature impulses. *Am. Heart J.* **4**: 49, 1951.
13. Jordan, J., Yamagudi, I., Mandel, W.J., and McCullen, A.E.: Comparative effects of overdrive on sinus and subsidiary pacemaker function. *Am. Heart J.* **93**: 367–374, 1977.
14. Mandel, W.J., Hayakawa, H., Allen, H.N., et al.: Assessment of sinus node function in patients with the sick sinus node syndrome. *Circulation* **46**: 761–769, 1972.
15. Benditt, D.G., Strauss, H.C., Scheinman, M.M., et al.: Analysis of secondary pauses following termination of rapid atrial pacing in man. *Circulation* **54**: 436–441, 1976.
16. Strauss, H.C., Saroff, A.L., Bigger, J.T., and Girardine, E.G.V.: Premature atrial stimulation as a key to the understanding of sinoatrial conduction in man. *Circulation* **47**: 86–93, 1973.
17. Gould, L., and Reddy, C.U.R.: Failure of cardiac conduction studies to detect the sick sinus syndrome. *Angiology* **26**: 467–470, 1975.
18. Rosen, K.M., Loeb, M.S., Simmo, M.Z., et al.: Cardiac conduction in patients with symptomatic sinus node disease. *Circulation* **43**: 836–869, 1972.
19. Narula, O.S., Samet, P., and Javier, R.P.: Significance of the sinus node recovery time. *Circulation* **45**: 140–158, 1972.
20. Gupta, P.K., Lichstein, E., Chadda, K.D., and Badni, E.: Appraisal of sinus nodal recovery time in patients with sick sinus syndrome. *Am. J. Cardiol.* **34**: 265–270, 1974.

21. Thery, C., Gosselin, B., Lebieffre, J., et al.: Pathology of sinoatrial node. Correlation with electrocardiographic findings in three patients. *Am. Heart J.* **93**: 735–740, 1977.
22. James, T.: Myocardial infarction and atrial arrhythmias. *Circulation* **24**: 761, 1961.
23. Gann, D., Tolentino, A., and Samet, P.: Electrophysiologic evaluation of elderly patients with sinus bradycardia. *Ann. Intern. Med.* **90**: 24–29, 1979.
24. Cohen, H.E.: Sick sinus syndrome. *Circulation* **48**: 671, 1973.
25. Vera, Z., Mason, S.T., Awan, N.A., et al.: Improvement of symptoms in patients with sick sinus syndrome by spontaneous development of stable atrial fibrillation. *Br. Heart J.* **39**: 160–167, 1977.
26. Kleinfeld, M.J., and Boal, B.H.: Symptomatic improvement in a patient with sick sinus syndrome after the onset of stable atrial flutter. *Pace* **1**: 472–475, 1978.
27. Boal, B.H., and Kleinfeld, M.J.: A study of patients with the sick sinus syndrome with long-term survival. *J. Chron. Dis.* **31**: 501–505, 1978.
28. Rubenstein, J.J., Schulman, C.L., Yurchak, P.M., and DeSanctis, R.W.: Clinical spectrum of the sick sinus syndrome. *Circulation* **46**: 5–13, 1972.
29. Nager, F., and Kappenberger, L: Sick sinus syndrome label for many cardiac problems. *J.A.M.A.* **239**: 597, 1978.
30. Kaplan, B.M.: Sick sinus syndrome (Editorial) *Arch. Intern. Med.* **138**: 28, 1978.
31. Radford, D.J., and Julian, D.G.: Sick sinus syndrome. Experience of a cardiac pacemaker clinic. *Br. Med. J.* **3**: 504–507, 1974.

13

The Surgical Treatment of Cardiac Arrhythmias

Guy Fontaine, M.D.

Chronic cardiac arrhythmias often pose a difficult therapeutic problem. They may be poorly tolerated from the psychological point of view and interfere with the patient's professional, social and family life. Prolonged attacks can give rise to heart failure and may be life-threatening—those with rapid rates may induce myocardial desynchronization leading to sudden death from ventricular fibrillation.

The introduction of new effective antiarrhythmic agents in recent years has improved the quality of life and probably the long-term survival of many of these patients. However, in some cases, medical treatment cannot be continued indefinitely because of intolerance, unacceptable side effects, or simply because the drug is not available in a particular country. It is in these cases that surgery should be considered.

Leaving aside the use of specialized pacemakers, this paper aims to describe the recent advances in cardiovascular surgery in its three applications:

1. His bundle interruption.
2. Interruption of abnormal accessory atrioventricular conduction pathways in the Wolff-Parkinson-White syndrome.
3. Interruption of reentry pathways in certain forms of chronic ventricular tachycardia with or without previous myocardial infarction.

HIS BUNDLE INTERRUPTION

From an electrophysiological point of view the heart may be considered as two entities: the atria, origin of normal activation which arises from the sinus node, and the ventricles which are activated by the His-Purkinje system. They are separated electrically by the atrioventricular rings. The atrial activation is transmitted to the ventricle via the nodo-Hisian system, the only normal conduction pathway. The most important electrophysiological characteristic of this structure is its ability to cause delay between atrial and ventricular contraction for optimal mechanical cardiac function. This delay at increasing atrial rates or prematurity filters rapid atrial rhythms.

The association of two pathological conditions may subject the ventricles to abnormal rapid rhythms: a congenital abnormality preventing the nodo-Hisian system from playing its role of filtering abnormal atrial rhythms, varying from extrasystoles to atrial tachycardia, flutter or fibrillation which are usually acquired with increasing age.

When antiarrhythmic therapy fails to slow nodo-Hisian conduction (digitalis, propranolol, or a combination of both) or fails to depress atrial excitability (quinidine, procainamide, verapamil, amiodarone) the alternate solution is the surgical section of the atrioventricular conduction pathway.[1,2] This raises two distinct problems: the location of the His bundle and its interruption.

Location of the His Bundle

The classical anatomical location of the His Bundle is at the insertion of the septal leaflet of the tricuspid valve. However, surgical section in this region is not always successful as the His bundle may have an abnormal trajectory and in particular, be deeply situated. Even with the association of an incision with a scalpel and cross suturing, complete reestablishment of atrioventricular conduction in the days or weeks following operation may be observed. The fibers of the nodo-Hisian system must be *completely interrupted* to interrupt successfully.

The location of the His bundle by electrophysiological methods was pioneered by the Hoffman school.[3] It involves the detection of the intrinsic deflection of the depolarization of the His bundle which in some areas is easily distinguished from the depolarization of the adjacent cavities. This may be performed intraoperatively using an exploratory bipolar electrode to detect potentials along the insertion of the septal leaflet of the tricuspid valve.[4] The appearance of the His bundle potential is monitored on the screen of a three-channel oscilloscope (Fig. 13-1). The top channel shows atrial depolarization which is detected by a hook-shaped bipolar electrode fixed on the atrial wall. Bottom channel shows potentials detected by a similar system attached to the ventricular wall. The third channel situated between the previous ones shows the potentials detected by the exploratory electrode. A specific electrical

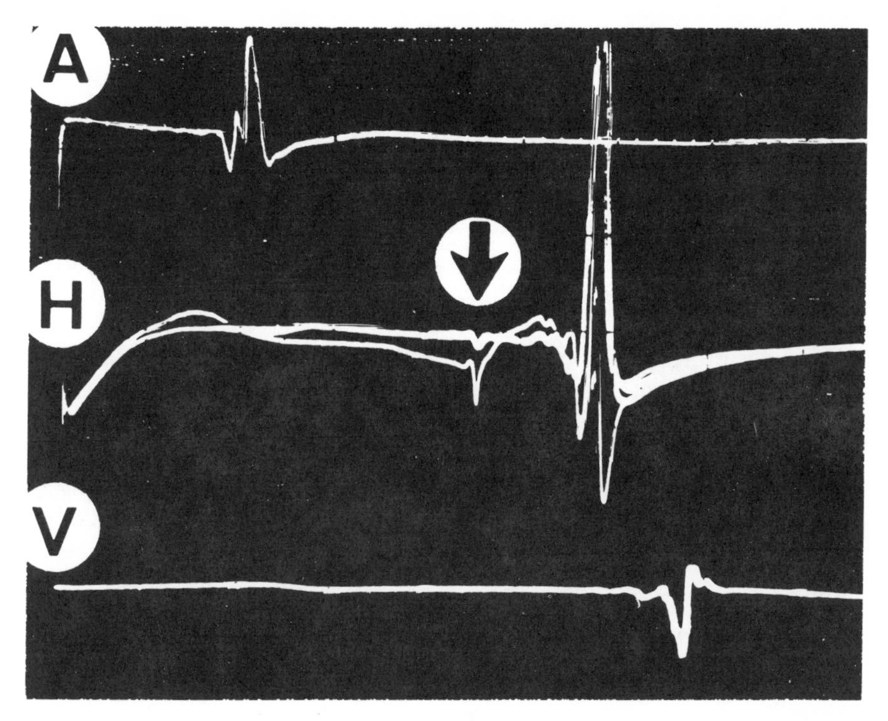

Figure 13-1. Peroperative recording of the His bundle potential. The atrial pacemaker triggers the oscilloscopic sweep on which the recordings are superimposed.

Top tracing: Atrial potential recorded from the anterior wall of the right atrium.

Bottom tracing: Ventricular potential recorded from the anterior wall of the right ventricle.

Middle tracing: Potentials recorded by the exploratory catheter which in this case is located near the ventricular cavity. The presence of a biphasic deflection of variable amplitude (position of the electrode) locates the His potential.

activity in the form of a bi- or triphasic deflection is recorded near the His bundle. Atrioventricular conduction defects which become more severe with increased pressure on the exploratory electrode are frequently observed.[5]

Interruption of the His Bundle

When the His bundle has been located, deliberate interruption of the atrioventricular conduction may be undertaken with greater chances of success. Cryosurgical techniques, using an appropriately shaped electrode to freeze a localized area identified beforehand by electrophysiological methods, appear to be more effective.[6] Cooling is produced by the rapid expansion of liquid nitrous oxide. Electronic controls allow variable degrees of cooling which is undertaken in two stages:

1. Initially the temperature is lowered to 0°. This interrupts conduction but spontaneous recovery occurs within seconds of stopping refrigeration.

2. Complete destruction of the conduction pathway is obtained by lowering the temperature to −60°. This creates a small ball of ice 1.5 cm in diameter at the tip of the electrode.

The advantage of this technique is that the conduction fibers are destroyed without altering the surrounding collagenous connective tissue so there is no residual scar.

Complete interruption of atrioventricular conduction necessitates the implantation of a permanent pacemaker; the epicardial electrodes are fixed during the same operation.

The surgical results cannot be assessed until several weeks after operation as the His bundle may only have been partially interrupted and the persistence of a few fibers may be enough to reestablish a conduction pathway once the edema and inflammation have subsided.

THE SURGICAL TREATMENT OF THE WOLFF-PARKINSON-WHITE SYNDROME

In this condition an embryological remnant constitutes an accessory conduction pathway across the atrioventricular junction in addition to the normal nodo-Hisian system. When operative its muscular anatomical structure enables rapid atrioventricular conduction with short-circuiting of the atrioventricular node. This gives rise to the delta wave of ventricular pre-excitation. The accessory pathway does not have the delaying properties of the normal nodo-Hisian system so that a pathological set up similar to that described above is realized when atrial arrhythmias occur. The one difference is that the activation is transmitted via the accessory pathway and not the nodo-Hisian system, thereby leading to very abnormal ventricular depolarization with increased pre-excitation.[7]

Location of the Accessory Pathway

This may be performed by a combination of different methods:

1. *ECG*: The electrical aspect of pre-excitation may help to locate an accessory pathway providing the heart is otherwise normal. Ventricular hypertrophy and intraventricular conduction defects may alter the topography of the delta wave and give an erroneous interpretation of the presumed site of pre-excitation.[8] In addition it is not always possible to distinguish between free wall and septal pre-excitation by this method.

2. *Endocavitary Mapping*: More precise information on the location of the zone of pre-excitation is available with endocavitary mapping.[9] For anatomical reasons it is easier to explore the atrial side of the atrioventricular rings. Ventricular pacing at a higher rate than the patient's spontaneous rhythm inhibits the sinus node, the activation being in most of the cases transmitted to the atria by the accessory pathway. Atrial endocardial mapping is then performed to determine the *earliest* point of atrial activation. On the right side the circumference of the tricuspid ring is explored with an exploratory bipolar catheter fitted with a preformed guide wire to facilitate manipulation. On the left side, a multi-electrode catheter is positioned in the coronary sinus. The earliest point of atrial activation may also be determined during reciprocating tachycardia as in this situation the circus movement passes down the nodo-Hisian system to the ventricles and then back to the atria by the accessory pathway.

3. *Epicardial Mapping*: This investigation consists of recording the passage of the intrinsic deflection at a number of predetermined points on the epicardium.[10] The ventricular aspect of the atrioventricular groove is explored first of all before moving progressively towards the apex when a global map of epicardial activation is desired. The interpolation of isochronic lines shows up the ventricular junction of the accessory pathway (Fig. 13-2 and 13-3).

In some cases, anterograde conduction through the abnormal pathway may suddenly stop during operation, and in others the pathway may never have been apparent in this direction. (These patients usually present with paroxysmal tachycardia with narrow QRS complexes and have no signs of pre-excitation in sinus rhythm). When this is the case it is possible to locate the pathway when retrograde conduction is preserved, as is usually the case. The earliest point of atrial activation is then the atrial epicardial pole of the accessory pathway, whether located during ventricular pacing as described above or during orthodromic tachycardia.

Atrial fibrillation poses a special problem as rapid, irregular ventricular rhythms with wide QRS complexes do not lead to stable atrioventricular sequences. Mapping must then be performed with a ventricular reference.

Interruption of the abnormal pathway is carried out with a scalpel shaving the endocardial wall of the atrial aspect of the atrioventricular ring opposite the zone of pre-excitation located by mapping. The incision should be transmural. The fascia in the atrioventricular groove is exposed and by displacing upwards the coronary vessels, the incision is continued over the edge of the ventricle.

The operation is relatively easy over the free wall of the ventricle but is more difficult when the septum is involved. This may be suspected when

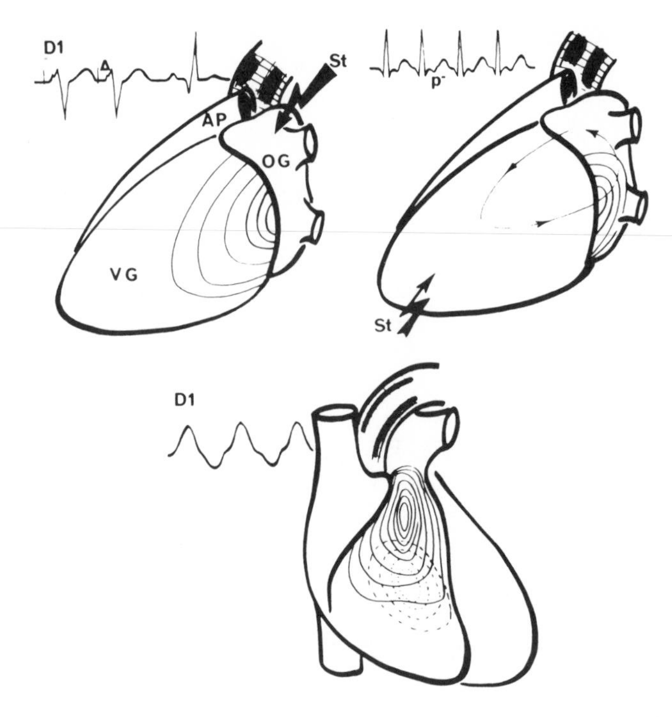

Figure 13–2. Principle of epicardial mapping in the WPW syndrome and ventricular tachycardia.

Mapping in a case of left lateral pre-excitation.

Upper left: During left atrial pacing the isochronic lines center around the left lateral region along the atrioventricular groove.

Upper right: Atrial map during orthodromic tachycardia with narrow QRS complexes or during pacing of the apex of the left ventricle, showing the isochronic lines centered around the adjacent zone of the left atrium.

Lower schematic: Epicardial mapping of ventricular tachycardia in a case of right ventricular dysplasia with dilatation of the infundibulum. *The origin of the normal activation* is shown in dotted lines. *The origin of the ventricular tachycardia* is shown by the continuous isochronic lines centered over the infundibular region.

the earliest point of epicardial activation is recorded before the start of the delta wave.[7]

Surgical section of an accessory pathway located in the upper part of the septum may endanger the His bundle. It is necessary to carry out mapping at the end of the operation to detect the presence of other abnormal pathways in other areas.[11]

The results of operation are generally good when performed by surgical teams specially trained in epicardial mapping and in the appropriate surgical techniques. In the majority of cases the delta wave is abolished

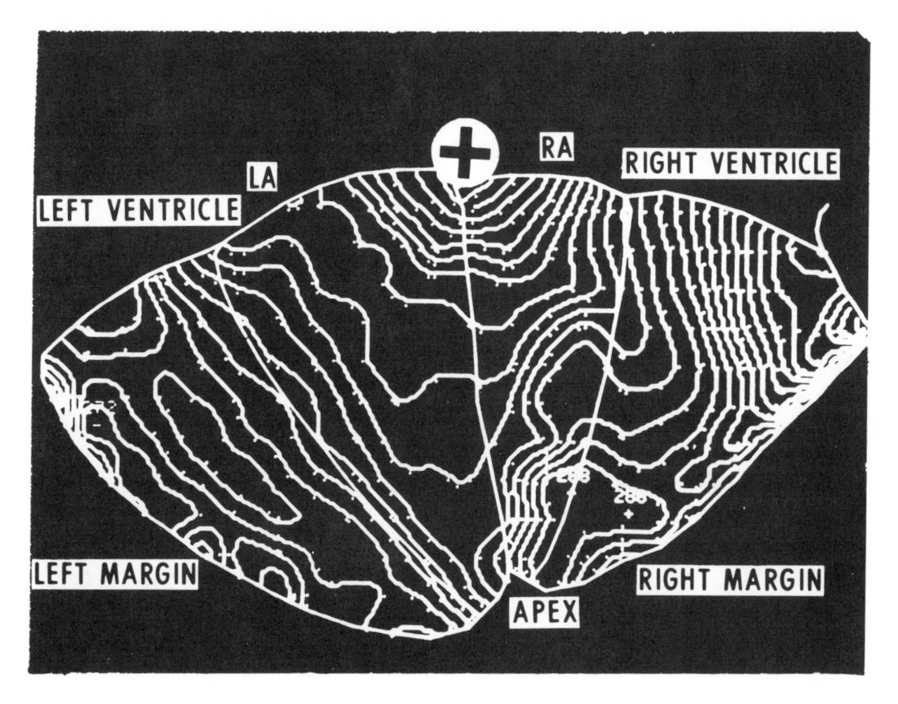

Figure 13-3. Mapping in a case of WPW syndrome. The heart is shown as if opened up along the *anterior* interventricular groove. The origin of the activation (+) is located at the crossing of the posterior atrioventricular and interventricular grooves.

and attacks of arrhythmia do not recur. When surgery is not completely successful, cases have been observed in which the delta wave has changed and the arrhythmias, when they recur, are sufficiently modified to be better tolerated or more amenable to medical treatment.

CHRONIC VENTRICULAR TACHYCARDIA

Up to now the surgical treatment of ventricular tachycardia had been mainly based on the excision of fibrous akinetic plaques, ventricular aneurysms complicating myocardial infarction, idiopathic ventricular aneurysms or myocardial tumors. Recent studies suggest that many cases of chronic VT are due to reentry phenomena, that is to say, a circus movement in a specific zone of myocardium which is then propagated to the rest of the ventricle.[12,13] In such cases, surgical section of the free ventricular wall (ventriculotomy) may interfere with the reentry pathway and prevent recurrent arrhythmias. It is not possible to map the exact pathway of the abnormal activation in the majority of cases so surgical section is guided by indirect data obtained during epicardial mapping.[14]

Location

Epicardial mapping in sinus rhythm demonstrates the epicardial breakthrough related to the distal branches of the His-Purkinje system (Fig. 13-2 and 13-5). The epicardial potentials recorded over fibrous scars of myocardial infarction show fragmentation with a notable reduction in amplitude. The points where activation is most delayed, especially when abnormally delayed and recorded during the ST segment are often the points of origin of VT and sites of ventriculotomy.

Epicardial mapping in VT is performed after inducing the arrhythmia by pacing techniques established during preoperative electrophysiological exploration (Fig. 13-4). Epicardial mapping in VT is then carried out providing the rhythm is not too rapid.

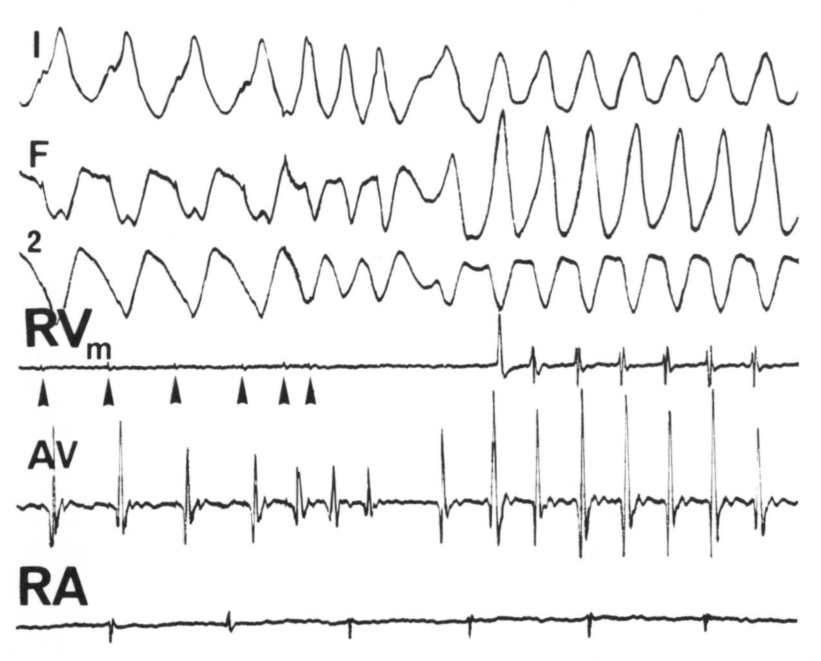

Figure 13-4. The induction of VT by programmed pacing from above below: S1, AVF, V2 potentials from the midzone of the right ventricle (at the end of the tracing) (RVm), atrioventricular junction (AV), right atrium (RA). The spikes are arrowed.

Mapping in VT shows the origin of the abnormal activation, either with VT with early breakthrough in two different myocardial zones or with two different VTs with different morphologies and rhythms. In many cases, these points of epicardial breakthrough are considered to be the nearest points to the reentry pathway and so ventriculotomy is performed at these sites.[14]

Ventriculotomies

The sample ventriculotomy is a transmural section of the ventricular wall at the point of origin of the abnormal activation during VT or in the zones where abnormally delayed potentials have been observed. It is carried out with a scalpel, respecting the underlying anatomical structures (coronary vessels, papillary muscles of the atrioventricular valves) (Fig. 13-5).

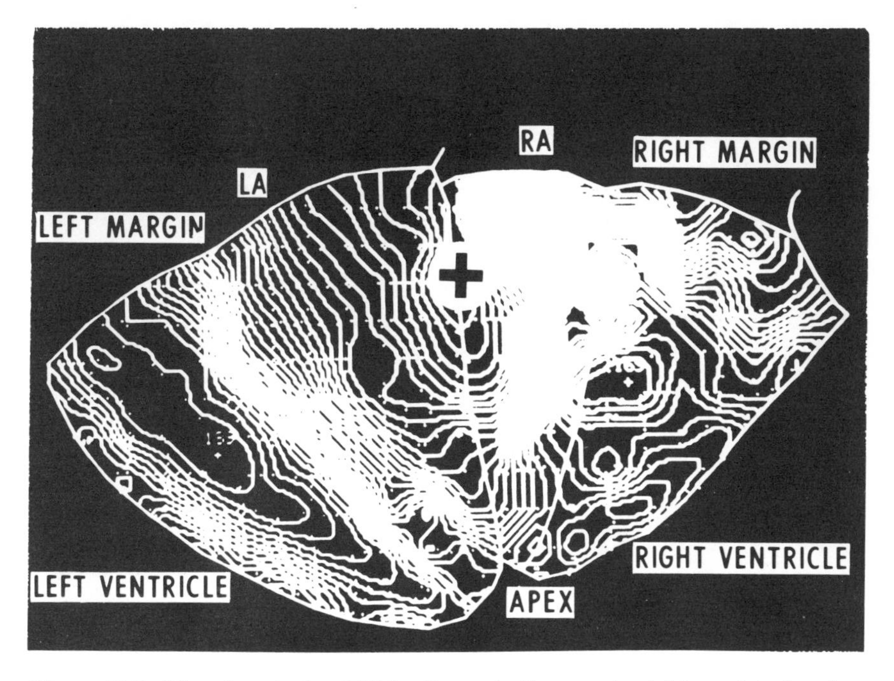

Figure 13-5. Mapping during VT in the arrhythmogenic right ventricular dysplasia syndrome. The origin of the activation (+) is in the posterior interventricular groove. During VT the isochrones are bunched up showing delay in the propagation of the activation especially over the diaphragmatic and lateral walls of the right ventricle.

When VT complicates myocardial infarction, the origin of the abnormal activation is often in the border zones between the area of necrosis and the healthy tissues where surviving bundles of fibers delay the activation, an essential condition for the induction of reentry phenomena. In these patients a new form of ventriculotomy called endocardial encircling ventriculotomy[15] has been developed which is performed within the ventricular cavity, sectioning from the endocardium to the epicardium and circumscribing the abnormal zone. This operation gives more coherent results than simple ventriculotomy in these patients.

CONCLUSION

The surgical management of cardiac arrhythmias is a rapidly expanding field. It is too soon yet to define its limits. However, one thing is certain: these new techniques require the use of fine electrophysiological methods in the operating theater such as epicardial mapping or the interpretation of certain potentials such as those recorded in the zone of the His bundle or delayed potentials where medicosurgical cooperation is most important. The selection of patients for surgery should be based on other clinical electrophysiological data obtained in the catheter laboratory. It is from these data that, for instance, the type of pre-excitation in the WPW syndrome may be defined as several possible anatomical dispositions or the mechanism of VT may be recognized; surgery for foci of increased automaticity is at present controversial.

These different surgical methods should only be resorted to when the patients have been shown to be untreatable from a medical point of view so that major cardiovascular surgery is avoided whenever possible.

REFERENCES

1. Slama, R., Coumel, P., Motte, G., et al.: Section volontaire du faisceau de His pour troubles du rythme grave. *Arch. Mal. Coeur* **64**: 27, 1970.
2. Giannelli, S., Ayres, S.M., and Comprecht, R.F.: Therapeutic surgical division of the human conduction system. *J.A.M.A.* **199**: 155, 1967.
3. Hoffman, B.F., Cranefield, P.F., Stuckey, J.H., et al.: Direct measurement of conduction velocity in the in situ specialized conducting system of the mammalian heart. *Proc. Soc. Exp. Biol. Med.* **102**: 55, 1959.
4. Kupersmith, J.: Electrophysiologic mapping during open heart surgery. *Prog. Cardiovasc. Dis.* **3**: 167, 1976.
5. Frank, R., Fontaine, G., and Vanetti, A.: Nouvelle technique di reperage a coeur couvert du faisceau de His. *Arch. Mal. Coeur* **70**: 213, 1977.
6. Harrison, L., Gallagher, J.J., Kasell, J., et al.: Cryosurgical ablation of the AV node-His bundle: A new method for producing A-V block. *Circulation* **55**: 463, 1977.

7. Gallagher, J.J. Prichett, E.L.C., Sealy, W.C., et al.: The pre-excitation syndromes. *Prog. Cardiovasc. Dis.* **20**: 285, 1978.
8. Frank, R.: Apport de investigations endocavitaires et des cartographies epicardiques dans l'etude des syndromes de pre-excitation ventriculaire. Thesis, Paris, 1974.
9. Gallagher, J.J., Sealy, W.C., Wallace, A.G., and Kasell, J.: Correlation between catheter electrophysiologic studies and findings on mapping of ventricular excitation in the WPW syndrome. In Wellens, H.J.J., Lie, K.I., and Janse, M.J. (eds.): *The Conduction System of the Heart.* Leiden, Stenfert Kroese B.V., 1976, p. 588.
10. Durrer, D., Van Dam, R.T., Freud, G.E., et al.: Total excitation of the isolated human heart. *Circulation* **41**: 899, 1970.
11. Gallagher, J.J., Sealy, W.C., Kasell, J., and Wallace, A.G.: Multiple accessory pathway in patients with the pre-excitation syndrome. *Circulation* **54 (IV)**: 571-591, 1976.
12. Wellens, H.J.J., Durrer, D.R., and Lie, K.I.: Observations on mechanisms of ventricular tachycardia in man. *Circulation* **54**: 237, 1976.
13. Josephson, M.E., Horowitz, L.N., Farshidi, A., and Kastor, J.A.: Recurrent sustained ventricular tachycardia. I. Mechanism. *Circulation* **57**: 431, 1978.
14. Fontaine, G., Guiraudon, G., Frank, R., et al.: Stimulation studies and epicardial mapping in ventricular tachycardia: Study of mechanisms and selection for surgery. In Kulbertus, H.E. (ed.): *Reentrant Arrhythmias.* Lancaster, MTP Press, 1977, p. 334.
15. Guiraudon, G., Fontaine, G., Frank, R., et al.: Encircling endocardial ventriculotomy. A new surgical treatment for life-threatening ventricular tachycardias resistant to medical treatment following myocardial infarction. *Ann. Thor. Surg.* **26**: 438, 1978.

14

Amiodarone: A New Antiarrhythmic Drug With Strong Cumulative Effect

Mauricio B. Rosenbaum, M.D., Pablo A. Chiale, M.D., M. Susana Halpern, M.D., Gerardo J. Nau, M.D., Julio Przybylski, M.D., Raúl J. Levi, M.D., Julio O. Lázzari, M.D., and Marcelo V. Elizari, M.D.

An excellent review on "new" antiarrhythmic drugs was recently published by Zipes and Troup,[1] including amiodarone, aprindine, disopyramide, ethmozin, mexiletine, tocainide, and verapamil. This reflects the present concern to obtain new antiarrhythmic agents. The pharmaceutical companies have developed many "new" agents and have flooded the market. The change of a single molecule may not be considered as the development of a new drug or congener. The position, not of the chemist, but of the clinical cardiologist is that a new antiarrhythmic agent is that in which the new molecule brings along a new useful antiarrhythmic property. Chemical agents which practically duplicate the properties of quinidine-like drugs with small variations in toxicity, tolerance, and duration of action cannot be considered to be real new antiarrhythmics. They do not fulfill our present expectations. These drugs are limited from the very outset. Pursuing this viewpoint, very few new antiarrhythmic drugs have been developed over the last year. Verapamil is certainly a new drug. Amiodarone is also a new drug, both because of their electrophysiologic properties as well as their strong cumulative effect. A genuinely new drug should be able to teach us new things. For example, until the appearance of amiodarone, with its extremely pro-

This work was supported in part by the Comisión para el Estudio Integral de la Enfermedad de Chagas and the Fundación de Investigaciones Cardiológicas Einthoven.

longed action, the importance of such a property for the chronic treatment of prophylaxis of arrhythmias was never so clearly appreciated as it is now.

A series of antiarrhythmic drugs, old and new, listed according to their approximate half-life is shown on Table 14-1. The top of the list shows "short-acting" drugs, suitable for treatment of acute situations (and for diagnostic purposes); the bottom, "long-acting" drugs, which are more convenient for the chronic treatment or prevention of arrhythmias. The half-life of amiodarone, which has been estimated as 28 days by some[2] and 60 days by others,[3] can be said to be "astronomical" as compared with all other drugs. Whatever its other properties, amiodarone can be conveniently analyzed as the prototype of long-acting antiarrhythmic agents.

Table 14-1. Approximate Half-life of Several Antiarrhythmic Drugs

Drug	Half-life
Ajmaline	5-8 min.
Verapamil	15 min.
Lidocaine	30 min.
Procainamide	3 hr.
Disopiramide	6 hr.
Quinidine	7 hr.
17 Monochloroacetylajmaline	10 hr.
Tocainide	12 hr.
Phenytoin	22 hr.
Aprinidine	28 hr.
Digoxin	40 hr.
Perhexiline	3 days
Digitoxin	7 days
Amiodarone	28 days

CLINICAL TRIAL

The drug was used in a series of 252 patients with persistent or repetitive atrial and ventricular arrhythmias.[4] Amiodarone was shown to have excellent clinical efficacy. The drug provided total control and protection in 96.6 percent of 89 patients with recurrent supraventricular tachycardia, atrial flutter, and/or fibrillation, regardless of the mechanism and etiology. Of particular importance was the fact that this effectiveness was generally achieved with small doses (200 to 400 mg/day). Patients with WPW syndrome were specially benefited.[4,5] However, in highly refractory cases, for example those showing the "incessant" forms of supraventricular tachycardias,[6] much higher doses (600 to 800 mg/day) were needed or the use of amiodarone with digitalis was required. Excellent results were also reported in 77.2 percent of 44 patients with recurrent refractory ventricular tachycardia (VT), and in 84.1 percent of 101 patients with persistent ventricular extrasystoles (VE). Special mention can be made of the results obtained in six of eight patients with repetitive VT related to postinfarction ventricular aneurysm, six of whom also had multiple episodes of ventricular fibrillation (VF). These results were also achieved with small or moderate doses, usually 400 to 600 mg per day. After the original experience, when doses of 600 to 1000 mg a day were administered to larger number of patients, the efficacy of amiodarone in controlling repetitive VT and/or VF increased to around 95 percent, and in persistent VE, to 95 to 99 percent.[7]

Confirmation of these results was recently provided by a new study on the effects of amiodarone on the malignant ventricular arrhythmias of chronic chagasic myocarditis.[8,9] The arrhythmias consist of frequent and multiform VE, repetitive couplets and VT, and a tendency for the occurrence of VF and sudden death. The persistence of the arrhythmia in this disease is remarkable and has been recently documented with repeated Holter monitoring at weekly or monthly intervals.[8] The effects of amiodarone (600 to 1000 mg per day) on 24 selected cases of chagasic myocarditis can be summarized as follows. In 23, the number of VE in 24 hours was reduced between 93.20 and 99.95 percent, three to 20 weeks after the beginning of treatment, and this effect was shown to persist during an average follow-up of 13 months. Couplets were totally suppressed in 22 cases. Six patients who prior to treatment could not be exercised beyond the warming up period because of the occurrence of repetitive bursts of VT, were able to complete a full test during treatment without such complication. Before treatment, seven of the 24 patients had between 26150 and 61733 VE in 24 hours, and the remaining cases, 3780 to 14861 VE. All the patients showed at least three different extrasystolic patterns, and all presented numerous or countless couplets associated in 20 with salvos of VT. The follow-up of the 24 patients ranged between two and 24 months, with an average of 13 months. One of the 24 patients died suddenly six months after the beginning of treatment, while receiving a daily dose of 600 mg. A Holter recording one day before still showed one episode of VT lasting 12 seconds.

ELECTROPHYSIOLOGIC PROPERTIES

Amiodarone prolongs refractoriness in all *normal* cardiac tissues, including atria, ventricles, His-Purkinje system, AV node and accessory pathways. Although a total prolongation of refractoriness in the human is likely, it seems that amiodarone prolongs more specifically the absolute refractory period at the expense of the relative refractory period, thus abbreviating the interval during which slowly conducted premature responses may occur.[10] In canine ventricular and Purkinje fibers, prolongation of the action potential duration is not a significant feature. In addition, amiodarone improves the rate of rise and increases the size of the overshoot of premature responses. At therapeutic doses, conduction velocity is not depressed or may be even increased during premature impulses. In *abnormal* cardiac tissues, particularly Purkinje fibers, amiodarone may greatly prolong the total duration of refractoriness, and may reduce conduction velocity by depressing membrane responsiveness. This effect is, however, less than the one caused by ajmaline, aprindine, dysopraimide, and procainamide. Amiodarone depresses automaticity in the SA node and conductivity in the AV node, probably through an antiadrenergic effect, although a direct effect on both nodes cannot be ruled out. Although amiodarone seems to delay initially the reactivation of the fast sodium channel, this appears to be followed by a more rapid reactivation of both the fast sodium and slow calcium channels. However, this is based only on indirect observations. The ionic basis of the electrophysiologic actions of the drug are still unknown. Amiodarone shares, at least partially, properties of the Class I, II, and III antiarrhythmic drugs,[11] and may possess a "new" or Class V effect not shared by other antiarrhythmic agents. The acute intravenous administration provokes rapidly some of the Class I and II effects, whereas the Class III and V actions can only occur, probably, during chronic or prolonged administration of the drug.

THE CUMULATIVE EFFECT

Amiodarone causes sinus bradycardia, prolongs the Q-T interval, and induces characteristic T-wave changes. All these changes persist up to four weeks or more from withdrawal of the drug, after continuous administration. It has been shown in a series of 67 patients with persistent or repetitive arrhythmias that, at the dose of 400 to 600 mg per day, it takes four to eight days for the drug to reach a therapeutic effect and a much longer time has been estimated for the effect to disappear when treatment is interrupted.[4] This interval is dependent on dosage and time of administration. Persistence of the antiarrhythmic effect for 10 to 20 days and even 30 and 45 days is common. Recently, we were able to document the antiarrhythmic effect for more than 90 days in three different patients, and similar results have been reported by others.[12]

This property contributes enormously to the clinical usefulness of amiodarone, because it liberates patients from compelling submission to a rigid hourly schedule, and provides them with more continuous sustained and effective antiarrhythmic protection. Dosage regimes in which the drug is discontinued either two days every week, or one week per month are equally effective. Patients prefer, however, to take the drug in divided doses (although this is irrelevant) and to discontinue the drug only on Saturdays and Sundays.

Due to its slowly cumulative effect, amiodarone is more likely to impregnate each cardiac cell more homogeneously, and this does not seem to occur with the short-acting drugs which must be administered frequently. Short-acting drugs probably cause inhomogeneities in the geometrical distribution of the electrophysiologic effects of a drug, which may become important in explaining why classical antifibrillatory drugs may potentially cause fibrillation. In any event, clinical evidence indicates that the likelihood of an arrhythmogenic effect with amiodarone is much less than with other antiarrhythmic drugs.

SAFETY MARGIN AND SIDE EFFECTS

The safety margin of a given drug is shown by the number of patients who have to discontinue the use of a given drug because of adverse effects. Intolerance to amiodarone occurs in a small number of patients in the order of 1 to 3 percent. While the half-lethal dose of quinidine or procainamide is 2.5 times the average therapeutic dose, this index rises to 12 to 35 when amiodarone is given parenterally, and there is no lethal dose at all when the drug is administered orally. In other words, it is just impossible to kill an animal with acute oral administration of amiodarone. Clinical observations are equally reassuring. While a commonly effective dose is 200 to 400 mg per day, we have administered up to 2000 mg per day to many patients with refractory arrhythmias in the presence of advanced heart failure or an acute myocardial infarction without apparent ill effects. Amiodarone may cause mild digestive problems, but the three most important side effects are the corneal microdeposits and the dermatologic and thyroid changes. The corneal microdeposits appear to stigmatize an extremely useful and promising drug psychologically rather than for any other reason. The benignity and reversibility of such deposits is well established, as well as the fact that no other structure of the eye is involved. The effects of amiodarone are totally different from those provoked by chloroquin and the 8-hydroxyquinolines, particularly iodochlorhydroxyquin, at least after the first 10 years of studies performed by European ophthalmologists.[7] The most annoying side effect of amiodarone is a bluish decoloration of the skin which occurs in 0.5 percent of the patients after prolonged periods of treatment (6 to 30 months) with high doses. Like the more common corneal deposits, this process is gradually reversible. One to two percent of the patients may develop either hypo- or hyperthyroidism, which can be controlled with conventional administration of thyroid or antithyroid drugs, and these changes are generally reversible.

PROSPECTS AND LIMITS

Figure 14-2 lists the main requirements which a drug must fulfill in order to offer good prospects for the chronic treatment and prevention of arrhythmias, including possibly ventricular fibrillation. The first property should be minimal cardiac and extracardiac toxicity. A wide therapeutic margin is desirable. In large series of patients, discontinuation of amiodarone due to adverse side effects occurs in 1 to 3 percent of the cases. This indicates that in this regard the drug compares favorably with most other antiarrhythmic agents. However, since the effects of a drug to be administered chronically or for life can be considered as being "another disease", a balance will have to be made in every case between the benefit produced by the drug and the detriment caused by its chronic administration. For example, when the side effects are highly annoying (such as a bluish decoloration of the skin) in a patient in whom the drug was indicated for the treatment of a relatively benign arrhythmia, amiodarone is not justified. On the other hand, in a case in which amiodarone prevents the occurrence of repetitive VT or VF, the same side effect, although still annoying, may not be such a high price to pay for keeping the patient alive. In some patients (but not in all) with repetitive supraventricular tachycardias, a dose of 150 to 200 mg per day may be sufficient to control the tachycardias completely. In such cases, the side effects will be naturally less, and the patient himself may look for the minimal dose which keeps him free of symptoms. At the other end of the spectrum, when trying to control malignant ventricular arrhythmias and particular repetitive VT and VF, the situation is more difficult.

Table 14-2. Main Requirements of a Drug Suitable for Chronic Treatment and Prevention of Arrhythmias

Wide therapeutic margin
Efficacy
Cumulative effect
Versatility
No negative inotropic effect

To start with, much higher doses may be needed in the order of 600 to 800 mg per day as maintainance, clearly increasing the possibility of side effects. This also requires the use of repeated and costly ambulatory monitoring in order to evaluate the effects of treatment. And in such cases, when the patient has been protected for several months from the occurrence of repetitive VT or VF, it may be hazardous to start looking for a minimal protective dose. It is, however, in this widely obscure area that the future of amiodarone or any other similar drug will be played. We know little about the average dose which will be required to prevent

VF in patients with ischemic heart disease. In a few selected cases, the dosage of 400 mg per day was sufficient to protect the patient from the occurrence of repetitive VT and VF after a follow-up of two to four years, but in some other cases, the required dose was much higher. If the suitable dose needed to achieve a high percentage of protection is close to 400 mg per day and not beyond 600 mg per day, the future of amiodarone will be bright. If the average dose is closer to 600 or 1000 mg per day, the future of the drug will be much less promising, even if some malignant ventricular arrhythmias are controlled for relatively long periods of time. Only well designed prospective randomized studies will provide the answer so badly needed to this crucial question.

The next requirement is "efficacy" and in this regard amiodarone is highly satisfactory, probably to levels not commonly achieved by other antiarrhythmic drugs. The most convincing results are probably those reported on the malignant ventricular arrhythmias of chagasic myocarditis.[9] Whether or not similar results will apply to patients with ischemic heart disease is another pressing question to be answered in the near future.

A third important property is the cumulative effect. Mechanisms related to this property have not been well defined since this is the first time that we have had to deal with an antiarrhythmic agent with a prolonged duration of action. A new methodology will have to be developed to evaluate this property. The fact that a single daily dose or even temporary withdrawal of the drug is feasible makes this drug very desirable in the prevention of VF; particularly if intended for wide-scale and long-range use.

Another important property is "versatility". In the case of amiodarone, this refers to the fact that the drug covers equally well the treatment of supraventricular and ventricular arrhythmias. But it applies also to the fact that its simplicity of dosage scheduling makes it the kind of drug which can be handled readily by the specialized arrhythmologist as well as the general practitioner. Plasma levels are not ever likely to become important for proper use of amiodarone.

The lack of negative inotropic effect is generally identified as an independent property, although it participates in providing better therapeutic safety margin. Available information has proven beyond any doubt that amiodarone does not depress ventricular function.

In conclusion, amiodarone possesses several properties which make it an excellent antiarrhythmic agent. The known side effects and its long range effects require further clarification.

The present, already wide, experience indicates that it offers very desirable features and the drug in its present form or a derivative may become useful for the prevention of sudden cardiac death.

REFERENCES

1. Zipes, D.P., and Troup, P.J.: New antiarrhythmic agents. Amiodarone, aprindine, ethmozin, mexiletine, tocainide, verapamil. *Am. J. Cardiol.,* **41**: 1005, 1978.
2. Broekhuysen, J., Laurel, R., and Sion, R.: Etude comparée du transit et du métabolism de I'amiodarone chez diverses especes animals et chez l'homme. *Arch, Int. Pharmacodyn.,* **177**: 340, 1969.
3. Massin, J.P., Thomopoulos, P., Karam, J., and Savoice, J.C.: Le risque thyroidien dún nouveau coronaro-dilatateur iodé: Iámiodarone (cordarone). *Ann. Endocrin. (Paris),* **32**: 438, 1971.
4. Rosenbaum, M.B., Chiale, P.A., Halpern, M.S., et al.: Clinical efficacy of amiodarone as an antiarrhythmic agent. *Am. J. Cardiol.,* **38**: 934, 1976.
5. Rosenbaum, M.B., Chiale, P.A., Ryba, D., and Elizari, M.V.: Control of tachyarrhythmias associated with Wolff-Parkinson-White syndrome. *Am. J. Cardiol.,* **34**: 215, 1974.
6. Coumel, P., Cabrol, C., Fabiato, A., et al.: Tachycardia permanente par rythme réciproque. *Arch. Mal. Coeur,* **60**: 1830, 1967.
7. Rosenbaum, M.B., Chiale, P.A., Halpern, M.S., et al.: Antiarrhythmic drugs of strong cumulative effect. In *Symposium of Cardiac Arrhythmias,* Manila, Philippines, January 25–27, 1979 (to be published).
8. Chiale, P.A., Halpern, M.S., Tambussi, A., et al.: Malignant ventricular arrhythmias in chronic chagasic myocarditis. (To be published).
9. Chiale, P.A., Halpern, M.S., Nau, G.J., et al.: The treatment of malignant ventricular arrhythmias in Chagas disease with amiodarone hydrochloride. (To be published).
10. Elizari, M.V., Levi, R.J., Novakosky, A.: Electrophysiological properties of amiodarone on canine Purkinje and ventricular fibers. (To be published).
11. Vaughan Williams, E.M.: Classification of anti-arrhythmic drugs. In Sandoe, E., Flensted-Jensen, E., and Olesen, K.H. (eds.): *Symposium on Cardiac Arrhythmias,* Elsinore, Denmark. Sodertalje, Sweden, AB Astrax, 1970, p. 449.
12. Fidelle, J.E., Attuel, P., Toumieux, M.C., and Coumel, P.: L'utilization de l'amiodarone dans les troubles rythmiques graves et revelles de l'enfant. A propos de 50 cas. *Ann. Cardiol.* (in press).

15

Prognostic Significance of Ventricular Arrhythmias in Relation to Sudden Death

Shlomo Stern, M.D. and Zvi Stern, M.D.

Ventricular arrhythmias are established as the most frequent precedent of ventricular fibrillation and sudden cardiac death.[1] This relationship has been firmly established in studies in which the ectopic activity was detected during the acute or subacute phase of myocardial infarction or in the immediate postinfarction period.[2,6–9] However, only a few investigations have dealt so far with the prognostic significance of ventricular arrhythmias in ambulatory patients with chronic ischemic heart disease[3] without previous infarction and even less is known concerning the significance of ventricular ectopic activity in subjects not suffering from overt ischemic heart disease.[1,4]

A review of the subject of ambulatory monitoring describing the history of this method, starting from its pioneering days, stressing that its origin preceded by 10 years the concept of in-hospital long-term ECG monitoring, its techniques, its use in detecting hidden, transitory arrhythmias, its importance in disclosing ischemic periods, with or without accompanying pain, and its significance in discovering transient ST elevation (the so-called Prinzmental angina), is presented elsewhere in this book. Similarly, in that chapter, the importance of avoiding artifacts, an occurrence not infrequent in any of the sophisticated methods used today in medicine, is stressed.

In collaboration with Dr. Dan Tzivoni, Dr. Andre Keren and Dr. Shmuel Penchas

MATERIALS AND METHODS

In this study, we investigated the prevalence of sudden cardiac death in a population of 888 patients who underwent 24-hour ambulatory ECG monitoring[5] during the years 1971–1974.[10] The age and sex distribution of the patients is given in Table 15-1.

Table 15-1. Age and Sex Distribution of 888 Subjects With 24-Hour Ambulatory ECG Monitoring

Born	Total	Females	Males
1960–1974	4	1	3
1940–1959	95	47	48
1930–1939	156	59	97
1920–1929	221	83	138
1910–1919	225	92	133
1900–1909	145	52	93
1899	42	17	25
Total	888	351	537

The indications for performing the ambulatory ECG monitoring in these 888 subjects were as follows:

Precordial pain, defined as the pain characteristic for angina pectoris, was the indication in 284 subjects; vague precordial symptoms, such as pressure or discomfort unrelated to effort in 189 subjects; palpitations, in subjects who had no arrhythmia in their resting ECG in 160 patients. Fifty-five subjects did have arrhythmia previously documented in routine ECG; 63 subjects suffered from cerebral manifestations, such as syncope, vertigo, or blackout; 55 were postmyocardial infarction patients; 25 patients had permanent pacemakers; seven had neurocirculatory asthenia. There were also 31 control subjects who were all under 40 years of age, without any apparent disease, and finally, the group of "others", which included 19 subjects with thyroid disorders, duodenal ulcer, malignant disease, etc.

Most of the patients were between the ages of 30 to 60. Less than two-thirds were males.

Premature ventricular contractions were classified according to the following grading system: rare—if less than 10 unifocal beats per any hours were found; moderate—if 10 to 60 unifocal beats per hour were found; frequent—if one or more unifocal beats per minute were found.

Ventricular tachycardia was diagnosed when three or more successive ventricular beats were seen.

The diagnosis of ischemic heart disease was made in those patients who fulfilled one or more of the following criteria:

1. Patients who exhibited ST-T alterations in their resting ECG typical for ischemia;

2. Patients in whom ST depression of more than 1 mm of the "ischemic type" was detected during ambulatory ECG monitoring;
3. Patients who had a documented previous myocardial infarction;
4. Patients who had an abnormal coronary arteriogram.

In none of the other patients was there any clinical or laboratory evidence or suspicion of ischemic heart disease. Incidentally, the number of patients with or without ischemic heart disease turned out to be equal: 444 subjects were in each group.

The Israel Bureau of Statistics provided information as to which of the 888 patients died before December 31, 1976, the antemortem diagnosis, the cause of death as it appeared on the death certificates, and whether the death occurred in or outside the hospital. The death certificates were filled out always by the treating physician who was present at the time of death, or who arrived at the scene immediately thereafter. The coding of the International Classification of Diseases was issued by the Israel Bureau of Statistics. We grouped together the different diagnoses that led to death as "cardiac" or "noncardiac". Moreover, the death cases were classified as "sudden" if they happened at home, at work or in the street, or as "hospital death" if they happened in the hospital, even when death occurred shortly after the arrival of the patient.

The statistical significance of the results was tested by a two-tailed chi-square method, as applied to 2 × 2 contingency table, with Yates' correction for continuity. All results held true with this correction, except for two instances, where it is stated clearly.

RESULTS

Seventy three out of the 888 patients died during the follow-up period. The age and sex distribution of these patients according to the cause of death is given in Table 15-2.

Ventricular arrhythmias were detected in 386 patients and among them 47 (12.2%) died, 14 from noncardiac causes and 33 from cardiac causes, of which 16—nearly one half—were sudden deaths. On the other hand, among the patients in whom ventricular arrhythmias were not detected, 26 patients (5.2%) died, 11 from noncardiac and 15 from cardiac causes; only slightly more than one-fourth of the cardiac deaths were sudden. The difference between the two groups as to the number of patients with cardiac deaths as well as the difference between the two groups as to the number of patients with sudden coronary deaths, was statistically significant (Table 15-3).

The resting twelve-lead ECG of the 47 patients who died from cardiac causes showed the following abnormalities: four patients had premature contractions; 13 were after myocardial infarction; five had right or

Table. 15-2. Age and Sex Distribution of the 73 Deceased Patients According to Cause of Death

Born	Total	19 Females Cardiac Deaths		Noncardiac Deaths	Total	54 Males Cardiac Deaths		Noncardiac Deaths
		Sudden death	Hospital death			Sudden death	Hospital death	
1960–1974	—	—	—	—	—	—	—	—
1940–1959	—	—	—	—	—	—	—	1
1930–1939	—	—	—	—	6	3	3	—
1920–1929	3	2	1	2	6	3	3	1
1910–1919	4	—	4	2	10	4	6	5
1900–1909	3	1	2	4	9	4	5	6
1899 or before	—	—	—	1	7	1	6	3
Total	10	3	7	9	38	15	23	16

Table 15-3. Number of Patients Deceased During the Two to Six Year Follow-up, From Cardiac or Noncardiac Causes, With or Without Ventricular Arrhythmias

	Total	Subjects Deceased		Noncardiac deaths			Cardiac deaths		
		Number	Percent	Number of Subjects	Sudden Death	Hospital Death	Number of Subjects	Sudden Death	Hospital Death
Without ventricular arrhythmia	502	26	5.2	11	2	9	15*	4†	11
With ventricular arrhythmia	386	47	12.2	14	1	13	33*	16†	17

*Difference statistically significant ($p < 0.001$).
†Difference statistically significant ($p < 0.001$).

left-bundle branch block and 14 had ischemic changes. The other 12 patients had a normal resting ECG.

The correlation between sudden coronary death, ischemic heart disease and ventricular arrhythmias is as follows:

Out of the 444 patients with ischemic heart disease, in those with ventricular arrhythmias, the number of deaths owing to cardiac causes was 22. In the group of 248 patients with ischemic heart disease, but no ventricular arrhythmias—only 10 died—a statistically significant difference ($p < 0.01$). In the 196 patients with ventricular arrhythmias there were 12 sudden coronary deaths, while among the 248 patients without ventricular arrhythmias, there were four sudden coronary deaths; this difference was also found to be statistically significant ($p < 0.05$) (Table 15-4).

In the 444 patients without ischemic heart disease, ambulatory ECG monitoring disclosed ventricular arrhythmias in 190, and among them 11 patients died from cardiac causes, while among the 254 subjects without ventricular arrhythmias only five patients (1.9%) died from cardiac causes, a difference statistically significant ($p < 0.05$). Four patients out of the 11 died suddenly. No sudden coronary deaths occurred among the five patients without ventricular arrhythmias ($p < 0.025$). These differences are statistically nonsignificant if the Yates correction is applied, but are significant without it (Table 15-4).

Table 15-5 shows that in the patients who had ventricular arrhythmias, but with and without ischemic heart disease, there was no significant difference between the mean age of the survivors and of those who died. Therefore, in these group an age difference would not account for the death cases. On the other hand, in the patients without ischemic heart disease and without ventricular arrhythmias, the age of the patients who died was significantly higher than the age of the survivors.

CONCLUSION

It is our conclusion that ventricular arrhythmias carry a high risk of sudden cardiac death not only in the postinfarction patient, as it has been documented previously, but also in patients with chronic ischemic heart disease without infarction.

Moreover, our study indicates that even in subjects without ischemic heart disease and who are apparently free from stigma of heart disease, sudden cardiac death is more frequent than in individuals without ventricular arrhythmias. It is a possibility that the ventricular arrhythmia detected in these patients was an early manifestation of coronary, ischemic or other type of heart disease, but at the time of the examination these individual were *not* classified as cardiac patients and were managed by their doctors as normal subjects.

Table 15-4. Total Number of Subjects Deceased During the Follow-up Period From Cardiac Causes and Number of Sudden Death Cases, in 888 Individuals With or Without Ischemic Heart Disease, With or Without Ventricular Arrhythmias

	Total Number of Subjects in Group	PVC's			VT	Total Number of Cardiac Deaths	Sudden Death
		Frequent	Moderate	Rare			
IHD with VA	196	75	47	67	6	22*	12†
IHD without VA	248	—	—	—	—	10*	4†
No IHD, with VA	190	84	55	58	11	11‡	4**
No IHD, without VA	254	—	—	—	—	5‡	0**

*Difference statistically significant ($p < 0.01$).
†Difference statistically significant ($p < 0.05$).
‡Difference statistically significant ($p < 0.05$) only without Yates correction, but nonsignificant with it.
**Difference statistically significant ($p < 0.025$) only without Yates correction, but nonsignificant with it.

Table 15-5. Number, Age Distribution, and Mean Age of Patients in Groups With or Without Ischemic Heart Disease, With or Without Ventricular Arrhythmias

	IHD, with VA		IHD, without VA		No IHD, with VA		No IHD, without VA	
	Total	Cardiac death	Total	Cardiac death	Total	Cardiac death	Total	Cardiac death
Below 40	5	—	8	—	38	—	75	—
40–49	32	3	50	—	38	3	69	—
50–59	44	7	75	4	49	2	59	—
60–69	66	6	75	4	41	3	36	2
Above 70	49	6	40	2	24	3	15	3
Total	196	22	248	10	190	11	254	5
Mean age of group, years	61.01	60.86	58.27	63.40	52.96	61.09	47.06	76.00
SD	±11.09	±11.52	±10.93	± 6.75	±15.66	±16.73	±14.02	±10.12
	Difference nonsignificant		p < 0.05*		Difference nonsignificant			

*Difference statistically significant at the 5 percent level (two-sided Welch test).

If the relationship between ventricular arrhythmias and sudden cardiac death would be established "beyond any reasonable doubt", this relationship could carry important significance as to the treatment of such arrhythmias in a so-called normal population. From our study, similarly from all presently available studies in the literature, no conclusion can be drawn as to the effect of antiarrhythmic therapy, but it is our suggestion that a more aggressive approach to the treatment of ventricular arrhythmias should be adopted.

Finally, it is our opinion that the routine 12-lead ECG is a poor indicator of the presence, or absence, of ventricular ectopic activity, and ambulatory monitoring of the ECG for longer periods is advocated for more exact diagnosis.

REFERENCES

1. Alexander, S., Desai, D.C., and Hershberg, P.I.: Clinical significance of ventricular premature beats in an outpatient population. (abst.) *Am. J. Cardiol.* **29**: 250, 1972.
2. Coronary Drug Project Research Group: Prognostic importance of premature beats following myocardial infarction. *JAMA* **223**: 1116, 1973.
3. Fisher, F.D., and Tyroler, H.A.: Relationship between ventricular premature contractions on routine electrocardiography and subsequent sudden death from coronary heart disease. *Circulation* **47**: 712, 1973.
4. Hinkle, L.E., Carver, S.T., and Argyros, D.C.: Antecedents of sudden death in middle aged men. *Circulation* **49–50 (Suppl.)**: 705, 1974.
5. Holter, N.J.: New method for heart studies by continuous electrocardiography of active subjects. *Science* **134**: 1214, 1964.
6. Kolter, M.D., Tabatznik, B., Mower, M.M., and Tominaga, S.: Prognostic significance of ventricular ectopic beats with respect to sudden death in the late post-infarction period. *Circulation* **47**: 959, 1973.
7. Moss, A.J., DeCamilla, J., and Davis, H.P.: Ventricular ectopic beats in the early posthospital phase of myocardial infarction: their clinical significance. *Am. J. Cardiol.* **39**: 635, 1977.
8. Oliver, G.C., Nolle, F.M., and Tiefendrunn, J.: Ventricular arrhythmias associated with sudden death in survivors of acute myocardial infarction.
9. Ruberman, W., Weinblatt, E., Goldberg, J.D., et al.: Ventricular premature beats and mortality after myocardial infarction. *N. Eng. J. Med.* **297**: 750, 1977.
10. Stern, Z., Penchas, S., Tzivoni, D., and Stern, S.: Computer generated patient files in a 24-hour ECG monitoring cardiac station. *Harefuah* **91**: 245, 1976.

16

Long-Term Monitoring of Lethal Arrhythmias

Ronald R. Hope, M.D.

Long-term monitoring and recording of the heart rhythm stems from pioneer studies performed by Dr. Norman J. Holter [1,2] approximately 20 years ago. Original monitors were large and cumbersome, their size being limited by the tape recording apparatus which originally recorded for a maximum of 10 hours. Today's units encompassing microrecorders are compact and most often record for a period of 24 hours.

ELECTROCARDIOGRAM VERSUS HOLTER MONITORING FOR ARRHYTHMIA DETECTION

The electrocardiogram is a pillar of modern cardiology and provides much morphological information about the heart. As a device to detect cardiac arrhythmias the electrocardiogram falls far short of long-term ambulatory monitoring. Unfortunately, as practicing cardiologists screening for arrhythmias in the individual patient, we still tend to use the electrocardiogram which records only 30 to 60 seconds of the patient's rhythm. The Coronary Drug Project[3] in studying survivors of myocardial infarction examined the long-term risks of death including sudden death, based on the incidence of ventricular premature beats detected on the standard electrocardiogram. In the study, the electrocardiogram recorded an average of 49 heart beats for each patient. Using the electrocardiogram, 11.5% of 2035 patients surviving myocardial infarction were seen to have ventricular premature beats. Chiang et al.[4] examined the relationship of premature systoles to coronary heart disease and sudden death in a population of 5129 persons aged 16 and over.

Using the standard electrocardiogram, they detected premature systoles in only 5.1 percent of the population (70% ventricular and 30% supraventricular). Even more recent studies have clung to the use of the electrocardiogram for arrhythmia screening. Crow et al.[5] used a two-minute, lead I electrocardiogram to screen 10,880 men between the ages of 35 and 57 years. Ventricular premature beats were detected in only 4.96 percent. Complex ventricular premature beats were detected in 0.7 percent. Detection of arrhythmias is markedly increased with long-term ambulatory monitoring of the electrocardiogram. In 1969 Hinkle and colleagues[6] examined a population of 283 asymptomatic men of median age 55 years. Holter monitoring was performed for six hours and 62 percent demonstrated ventricular premature beats, 19 percent of which were complex ventricular arrhythmias. Approximately 20 percent of their population had known coronary disease. Monitoring for 12 hours by Kotler and colleagues[7] disclosed ventricular arrhythmias in 85 percent of 160 patients who had previously experienced myocardial infarction. Even in young asymptomatic males studied for 24 hours with ambulatory monitoring, ventricular premature beats were detected in 50 percent.[8] The latter study contrasts markedly with earlier classical studies by Lamb and co-workers. Hiss and Lamb,[9] using only the electrocardiogram found ventricular premature beats in a few as 0.78 percent of 122,043 relatively healthy young males.

Arrhythmia detection depends on the sampling time and upon the true occurrence of the arrhythmias. Rydén and colleagues[10] examined the reliability of intermittent ECG sampling in arrhythmia detection. They concluded that intermittent ECG sampling offers both a low detection rate for infrequent arrhythmias and short ECG samples, and brought about a risk of underestimating or overemphasizing the arrhythmia occurrence. Even with long-term ambulatory monitoring the sampling time is important. Differences in the frequency of arrhythmias detected may in part be explained on the population sample under scrutiny but is also influenced by the duration of monitoring.[6,7] Kennedy and colleagues[11] specifically addressed the question as to effectiveness of increasing hours of continuous ambulatory monitoring. They examined the effectiveness of 1, 6, 12, 24, 36 and 48 hours of continuous monitoring both in patients with coronary heart disease and in normal subjects. Their study found continuous 6 and 12-hour examinations to be from one to three times less effective than the 24-hour examination which detected the maximum grade of ventricular ectopy in 71 to 74 percent and the maximal frequency in 58 to 83 percent of patients with coronary heart disease. Kennedy and colleagues found that examination of the initial hour of the ambulatory recording or any single hour of dynamic activity, frequently failed to reveal maximal ventricular ectopy, particularly in regard to complex types of arrhythmia occuring with high frequency. Nevertheless, other authors[12] have reported favorably on short-term continuous electrocardiographic studies using the initial hour of long-term ambulatory monitoring. However, even in this study, less than 25 percent of patients who manifested complex ventricular arrhythmias were detected by such brief examinations. More recently Graboys and Lown[13] have advocated a 30-minute period of on-line ECG monitoring to serve as a rapid screening method for advanced grades of ventricular dysrhythmias. They studied 145 patients and concluded that a 30-minute period of initial observation provided adequate monitoring for about 95 percent of patients in whom extended (24 hours) monitoring was to be considered for arrhythmia detection. It is difficult to see how the authors arrived at this conclusion from their own data. Forty-five percent of their patients were shown to have ventricular premature beats during abbreviated monitoring compared with almost 80 percent during 24-hour monitoring and detection of high grade arrhythmias (grades III, IVa and IVb) were approximately doubled by 24-hour monitoring as compared with 30-minute screening. The findings of Kennedy and colleagues supports the use of long-term ambulatory monitoring for a duration of approximately 24 hours and this confirms the work of Lopes et al.[14] by emphasizing the superiority of 24 hours versus 12 hours of monitoring. A continuous or 36 to 48 hour recording may be more appropriate for some patients with a high risk of serious ventricular arrhythmias such as survivors of primary ventricular fibrillation.[10,15]

Finally, in order to emphasize the poor rate of detection of ventricular arrhythmias by the standard electrocardiogram in comparison with continuous ambulatory monitoring, the work of Vismara and colleagues should be considered.[16] These authors examined 101 patients with stable coronary artery disease. Each patient had Holter monitoring for ten hours and the results of the single ten-hour tracing was compared with multiple 12-lead electrocardiograms performed on these patients within two years of dynamic monitoring. A total of 1414 such electrocardiograms were obtained on the 101 patients. The ten hours of Holter monitoring detected premature ventricular contractions in 77 patients. In 50 percent of these the premature ventricular contractions were considered serious (multifocal, paired, more than 5 per minute, or R on T phenomenon) and 9 percent of all patients showed ventricular tachycardia. One thousand four hundred fourteen standard ECG's performed on the same patients detected premature ventricular contractions in 49 percent of patients in which serious premature ventricular beats were seen in 25 percent and ventricular tachycardia in 1 percent. Single ECG's recorded within twelve hours of Holter monitoring, or several ECG's recorded within two weeks of Holter monitoring, recorded even lower incidences of premature ventricular beats and of ventricular tachycardia. Conversely, any ventricular ectopy present on the standard ECG within three months of ambulatory monitoring was associated with a high prevalance of hazardous premature beats on portable Holter monitoring (serious premature ventricular beats 92%, ventricular tachycardia in 17%). Significantly even those patients free of ventricular arrhythmias as measured by two years' serial and repeated electrocardiograms were shown on a single ten-hour Holter recording to have serious premature ventricular beats in 62 percent and ventricular tachycardia in 6 percent.

Thus it becomes apparent that the standard electrocardiogram is unacceptable in the evaluation of patients for cardiac arrhythmia. Ambulatory monitoring of the cardiac rhythm must be performed under these circumstances. Vismara and colleagues have indicated that patients with no ventricular premature beats detected on serial ECG's over two years still show a remarkably high incidence of ventricular arrhythmias on Holter monitoring. The same authors, however, emphasize that any premature ventricular contractions seen on any electrocardiogram may connote serious ventricular arrhythmias on long-term monitoring; for example, patients showing as few as one to three premature ventricular contractions in total, on serial ECG's over three months, had a 62 percent incidence of serious ventricular arrhythmias and a 12 percent incidence of ventricular tachycardia. Those patients showing greater than ten premature ventricular contractions on electrocardiograms over three months had a 25 percent incidence of ventricular tachycardia.

It should be stressed at this point that the value of Holter monitoring lies not simply in the detection of ventricular tachyarrhythmias but in a multitude of uses in the detection of bradyarrhythmias in patients with history of syncopal episodes or transient ischemic episodes. Lipski and colleagues[17] examined 55 symptomatic patients with syncope, palpitations, or dizziness and uncovered significant arrhythmias in 55 percent. Bradyarrhythmias accounted for the majority of arrhythmias detected in this population and six patients had episodes of sinus arrest of up to five seconds in duration. Lipski and colleagues[17] noted that long periods of monitoring may be needed to make a diagnosis in this type of patient and that a period of sleep should be included in the observation period.

Long-term recording of cardiac rhythm must, on occasion, be extended to the coronary care monitoring equipment. Certain arrhythmias, particularly ventricular premature beats and paroxysmal ventricular tachycardia, are completely undetected in an astoundingly high proportion of cases.[18,19]

REPRODUCIBILITY OF HOLTER MONITORING

Calvert, Lown and Gorlin[20] examined the reproducibility of a single

24-hour monitoring session in a repeat study of 65 patients. Approximately 83 percent of all patients showed ventricular ectopic activity on one 24-hour recording. This was increased to nearly 95 percent when two 24-hour sessions were combined. Significantly, frequent and multiform ventricular arrhythmias were highly reproducible, although repetitive grade IV arrhythmias (repetitive ventricular responses) were reproducible in only 40 percent of patients. Severity of heart disease was an important factor in reproducibility. Repetitive ventricular activity was most often reproduced in those patients with multivessel coronary disease in contrast to those with single or no coronary disease, and in patients with asynergy as compared to those without asynergy. Schroeder and Fitzgerald[21] examined 57 ambulatory electrocardiogram recordings in 18 patients, each of whom had two or more recordings. They concluded that the presence or absence of premature ventricular beats and frequency of more or less than ten premature ventricular beats per 15 minutes was highly reproducible. The frequency range of premature ventricular beats, however, varied greatly from week to week. Spontaneous decreases in frequency of premature ventricular beats of more than 50 percent and increases as high as 1200 percent were noted. Morganroth and colleagues[22] examined 15 clinically stable patients with different cardiac disorders during three consecutive 24-hour ECG monitoring periods. There were spontaneous variations in arrhythmia frequency of 23 percent from one day to the next, 29 percent between 8-hour hour periods within one day, and 48 percent from hour to hour. The variability in frequency of premature ventricular beats between repeated three-day monitoring periods was assessed in five patients and found to be 37 percent. These authors concluded that in order to distinguish between therapeutically induced reductions in ventricular premature beats and spontaneously occuring variations, it would require a reduction greater than 83 percent if two 24-hour monitoring periods were compared (and 65 percent if two 72-hour periods were compared). Schroeder and Fitzgerald[21] in their study similarly estimated that at least a 75 percent decrease in premature ventricular beat frequency must be achieved before efficacy of antiarrhythmic therapy can be concluded. Such criteria have been adhered to, for example, in the study of a sustained-release procaineamide preparation by Bauer and co-workers.[23]

SUDDEN DEATH DURING AMBULATORY MONITORING

In spite of the increasing usage of Holter monitoring, only a handful of case reports of death during ambultory monitoring are available. Ventricular fibrillation is usually the terminal rhythm in most patients. Liberthson and colleagues[24] indicate that other arrhythmias are responsible for 28 percent of terminal rhythms. Bleifer,[25] and Hinkle and colleagues[26] have reported sudden death during ambulatory monitoring attributable to short-cycled ventricular ectopic beats resulting in induction of ventricular tachycardia and fibrillation. In the case report by Hinkle and colleagues[26] early cycle ventricular premature contractions had been noted in electrocardiogram recordings from the same patient for four years prior to the terminal event. The coupling interval remained constant until five minutes before death when the ventricular premature depolarization began to encroach on the T-wave and fibrillation resulted. Gradman and colleagues[27] reported death during ambulatory monitoring in a man who became excited while watching a televised basketball game. The ventricular premature beat initiating ventricular fibrillation in this case was late coupled and appeared after the T-wave of the preceding sinus beat. Gradually increasing sinus rate during the two hours prior to death was documented. Our own case of sudden death herein reported may represent a different mechanism for initiation of ventricular fibrillation. The figures are from a Holter recording on a 56-year-old patient with known coronary artery disease. In panel *A* (Fig. 16-1) frequent premature ventricular beats are seen at 12:26 P.M. The first premature beat has a coupling interval of approximately 0.36 seconds and falls just beyond the T-wave of the preceding sinus beat. Panel *B* shows more complex couplets of ventricular premature beats occuring at 2:28 P.M. During the Holter recording the patient showed frequent premature ventricular beats of similar morphology to those shown in panels *A* and *B* and occurring with a frequency of one to ten per minute over a four-hour period. Panel *C* shows the induction of ventricular tachycardia at 5:28 P.M. The coupling interval of the ventricular premature beat initiating the ventricular tachycardia is identical to the first premature ventricular beat shown in panel *A*. The preceding sinus cycle is, however, slightly shorter. Panel *D* is not continuous and shows the ventricular tachycardia 30 seconds later. Ventricular tachycardia persisted and panel *E* (Fig. 16-2) shows the progression of the ventricular tachycardia six minutes later. The patient was not observed during this period and it is not known if he was conscious during this long sequence of ventricular tachycardia. Panel *F* was recorded 20 seconds later and shows some further change in morphology with rate variation of the tachycardia towards the end of the strip and seven seconds later in panel *G*, the ventricular tachycardia or flutter abruptly terminates spontaneously. There is an asystolic pause of approximately 2.2 seconds, perhaps due to over-drive suppression by the ventricular tachycardia and this is terminated by a ventricular beat of very similar morphology to those seen during the tachycardia. The next beat, also ventricular, occurs 0.6 seconds later, i.e., well after the T-wave of the preceding complex, but immediately initiates the terminal ventricular fibrillatory episode. It would seem from this series of events that the patient was able to sustain a long episode (greater than 6 minutes) of ventricular tachycardia. Immediately following a pause in this rhythm, two ventricular depolarizations, not closely coupled, induced ventricular fibrillation. We have previously reported on the significance of pauses during acute ischemia[28] and during healing myocardial infarction[29] and have indicated the mechanisms whereby such events may initiate ventricular tachycardia and ventricular fibrillation. Recovery of both ventricular activation delay and dispersion of repolarization has been noted to occur after a pause following rapid heart rates. Activation of the second beat, however, is markedly delayed as is repolarization and is heterogeneous within different areas of the ischemic area. In particular, postrepolarization refractoriness may be the crucial factor responsible for the initiation of ventricular fibrillation under these circumstances.[28,29]

VENTRICULAR ARRHYTHMIAS IN ACUTE MYOCARDIAL INFARCTION

The incidence of cardiac rhythm disturbances among patients seen immediately following myocardial infarction has increased with the increased use of Holter monitoring versus intermittent ECG sampling for arrhythmia documentation. Bigger and colleagues[30] have comprehensively summarized the literature relating to ventricular arrhythmias in acute myocardial infarction. In the prehospitalization period of acute infarction, ventricular premature beats have been detected in as few as 10 percent of patients when intermittent rhythm strips were used in a mobile coronary care unit. However, Pantridge et al.[31] used continuous monitoring in their mobile unit and detected premature ventricular beats in 58 percent of patients in the first hour of infarction and in 93 percent of patients in the first four hours of infarction preceding coronary care admission. Similarly, Moss et al. [32] used continuous recordings and found ventricular premature beats in 74 percent of patients observed within an hour of the onset of symptoms of myocardial infarction.

Most patients with acute myocardial infarction are not admitted to coronary care units until several hours after the onset of infarction. The frequency of ventricular arrhythmias in the coronary care setting has been controversial. Recent studies [18,19] have utilized continuous monitoring of the cardiac rhythm rather than intermittent ECG sampling or conventional coronary care monitoring equipment. These studies have strikingly demonstrated the nearly ubiquitous occurrence of ventricular arrhythmias during the acute in-hospital phase of myocardial infarction. In fact Abjörn and colleagues,[33] using continuous ECG recordings demonstrated ventricular arrhythmias in all 31 patients studied with acute myocardial infarction.

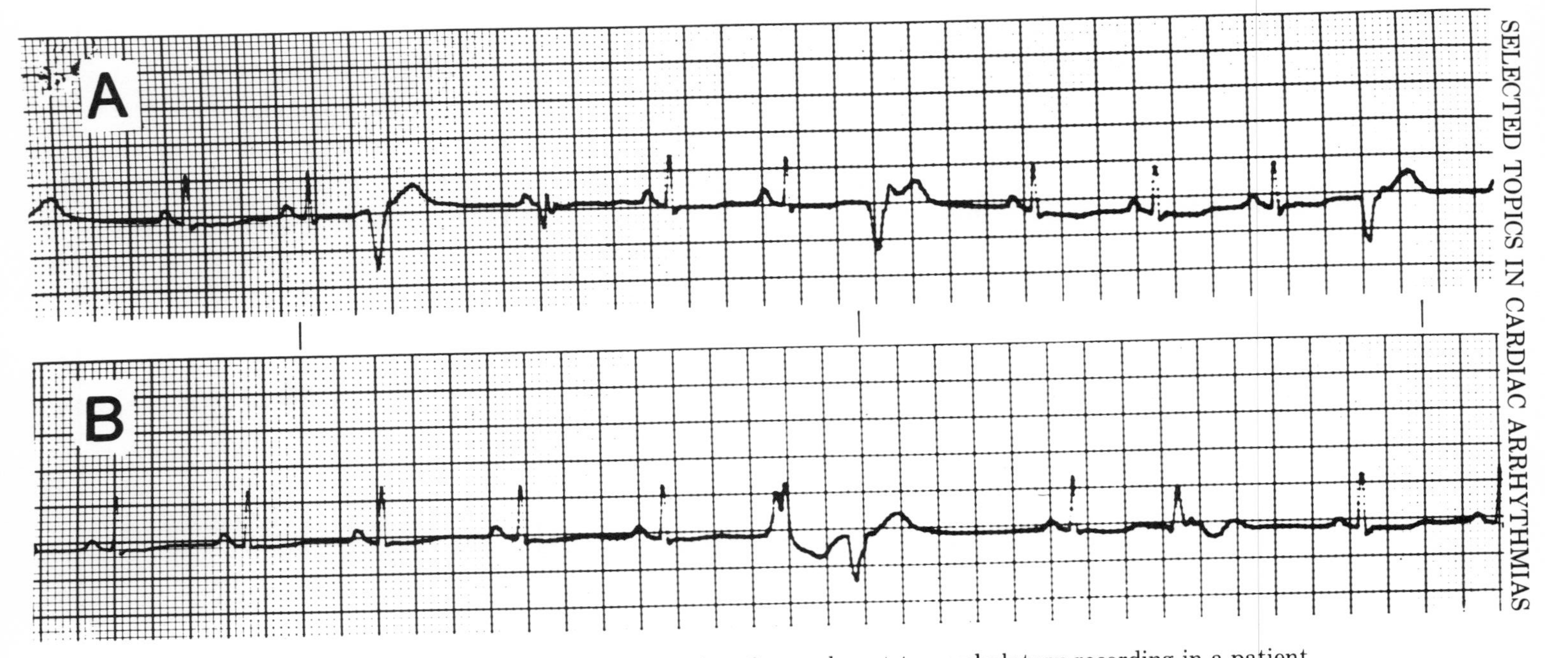

Figure 16-1. Nonconsecutive monitor recording strips taken from a long-term ambulatory recording in a patient at 12:26 P.M. (panel A), at 2:28 P.M. (panel B), and at 5:28 P.M. (panels C and D). See text for explanation.

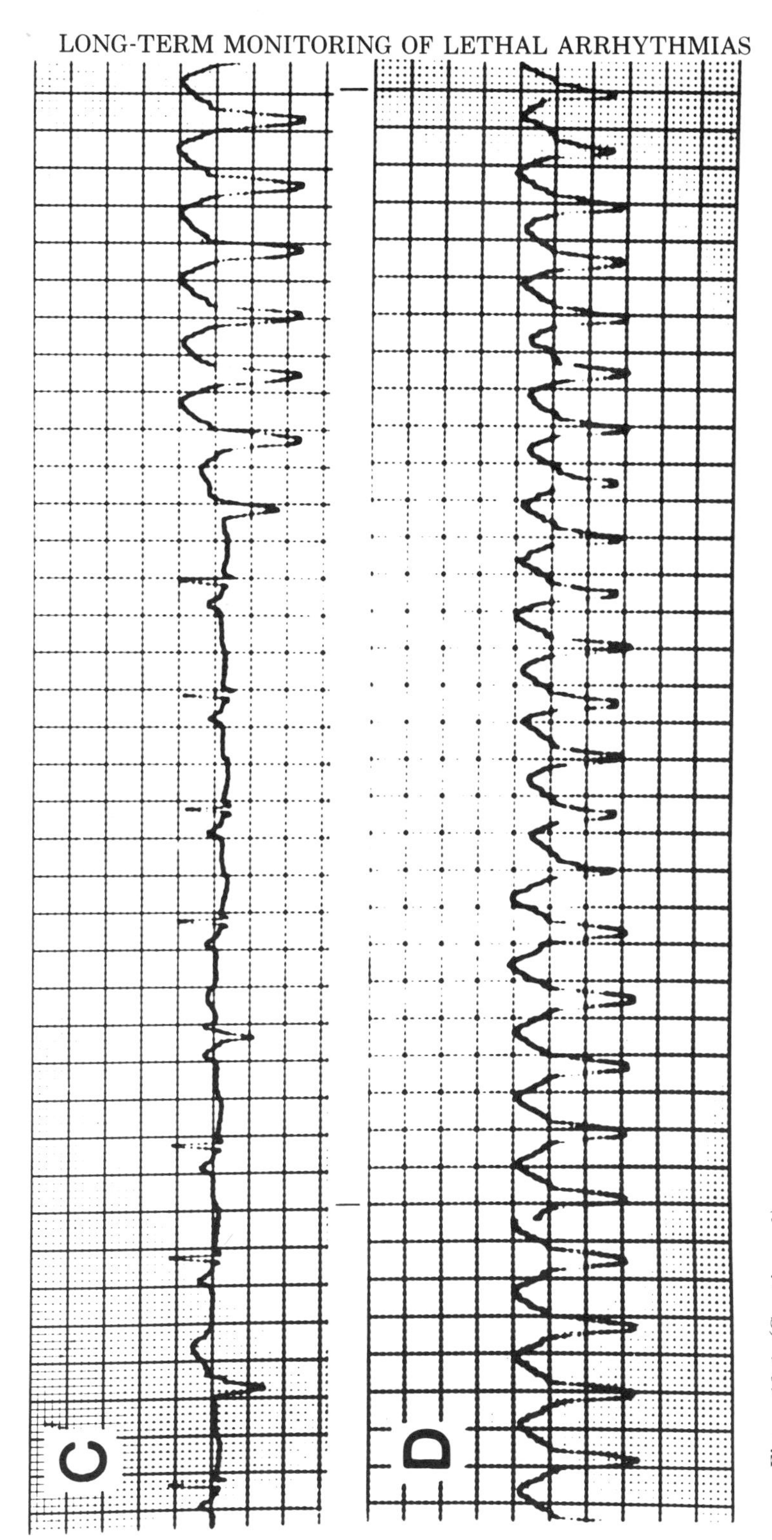

Figure 16–1. *(Continued).*

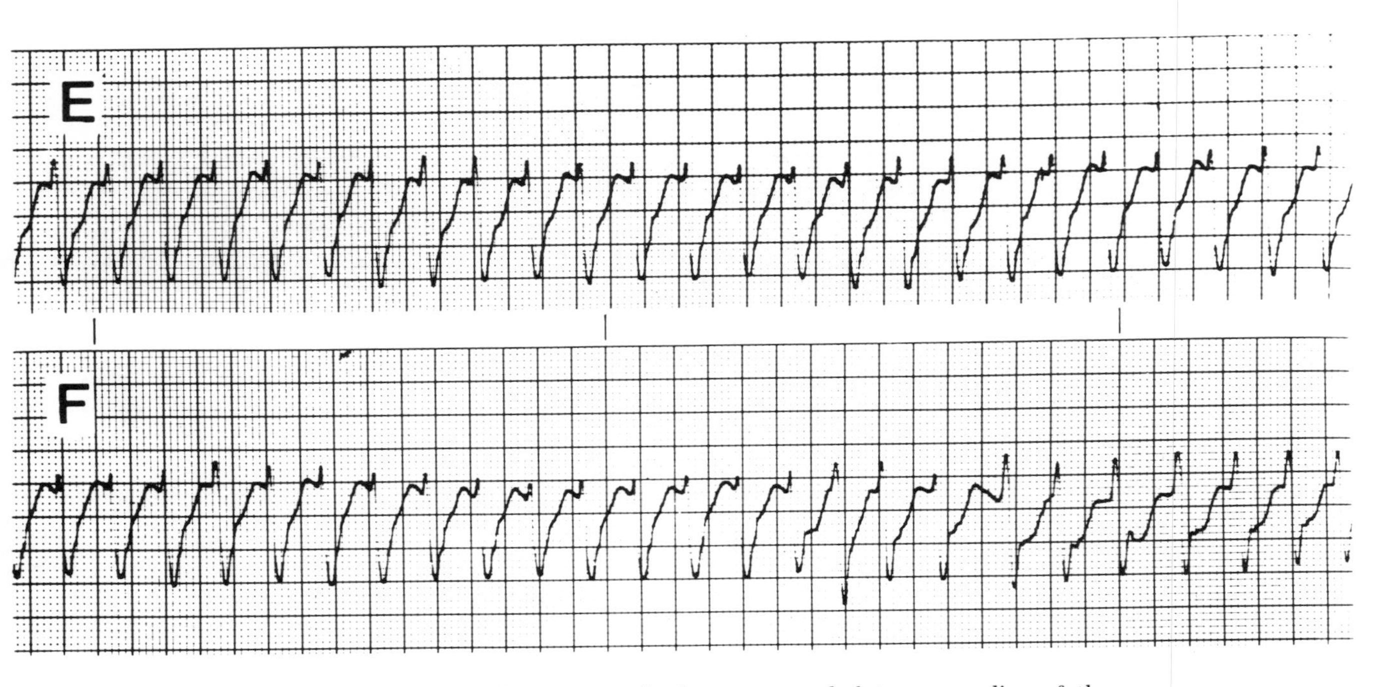

Figure 16-2. Further monitoring strips are shown from the long-term ambulatory recording of the same patient in Figure 16-1. Panel E is recorded approximately 6 minutes after panel D in the preceding figure. For full explanation see text.

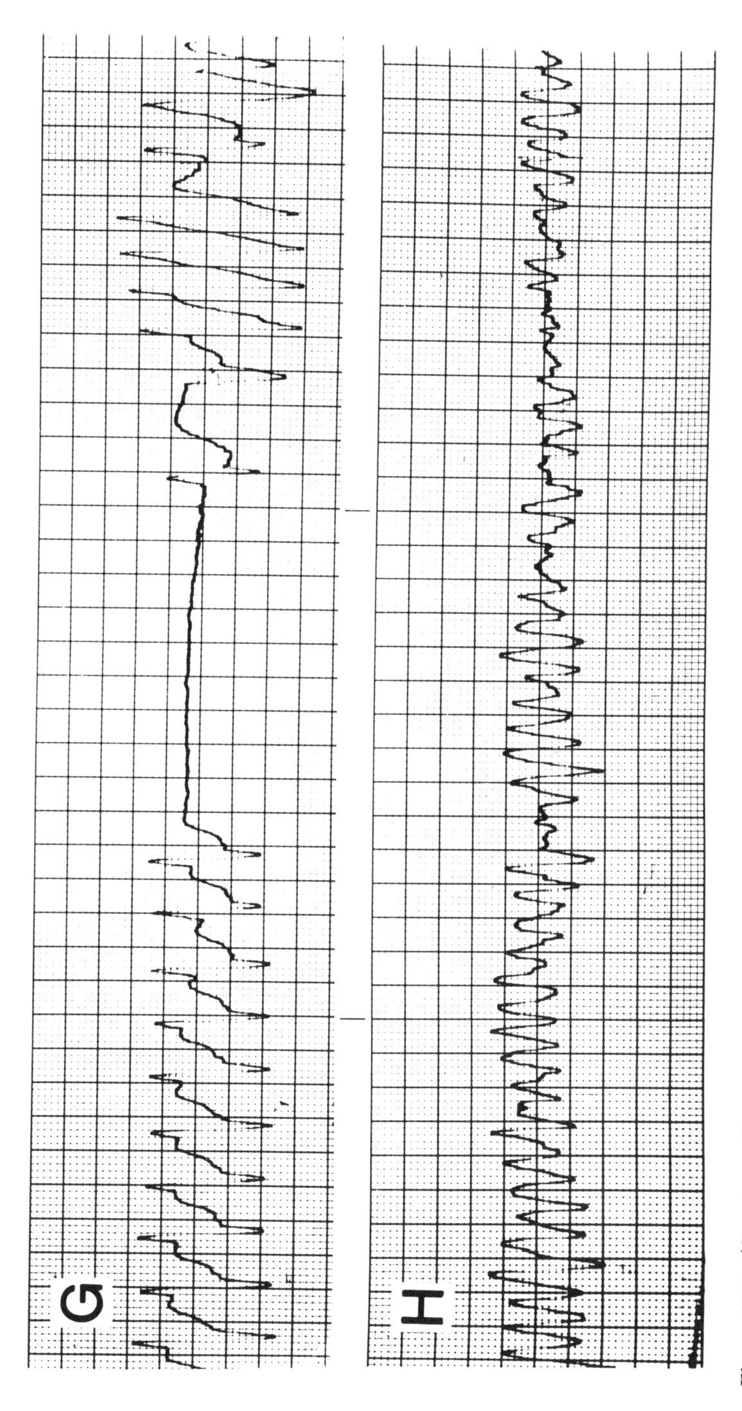

Figure 16–2. *(Continued).*

Continuous recordings of cardiac rhythms during the early phase of hospital admission has allowed us to make comments as to the prognostic value of dysrhythmias occurring at this time. Abjörn et al.[33] used continuous ECG recordings in 31 patients with acute myocardial infarction during the early hospitalization and compared with a 20-hour recording performed just prior to discharge from hospital at a later date. Frequency and severity of arrhythmias during the first day after the infarction correlated poorly with a persistent tendency to arrhythmias or to the risk of sudden death during the following two years. Other studies have tended to confirm that in those patients who survive the acute phase of myocardial infarction, early ventricular arrhythmias bear little relationship to later arrhythmias[34] or to overall long-term prognosis.[35] Paroxysmal ventricular tachycardia during the acute phase of myocardial infarction was studied by de Soyza and colleagues.[36] They demonstrated that in surviving patients, early paroxysmal ventricular tachycardia correlated poorly with subsequent long-term mortality. Vismara and colleagues[34] found surprisingly that ventricular arrhythmias were detected about as frequently in the acute phase of myocardial infarction (84.3%) as in the period during hospitalization after the coronary care unit period (85.5%). Complicated ventricular arrhythmias were about the same in both groups. Importantly, the absence of complicated ventricular arrhythmias including ventricular tachycardia in the coronary care unit did not exclude their subsequent occurrence in the late hospital period. The frequency of ventricular fibrillation did, however, decrease during hospitalization.

For many years cardiologists have directed their attention to so-called "warning arrhythmias", particularly during acute myocardial ischemia and infarction. Frequent ventricular premature beats, multiform ventricular premature beats, and R-on-T phenomena have perhaps been most widely accepted as warning arrhythmias. Careful analysis of continuous long-term recordings of cardiac rhythm during early myocardial infarction has cast some doubts on the classic concept of warning arrhythmias in this setting. For example, several well documented studies[37-41] have demonstrated that between 83 and 40 percent of patients developing primary ventricular fibrillation fail to demonstrate warning arrhythmias that can be treated before the occurrence of ventricular fibrillation. In a study of 417 consecutive cases of acute myocardial infarction, Saunamaki and Pedersen[42] compared the cardiac rhythm monitored in 41 patients who later developed cardiac arrest and compared the heart rhythms monitored over five days in 100 consecutive patients with acute myocardial infarction without complicating cardiac arrest. No significant difference in the frequency of cardiac arrhythmias could be demonstrated between the two groups with cardiac arrest and the control series. Moreover, the complete absence of rhythm disturbance right up to the beginning of the cardiac arrest was more frequently observed in those with cardiac arrest than in the control series. This has led to opposing schools of thought in regard to the prophylactic management of arrhythmias during the acute myocardial infarction. Because neither "warning arrhythmias" nor their absence can be safely relied upon to accurately predict the need for antiarrhythmic therapy, some workers have postulated that all patients with myocardial infarction potentially may benefit from prophylactic antiarrhythmic therapy, particularly lidocaine.[39,43] On the other hand, others have severely curtailed prophylactic antiarrhythmic therapy. Lofmark and Orinius[44] believe that ventricular tachycardia is the only acceptable warning arrhythmia for ventricular fibrillation. Using this strict criteria for warning arrhythmias they have published their results using limited prophylactic lidocaine therapy in 274 cases of acute myocardial infarction.

COMPARISON OF LONG-TERM AMBULATORY MONITORING WITH THE EXERCISE ELECTROCARDIOGRAM

Detection of Arrhythmias

Treadmill exercise testing and prolonged ambulatory electrocardiographic monitoring have been compared in their abilities to detect cardiac arrhythmias. Although controversy exists as to which method is most effective in detecting ventricular arrhythmias, it would appear that ambulatory monitoring results in a higher yield of arrhythmias detected.[45-47] Ryan and colleagues[47] demonstrated more frequent detection of arrhythmias with monitoring compared with exercise, and also showed that coupled premature ventricular beats were more frequently displayed with monitoring. They discerned that increased persistence of any particular grade of arrhythmia during monitoring enhanced its demonstration with exercise. These authors concluded that the two methods of arrhythmia detection may divulge different information regarding the electrophysiological state of the myocardium. It would thus seem reasonable not to look upon the two methods of arrhythmia detection as being mutually exclusive but rather a complementary. The pathophysiological mechanisms of ventricular arrhythmias observed during treadmill testing may differ from the mechanisms seen during routine ambulatory monitoring of the same patient and may not necessarily have the same prognosis. Further clinical studies are necessary in this area. Winkle and colleagues[48] compared the standard electrocardiogram, treadmill testing, and 24-hour ambulatory monitoring for arrhythmia detection in patients with mitral valve prolapse. In their study, both the treadmill and the

24-hour ambulatory recording were far superior to the 12-lead ECG in arrhythmia detection. While ventricular premature beats were detected with approximate equal frequency by both treadmill and 24-hour monitoring, the latter method resulted in greater frequency of detection for high grade ventricular arrhythmias as well as atrial arrhythmias.

ST-Segment Depression

As long as Holter monitoring has been used, investigators have been aware of transient episodes of ST-segment depression occurring during recording. Various explanations have been given, including postural changes of the patient, and poor frequency response of the recording apparatus. Almost certainly, both explanations have been correct on occasion and in the past, Holter monitoring equipment lacked the frequency response of modern equipment. However, modern Holter techniques may be used to study ST-segment depression during normal daily activity in patients with angina. Allen and colleagues[49] investigated 33 patients with angina and abnormal stress test in order to determine the frequency with which myocardial ischemia manifested by painless ST-segment activity during normal daily activity. Twenty-four patients showed ST-depression during the monitoring period. In twenty-one this occurred solely in the absence of pain or both with and without pain. Overall 61 percent of 109 episodes of ST-segment depression recorded were painless. These painless episodes of ST-segment depression were independent of activity other than automobile driving. In patients who smoke cigarettes, ST-segment was more common during smoking, but the overall incidence of ST-depression was not changed. The major thrust of their study was to emphasize that transient ST-segment depression occurred more commonly in the absence than in the presence of chest pain. Continuous ten-hour Holter recordings were performed in twenty patients with coronary heart disease by Schang and Pepine.[50] All patients had previously demonstrated ischemic type ST-depression with angina during treadmill exercise. Of more than 400 episodes of transient ST-depression recorded, only 25 percent were associated with angina. These results are very similar to the above-mentioned results of Allen and colleagues.[49] Schang and Pepine pointed out that all episodes of painless ST-segment depression occurred at heart rates significantly lower than those observed at the onset of angina during treadmill exercise testing. In addition, 72 percent of the painless episodes of ST-depression occurred only at rest or during minimal activity such as walking or sitting. Nitroglycerin administration hourly significantly reduced the frequency of the episodes supporting the concept that the episodes were in fact due to painless ischemia. Thus it is obvious that

Holter monitoring may be used to study painless ischemia during normal daily activity. It is conceivable that the effects of drugs or coronary artery surgery in relation to cardiac arrhythmia might be assessed in this fashion.

PROGNOSTIC IMPLICATIONS OF ARRHYTHMIAS FOLLOWING MYOCARDIAL INFARCTION

In those patients who survive myocardial infarction, long-term ambulatory monitoring has been used in an attempt to discern which patients are at risk from sudden death in the months or years following the myocardial infarction. In recent years several groups of researchers have used Holter monitoring in this area and rewarding information has been gained. Moss and his colleagues have been particularly interested in this field and in 1971 [51] they examined, in 100 patients, six-hour ambulatory ECG tape recordings made just prior to discharge from hospital following myocardial infarction. Ventricular arrhythmias were counted and classified. Altogether 72 percent of the patients had ventricular premature beats and 36 percent of the total number had what they termed "disturbing degree or type" of ventricular irritability. Moss and colleagues were surprised to find that this incidence of arrhythmias in their patients convalescing from infarction was not dissimilar to that reported by Hinkle et al.[6] in their study of a normal middle-aged ambulatory male population. Subsequently Moss and co-workers tried to identify more specifically those patients at high risk from sudden death following infarction. In a prospective follow-up study[52] involving 100 patients, they attempted to develop a step-wise discriminant analysis program to predict the likelihood of surviving two years after myocardial infarction. Variables recorded included rhythm parameters from a six-hour Holter recording, indices of the severity of myocardial infarction as well as other variables during hospitalization. Ventricular premature beats, particularly bigeminal rhythm and/or pairs of ventricular beats and patient age were by far the most important variables. In a complementary study, Luria and colleagues[53] used dynamic eight-hour Holter recordings in the late hospitalization period after myocardial infarction. They demonstrated that paired or multiform ventricular ectopic beats as well as ventricular ectopic beats occurring with frequency greater than one per hour were more often found in those patients who did not survive the two-year period after myocardial infarction. In a further study[54] Moss and co-workers tried to identify patients who would later develop a complicated course following myocardial infarction. A complicated course was defined as cardiac death or myocardial re-infarction within four months after hospital discharge. One hundred and ninety-three patients less than sixty-six years of age were studied and ventricular premature beats with the characteristics of either multiform pattern, bigeminal rhythm and/or frequency of greater than twenty per hour were significantly associated with a four-month posthospital complicated course. Once again, Holter data was recorded from six-hour recordings during ordinary daytime ambulatory in-hospital activity in the last few days before discharge following myocardial infarction. In this study the presence of absence of ventricular premature beats alone, late coupling versus early coupling and the presence or absence of paired ventricular beats was not of significant prognostic value in determining a complicated course after release from hospital. In another study, Moss and colleagues[55] used their prognostic indices in 518 patients less than 65 years of age who were discharged from the hospital following myocardial infarction and followed for four months. Four-month posthospital cardiac mortality rate was 3 percent in the low-risk and 14 percent in the high-risk group. The high-risk group was characterized by two or more of the following characteristics: (1) history of angina at ordinary levels of activity or at rest, (2) hypotension while in the coronary care unit and/or congestive heart failure and (3) ventricular premature beat frequency of more than twenty per hour on a six-hour ambulatory electrocardiogram tape recording prior to hospital discharge. Using this stratification scheme, the prognostic ability was such that 15 percent of the postmyocardial infarction survivors could be identified as high risks. This small subgroup contained almost half the patients who died of cardiac causes in the four-month posthospital interval. In a more recent study, Moss and colleagues[56] attempted to extend this type of analysis to the period extending up to one year after myocardial infarction. They examined 272 patients age 65 or less and once again studied prognosis in relation to ventricular ectopic beats identified in a six-hour Holter recording obtained before hospital discharge. The six-hour recording was repeated in each patient five months after discharge from hospital. They found that ventricular ectopic beats occurring at a rate of twenty or more per hour recorded prior to discharge were associated with complex ventricular ectopic beats in the same six-hour recording made five months later. Complex and high grade ventricular arrhythmias in this group appeared to worsen during the five months. This group of patients had an increased cardiac mortality in the first four months after discharge but not in the subsequent eight months. Ventricular arrhythmias recorded at the five-month follow-up study were not associated with an increased cardiac mortality in the subsequent period of the study. Interestingly, the finding of complex ventricular arrhythmias in follow-up examination was associated with concommitant use of antiarrhythmic agents but not with the use of digitalis, propranolol or tranquilizers. The authors, however, felt this represented an attempt at therapeutic intervention by the physicians treating these patients rather than an etiological relationship between antiarrhythmic agents and arrhythmias. Moss and colleagues[56] also commented upon, but could not explain the apparent progressive loss of prognostic specificity of ventricular arrhythmias over time following infarction. The problems of sudden cardiac death in the first six months after myocardial infarction together with the potential for mortality reduction in the early posthospital period has been addressed in a separate publication by the same authors.[57]

The predictive value of Holter recordings in postmyocardial infarction patients is further emphasized by studies of Vismara and colleagues[58] of 64 patients recovering from acute myocardial infarction in whom ten-hour Holter recordings were made just prior to hospital discharge. The follow-up period was approximately 26 months. All patients who died suddenly during the follow-up period demonstrated ventricular ectopy on the Holter recording prior to discharge. There were no sudden deaths in the patients without ventricular arrhythmias. Both those who died suddenly and survivors were similar in respect to age, sex, location of infarction, presence of coronary risks factors, severity of acute myocardial infarction (measured by cardiac enzymes), serum cholesterol level, evidence of cardiomegaly on x-rays, presence of ventricular gallop and drug therapy. The same study re-emphasized that the presence of acute arrhythmias in the coronary care unit did not separate patients who were later to die suddenly from those who survived; i.e., there were no differences between the two groups in ventricular tachycardia, ventricular fibrillation or complicated ventricular ectopy, while in the coronary care unit. In a separate study[59] these workers used continuous portable electrocardiographic monitoring throughout the three-week hospitalization period after acute myocardial infarction. They again demonstrated that the absence of premature ventricular contractions (including serious forms) in the coronary care unit did not exclude their high incidence rate in the late hospital phase. Late phase ventricular arrhythmias correlated with arterial hypoxia and elevated left ventricular filling pressure in the coronary care unit and with persistent ST abnormalities. Thus the authors believed that the extent of left ventricular dysfunction and ischemia associated with acute myocardial infarction appeared to correlate with late-phase ventricular arrhythmias. In their opinion, the prognostic significance of late-phase ventricular arrhythmis and their underlying causes, particularly ischemia, fibrosis, pump dysfunction and hypertrophy, were particularly related to sudden death after hospital discharge. These conclusions are approximately in agreement with observations of Schulze and colleagues.[60,61] In their studies, 24-hour Holter recordings were performed on patients within two to four weeks after myocardial infarction. Those patients with complex ventricular arrhythmias on Holter recording had a greater number of proximal narrowed major coronary arteries, a higher coronary score, a greater incidence of previous myocardial infarction, increased percentage of abnormal left ventricular segmental wall motion, and lower ejection fractions. Schulze and co-workers[60,61] thus suggested ventricular premature beats alone were not an independent risk factor for sudden cardiac death in the convalescent period of myocardial infarction, but simply reflected increased myocardial damage and extensive cardiac disease. A brief communication by Rehnqvist and Sjögren[62] similarly suggested that the occurrence of late ventricular ectopic beats was significantly associated with larger infarctions and with re-infarction. Of interest and in contrast to most of the studies discussed above, these authors found that ventricular tachycardia or ventricular fibrillation during the acute phase also correlated with late phase ventricular arrhythmias.

LONG-TERM PROGNOSIS AFTER MYOCARDIAL INFARCTION

Use of Holter Recordings

The increasing use of ambulatory monitoring in the late hospitalization period following myocardial infarction and in the months after myocardial infarction has led to a gradually accumulating data base from which some predictions can be made about long-term prognosis based on recorded arrhythmias following myocardial infarction. As previously discussed, Moss and colleagues[56] believe that the prognostic implications of ventricular arrhythmias detected prior to discharge from hospital after myocardial infarction are no longer valid after five months. Other workers would not agree with this. Rehnqvist and colleagues[63] followed 160 patients for two years after myocardial infarction. In their opinion ventricular arrhythmias retained their prognostic significance for one year. The appearance of ventricular ectopic beats among survivors in the second year was not of prognostic value. Kotler et al.[7] also studied 160 survivors of myocardial infarction and followed them for between 30 and 54 months. Twelve-hour electrocardiographic recordings were repeated in all patients at serial intervals and 80 percent showed ventricular ectopic beats. In this study only patients with New York Heart Association functional class I or II were followed. Thus no patients, including the fourteen who were later to develop sudden cardiac death, had severe functional cardiac disease at entry to the study. Kotler and colleagues found that, for the duration of their study, all complex forms of ventricular ectopic activity were associated with an increased risk of sudden cardiac death. The only exception was ventricular parasystole which was not associated with sudden cardiac death. One of the co-authors, Tabatznik, in a separate publication[64] again re-emphasized the apparently less malignant implications of parasystolic ventricular activity. He also suggested that severity of the underlying heart disease is the most important determinant of total mortality but believes there is still an independent relationship between sudden death and ventricular ectopic beats. Ruberman and colleagues[65] took a somewhat different approach in their attempt to assess the effects of ventricular premature beats on mortality after myocardial infarction They examined 1739 men with a history of prior myocardial infarction and monitored them for ventricular ectopic activity over a one-hour period in a standard baseline examination. Fifty percent were examined within three months of the infarction and a further 30 percent examined up to nine months after infarction. The remaining 20 percent were examined at even later dates in respect to their myocardial infarction. The follow-up period averaged approximately 25 months. They found that the presence of complex premature beats (R on T, runs of two or more, multiform or bigeminal premature beats) in the monitoring hour was associated with a risk of sudden coronary death three times that of complex ventricular premature beats. They concluded that such arrhythmias were an independent risk factor for sudden death. The heterogeneous time of entry of patients into their study is not helpful in allowing conclusions to be drawn as to the length of time for which ventricular beats may or may not have prognostic import following myocardial infarction. A comprehensive and large study was undertaken by Anderson, DeCamilla and Moss[66] involving 915 patients under the age of 66 years who were followed for periods ranging from four to forty-eight months following myocardial infarction. Six-hour Holter recordings were performed every four months during the follow-up and 199 episodes of ventricular tachycardia identified in 66 patients. Most had only one episode of ventricular tachycardia and in half of these, the longest run consisted of three premature ventricular beats in a row. Patients with ventricular tachycardia and those without ventricular tachycardia were similar in most clinical characteristics. Among those who died the age, sex, cause of death, suddenness of death, and mechanism of death were similar in those patients previously detected to have ventricular tachycardia and in those survivors of myocardial infarction without ventricular tachycardia. Percentage mortality rates in the ventricular tachycardia group was double the rate of myocardial infarction survivors without ventricular tachycardia but was not statistically significant. However, those patients with ventricular tachycardia were found to have a significantly greater incidence of more severe cardiac disease. From this study it could be concluded that the occurrence of ventricular tachycardia in the posthospital phase of myocardial infarction may be associated with a somewhat lower survival rate, but this difference is not striking. If such a reduction in survival rate is present, underlying severe cardiac disease rather than ventricular tachycardia appears to be responsible.

It is apparent from the studies discussed that long-term ambulatory monitoring of patients electrocardiograms performed just prior to discharge from hospital has an important role in the follow-up management of myocardial infarction. Controversies and uncertainties in several areas persist and further work is yet to be done. For example, it seems paradoxical that the frequency of ventricular arrhythmias in the postinfarction group of patients is similar to that in an age-matched population without myocardial infarction. Complex ventricular arrhythmias may be more frequent in the former group but definitive studies are yet to be carried out. Similarly, the length of time for which ventricular arrhythmias detected by Holter monitoring are of prognostic value remains controversial. Complex ventricular arrhythmias seen three weeks after myocardial infarction on Holter monitoring indicate a high risk of sudden death. Yet similar arrhythmias recorded at five months, or one year after infarction no longer seem to be prognostically significant. Explanations at this stage are largely conjectural. Until answers to these questions are known it is difficult to evaluate the effects of therapy on postmyocardial infarction arrhythmias and/or frequency of sudden death. In particular the influence of coronary artery bypass surgery on postmyocardial infarction arrhythmias or for that matter arrhythmias related to coronary artery disease without infarction has yet to be determined.

CONCLUSION

The increasing use of long-term ambulatory recording of cardiac rhythms attest to its value as a clinical tool in the hands of internists and cardiologists in particular. The time has long since past when the electrocardiogram can be used for the purposes of arrhythmia monitoring. The obvious superiority of the Holter over the electrocardiogram in arrhythmia detection has been discussed. Increasing use of Holter monitoring in many clinical areas beyond the scope of this chapter have been comprehensively discussed in a recent monograph edited by Stern.[67] Stern and co-authors have addressed subjects including ambulatory long-term electrocardiogram recording and blood pressure monitoring, Holter monitoring in pediatrics and neonatology, and ambulatory monitoring in patients with Prinzmetal angina. Finally, for those who interpret Holter monitors it is important that the work of Krasnow and Bloomfield[68] be cited. These authors classified and summarized fifteen different types of artifacts observed during ambulatory monitoring. These artifacts mimicked supraventricular arrhythmias of all types as well as dissociative rhythms. Other artifacts detected were misleading in interpretation of Q-waves, ST-segments and T-waves. In the opinion of the authors, at least half of the artifacts had potentially serious consequences if they had been misdiagnosed.

REFERENCES

1. Holter, N.J.: Radio-electrocardiography: A new technique for cardiovascular studies. *Ann. N.Y. Acad. Sci.* **65**: 913–923, 1957.
2. Holter, N.J.: New methods for heart studies. *Science* **134**: 1214–1220, 1961.
3. The Coronary Drug Project Research Group: Prognostic importance of premature beats following myocardial infarction. Experience in the Coronary Drug Project. *J.A.M.A.* **223**: 1116–1124, 1973.
4. Chiang, B.N., Perlaman, L.V., Ostrander, L.D., and Epstein, F.H.: Relationship of premature systoles to coronary heart disease and sudden death in the Tecumseh Epidemiologic Study. *Ann. Int. Med.* **70**: 1159–1166, 1969.
5. Crow, R.S., Prineas, R.J., Dias, V., et al.: Ventricular premature beats in a population sample. Frequency and associations with coronary risk characteristics. *Circulation* **III**: 211–215, 1975.
6. Hinkle, L.E., Carver, S.T., and Stevens, M.: The frequency of asymptomatic disturbances of cardiac rhythm and conduction in middle-age men. *Am. J. Card.* **24**: 629–650, 1969.
7. Kotler, M.N., Tabatznik, B., Mower, M.M., and Tominaga, S.: Prognostic significance of ventricular ectopic beats with respect to sudden death in the late postinfarction period. *Circulation* **47**: 959–966, 1973.
8. Brodsky, M., Wu, D., Denes, P., et al.: Arrhythmias documented by 24-hour continuous electrocardiographic monitoring in 50 male medical students without apparent heart disease. *Am. J. Card.* **39**: 390–395, 1977.
9. Hiss, R.G., and Lamb, L.: Electrocardiographic findings in 122,043 individuals. *Circulation* **25**: 947–961, 1962.
10. Rydén, L., Walderström, A., and Holmberg, S.: The reliability of intermittent ECG sampling in arrhythmia detection. *Circulation* **52**: 540–545, 1975.
11. Kennedy, H.L., Chandra, V., Sayther, K.L., and Garalis, D.G.: Effectiveness of increasing hours of continuous ambulatory electrocardiography in detecting maximal ventricular ectopy. *Am. J. Card.* **42**: 925–930, 1978.
12. Lown, B., and Wolf, M. Approaches to sudden death from coronary heart disease. *Circulation* **44**: 130–142, 1971.
13. Graboys, T.B., and Lown, B.: Abbreviated ECG monitoring for exposing ventricular ectopic activity. *Card. Med.* **4**: 795–800, 1979.
14. Lopes, M.G., Runge, P., Harrison, D.C., and Schroeder, J.S.: Comparison of 24 versus 12 hours of ambulatory ECG monitoring. *Chest* **67**: 269–273, 1975.
15. Schaffer, W.A., and Cobb, L.A.: Recurrent ventricular fibrillation and modes of death in survivors of out-of-hospital ventricular fibrillation. *N. Eng. J. Med.* **293**: 259–262, 1975.

16. Vismara, L.A., Pratt, C., Price, J.E., et al.: Correlation of the standard electrocardiogram and continuous ambulatory monitoring in the detection of ventricular arrhythmias in coronary patients. *J. Electro.* **10**: 299–304, 1977.
17. Lipski, J., Cohen, L., Espinoza, J., et al.: Value of Holter monitoring in assessing cardiac arrhythmias in symptomatic patients. *Am. J. Card.* **37**: 102–107, 1976.
18. Romhilt, R.W., Bloomfield, P.S., Chou, C., and Fowler, O.: Unreliability of conventional electrocardiographic monitoring for arrhythmia detection in coronary care units. *Am. J. Card.* **31**: 457–461, 1973.
19. Vetter, N.J., and Julian, D.G.: Comparison of arrhythmia computer and conventional monitoring in coronary care unit. *Lancet* **1**: 1151–1154, 1975.
20. Calvert, A., Lown, B., and Gorlin, R.: Ventricular premature beats and anatomically defined coronary heart disease. *Am. J. Card.* **39**: 627–634, 1977.
21. Schroeder, J.S., and Fitzgerald, J.W.: Indications and techniques for ambulatory electrocardiogram monitoring. *Heart & Lung* **4**: 540–545, 1975.
22. Morganroth, J., Michelson, E., Horowitz, L.N., et al.: Limitations of routine long-term electrocardiographic monitoring to assess ventricular ectopic frequency. *Circulation* **58**: 408–414, 1978.
23. Bauer, G.E., Mitchell, A.S., Bates, F., and Hellestrand, K.: The assessment of an antiarrhythmic agent, sustained-release procainamide, with the aid of Holter monitoring. *Med. J. Aust.* **2**: 733–735, 1977.
24. Liberthson, R.R., Nagel, E.L., Hirschman, J.C., et al.: Pathophysiologic observations in prehospital ventricular fibrillation and sudden cardiac death. *Circulation* **49**: 790–798, 1974.
25. Bleifer, S.B., Bleifer, D.J., Hansmann, D.R., et al.: Diagnosis of occult arrhythmias by Holter electrocardiography. *Prog. Card. Dis.* **16**: 569–599, 1974.
26. Hinkle, L.E., Argyros, D.C., Hayes, J.C., et al.: Pathogenesis of an unexpected sudden death role of early cycle ventricular premature contractions. *Am. J. Card.* **39**: 873–879, 1977.
27. Gradman, A.H., Bell, P.A., and DeBusk, R.F.: Sudden death during ambulatory monitoring. Clinical and electrocardiographic correlations—Report of a case. *Circulation* **55**: 210–211, 1977.
28. Hope, R.R., Scherlag, B.J., and Lazzara, R.: The induction of ventricular arrhythmias in acute myocardial ischemia by atrial pacing with long-short cycle sequences. *Chest* **71**: 651–658, 1977.
29. Hope, R.R., Scherlag, B.J., El-Sherif, N., and Lazzara, R.: Ventricular arrhythmias in healing myocardial infarction. *J. Thor. Cardiovasc. Surg.* **75**: 458–466, 1978.
30. Bigger, J.T., Dresdale, R.J., Heissenbuttel, R.H., et al.: Ventricular arrhythmias in ischemic heart disease: Mechanism, prevalence, significance, and management. *Prog. Card. Dis.* **19**: 255–300, 1977.
31. Pantridge, J.F., Adgey, A.A.J., Geddes, J.S., et al.: *The Acute Coronary Attack.* N.Y., Grune and Stratton, 1975, pp. 27–42.
32. Moss, A.J., Goldstein, S., Greene, W, and DeCamilla, J.: Prehospital precursors of ventricular arrhythmias in acute myocardial infarction. *Arch. Intern. Med.* **129**: 756–762, 1972.

33. Abjörn, C., Karlsson, E., and Sonnhag, C.: Ventricular arrhythmias in acute myocardial infarction. *Acta Med. Scand.* **201**: 119–125, 1977.
34. Vismara, L.A., DeMaria, A.N., Hughes, J.L., et al.: Evaluation of arrhythmias in the late hospital phase of acute myocardial infarction compared to coronary care unit ectopy. *Br. Heart J.* **37**: 598–603, 1975.
35. Oliver, G.C., Nolle, F.M., Tiefenbrunn, A.J., et al.: Ventricular arrhythmias associated with sudden death in survivors of acute myocardial infarction. *Am. J. Card.* **33**: 160, 1974.
36. deSoyza, N., Bennett, F.A., Murphy, M.L., et al.: The relationship of paroxysmal ventricular tachycardia complicating the acute phase and ventricular arrhythmia during the late hospital phase of myocardial infarction to long-term survival. *Am. J. Med.* **64**: 377–381, 1978.
37. Jones, D.T., Kostuck, W.J., and Gunton, R.W.: Prophylactic quinidine for the prevention of arrhythmias after acute myocardial infarction. *Am. J. Card.* **33**: 655–660, 1974.
38. Dhurandhar, R.W., MacMillan, R.L., and Brown, W.G.: Primary ventricular fibrillation complicating acute myocardial infarction. *Am. J. Card.* **27**: 347–351, 1971.
39. Wyman, M.G., and Hammersmith, S.: Comprehensive treatment plan for the prevention of primary ventricular fibrillation in acute myocardial infarction. *Am. J. Card.* **33**: 661–667, 1974.
40. Lie, K.I., Wellens, H.J., van Capelle, F.J., and Durrer, D.: Lidocaine in the prevention of primary ventricular fibrillation. A double-blind randomized study of 212 consecutive patients. *N. Eng. J. Med.* **291**: 1324–1326, 1974.
41. Lie, K.I., Wellens, H.J., Downar, E., and Durrer, D.: Observations on patients with primary ventricular fibrillation complicating acute myocardial infarction. *Circulation* **52**: 755–759, 1975.
42. Saunamäki, K.I., and Pedersen, A.: Significance of cardiac arrhythmias preceding first cardiac arrest in patients with acute myocardial infarction. *Acta Med. Scand.* **199**: 461–466, 1976.
43. Harrison, D.C.: Should Lidocaine be administered routinely to all patients after acute myocardial infarction? *Circulation* **58**: 581–584, 1978.
44. Löfmark, R., and Orinius, E.: Restricted Lignocaine prophylaxis in acute myocardial infarction. *Acta Med. Scand.* **201**: 89–91, 1977.
45. Kosowsky, B.D., Lown, B., Whiting, R., and Guiney, T.: Occurrence of ventricular arrhythmias with exercise as compared to monitoring. *Circulation* **44**: 826–832, 1971.
46. Crawford, M., O'Rourke, R.A., Ramakrishna, N., et al.: Comparative effectiveness of exercise testing and continuous monitoring for detecting arrhythmias in patients with previous myocardial infarction. *Circulation* **50**: 301–305, 1974.
47. Ryan, M., Lown, B., and Horn, H.: Comparison of ventricular ectopic activity during 24-hour monitoring and exercise testing in patients with coronary heart disease. *N. Eng. J. Med.* **292**: 224– 229, 1975.
48. Winkle, R.A., Lopes, M.G., Fitzgerald, J.W., et al. Arrhythmias in patients with mitral valve prolapse. *Circulation* **52**: 73–81, 1975.

49. Allen, R.D., Gettes, L.S., Phalan, C., and Avington, M.D.: Painless ST-segment depression in patients with angina pectoris. *Chest* **69**: 467–473, 1976.
50. Schang, S.J., and Pepine, C.J.: Transient asymptomatic S-T segment depression during daily activity. *Am. J. Card.* **39**: 396–402, 1977.
51. Moss, A.J., Schnitzler, R., Green, R., and DeCamilla, J.: Ventricular arrhythmias 3 weeks after acute myocardial infarction. *Ann. Int. Med.* **75**: 837–841, 1971.
52. Moss, A.J., DeCamilla, J., Engstom, F., et al.: The posthospital phase of myocardial infarction. Identification of patients with increased mortality risk. *Circulation* **49**: 460–466, 1974.
53. Luria, M.H., Knoke, J.D., Margolis, R.M., et al.: Acute myocardial infarction: Prognosis after recovery. *Ann. Int. Med.* **85**: 561–565, 1976.
54. Moss, A.J., DeCamilla, J., Mietlowski, W., et al.: Prognostic grading and significance of ventricular premature beats after recovery from myocardial infarction. *Circulation* **51–52 (III)**: 204–210, 1975.
55. Moss, A.J., DeCamilla J., Davis, H., and Bayer, L.: The early posthospital phase of myocardial infarction. Prognostic stratification. *Circulation* **54**: 58–64, 1976.
56. Moss, A.J., DeCamilla, J.J., Davis, H.P., and Bayer, L.: Clinical significance of ventricular ectopic beats in the early posthospital phase of myocardial infarction. *Am. J. Card.* **39**: 635–640, 1977.
57. Moss, A.J., DeCamilla, J., and Davis, H.: Cardiac death in the first 6 months after myocardial infarction: Potential for mortality reduction in the early posthospital period. *Am. J. Card.* **39**: 816–820, 1977.
58. Vismara, L.A., Amsterdam, E.A, and Mason, D.T.: Relation of ventricular arrhythmias in the late hospital phase of acute myocardial infarction to sudden death after hospital discharge. *Am. J. Med.* **59**: 6–12, 1975.
59. Vismara, L.A., Vera, Z., Foerster, J.M., et al.: Identification of sudden death risk factors in acute and chronic coronary artery disease. *Am. J. Card.* **39**: 821–828, 1977.
60. Schulze, R.A., Rouleau, J., Rigo, P., et al.: Ventricular arrhythmias in the late hospital phase of acute myocardial infarction. Relation to left ventricular function detected by gated cardiac blood pool scanning. *Circulation* **52**: 1006–1011, 1975.
61. Schulze, R.A., Humphries, J.O., Griffith, L.S.C., et al.: Left ventricular and coronary angiographic anatomy. Relationship to ventricular irritability in the late hospital phase of acute myocardial infarction. *Circulation* **55**: 839–843, 1977.
62. Rehnqvist, N., and Sjögren, A.: Ventricular arrhythmias three weeks and one year after acute myocardial infarction (AMI). *Br. Heart J.* **38**: 532, 1976.
63. Rehnqvist, N., Lundman, T., and Sjögren, A.: Prognostic implications of ventricular arrhythmias registered before discharge and one year after acute myocardial infarction. *Acta Med. Scand.* **204**: 203–209, 1978.
64. Tabatznik, B.: Ambulatory monitoring in the late post-myocardial infarction period. *Postgrad. Med. J.* **52 (7)** 56–59, 1976.

65. Ruberman, W., Weinblatt, E., Goldberg, J.D., et al.: Ventricular premature beats and mortality after myocardial infarction. *N. Eng. J. Med.* **297**: 750–757, 1977.
66. Anderson, K.P., DeCamilla, J., and Moss, A.J.: Clinical significance of ventricular tachycardia (3 beats or longer) detected during ambulatory monitoring after myocardial infarction. *Circulation* **57**: 890–897, 1978.
67. Stern, S.: *Ambulatory ECG Monitoring*: Chicago, Year Book Medical Publishers, Inc., 1978.
68. Krasnow, A.Z., and Bloomfield, D.K.: Artifacts in portable electrocardiographic monitoring. *Am. Heart J.* **91**: 349–357, 1976.

17

Mechanical Stimulation of the Heart

Benjamin Befeler, M.D.

Technological advancements in the post Second World War period have provided physicians with numerous new techniques and equipment which have facilitated and expanded the understanding of cardiac electrophysiology, and the treatment of rhythm disturbances.[1–3]

The application of these numerous new techniques and equipment are part of our everyday life. The level of sophistication in the use of these techniques and equipment has been such that simple methods for the treatment of various illnesses have been falling into disuse or in some instance discredit. Despite the sophisticated techniques and equipment available, if an abnormality of rhythm can be treated by a simple and safe technique, it would appear that as long as the objective can be accomplished without risk to the patient and with a reasonable chance of success, it would be desirable to utilize such a technique. Mechanical stimulation of the heart in the treatment of ventricular as well as supraventricular arrhythmias falls into this category.

We have utilized mechanical stimulation of the heart directly through the chest wall or with an endocardial catheter for the purpose of converting various tachycardias.[4–6] We have been particularly impressed by the ability to convert ventricular tachycardia in patients with left ventricular aneurysms when the thump is applied to the area of paradoxical pulsation.[5] Previous reports[7] have advocated chest thump for ventricular tachycardia in general, and our report was the first to present successful results with the thump applied directly to the area of paradoxical pulsation of a ventricular aneurysm.

The problem of conversion of tachyarrhythmias is twofold: (1) interruption of the sustaining mechanism, i.e., reentry or increased automaticity; and (2) prevention of its recurrence. At the present time, prevention of recurrence is best accomplished by therapy with drugs or by increasing the heart rate via electrical stimulation. Interruption of the arrhythmias requires interference with the sustaining mechanism. This can be accomplished by an atrial or ventricular premature beat[7–10] induced electrically or, presumably, mechanically which interrupts the reentrant pathway or drastically depresses an ectopic focus. Extensive experience exists with electrical stimulation. This paper deals with the clinical application of low energy mechanical stimulation in the treatment of tachyarrhythmias. This technique has also been used to initiate a cardiac rhythm during cardiopulmonary resuscitation due to cardiac arrest and has been recently suggested as a mode of temporary cardiac pacing.[11]

ILLUSTRATIVE CASES

Case 1

A 44-year-old, insulin-dependent, diabetic male had angina pectoris for one year and congestive heart failure for several months. He was treated with digoxin furosemide and coronary vasodilators. Two months prior to admission, he developed increasing angina and worsening dyspnea. He was admitted to another hospital after developing prolonged angina and an acute anterior wall myocardial infarction was diagnosed. He initially improved. On the tenth day he had a cardiac arrest with ventricular fibrillation. Post resuscitation, he was hypotensive and developed right lower lobe pneumonia. Three days later the patient again had another cardiac arrest with ventricular fibrillation and was defibrillated successfully. Post cardiac arrest, he had frequent extrasystole and was treated with procaineamide and quinidine. On the day prior to transfer to our hospital, the patient had frequent runs of ventricular tachycardia with hypotension, abolished by intravenous lidocaine. The patient was admitted to our hospital for further evaluation and management. On examination he was afebrile, pulse 114, slightly irregular, blood pressure 100/80, respiratory rate 40. Chest disclosed diffuse, coarse bronchi, dullness and decreased breath sounds at the right base, and bibasilar rales. The heart was not enlarged, but a double apical impulse was noted. S3 and S4 gallops were noted and no murmurs. The pulses were full with no cyanosis, edema or clubbing. Chest x-ray revealed slight cardiomegaly with right pleural effusion. The impression was arteriosclerotic heart disease with recent anterior wall myocardial infarction, recurrent ventricular tachycardia, early anterior left ventricular aneurysm. Upon admission to our Coronary Care Unit, he was found to have ventricular tachycardia at a rate of 120 beats per minute (Fig. 17-1). A chest thump

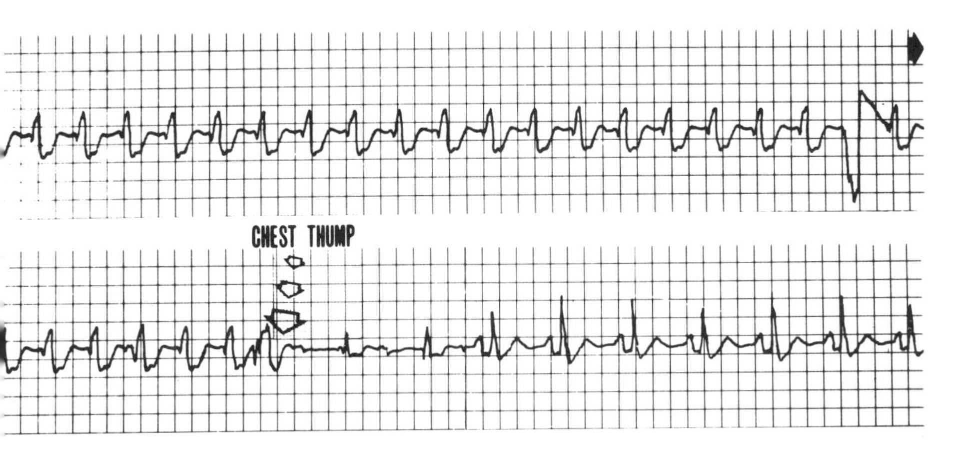

Figure 17-1. *(Case 1).* Shows a monitor lead demonstrating ventricular tachycardia with one premature beat towards the end of the first strip and then the arrow indicates where a chest thump was applied to the area of paradoxical pulsation with conversion to sinus rhythm. The first post-thump beat is a junctional escape beat followed by a blocked ectopic P, followed by another junctional beat, and then resumption of normal sinus rhythm.

over the area of paradoxical pulsation converted the rhythm to sinus. These episodes repeated several times and he was converted each time with chest thump. Patient was then started on a combination of procainamide, 500 mg every four hours and quinidine sulphate 300 mg every six hours with improvement. Two months later he underwent angiography. An anteroapical left ventricular aneurysm was found. The patient then underwent successful aneurysmectomy. The patient has done well after surgery on daily digoxin and procainamide 500 mg every six hours.

Case 2

A.F., a 78-year-old man was admitted to the hospital with a chief complaint of epigastric pain not relieved by nitroglycerine. He denied palpitation, diaphoresis, dizziness, nausea or shortness of breath. There was a history of previous anterior wall myocardial infarction. The electrocardiogram taken in the Emergency Room revealed ventricular tachycardia at a rate of 170 per minute. He was given intravenous lidocaine in boluses of 100 mg to a total of 400 mg and intravenous phenytoin 100 mg without success and was finally cardioverted with 100 watt-seconds to normal sinus rhythm. When in sinus rhythm, the electrocardiogram showed evidence of an anterior wall myocardial infarction and ST elevation suggestive of a ventricular aneurysm. Physical examination with the patient in sinus rhythm revealed a paradoxical pulsation at the cardiac apex and loud S3 and S4 gallops. Chest roentgenogram revealed a calcific aneurysm of the left ventricle. The patient was digitalized and placed on procainamide, 500 mg every six hours and remained in sinus rhythm without premature ventricular contractions. On the fifteenth hospital day, he exhibited bigeminal rhythm and digoxin was withheld because of the possibility of digitalis intoxication. On the following day, the patient was found to have a heart rate of 160 per minute. The electrocardiogram showed ventricular tachycardia. Carotid sinus pressure was applied in succession to the right and left carotid bodies with no change in the arrhythmias. Then a blow to the precordium was given with no effect on the arrhythmias. The area of paradoxical pulsation was then delineated and a sharp blow to this area abruptly converted the ventricular tachycardia to normal sinus rhythm, as shown in Figure 17-2. The arrow points to the timing of the blow. The stimulus to the chest evoked an early ventricular depolarization distinctly different in morphology from the preceding QRS. The first atrial beat had a shorter PR interval followed by normal sinus rhythm. The same afternoon the patient had another episode of ventricular tachycardia, despite intravenous lidocaine. This episode was successfully terminated with a similar blow over the area of paradoxical pulsation. He was then started on oral disopyramide phosphate with good results. The patient refused further evaluation and was discharged home.

Case 3

A.G., a 51-year-old man was in his usual state of good health until approximately six months prior to admission when he sustained severe excruciating midsternal chest pain. He was admitted to the hospital where he evolved an extensive anterior wall myocardial infarction. After four weeks of hospitalization, he was discharged on digoxin, intermittent diuretics, quinidine sulphate and persantine. While in the hospital, he convalesced slowly and had sinus tachycardia with frequent premature beats which decreased in number after the quinidine was started. After discharge he started to complain of tiredness and dyspnea on exertion. The symptoms progressed to nocturnal dyspnea. He was readmitted, stabilized, and then he had angiographic studies. On physical examination he was a middle-aged man, somewhat wasted, and appeared to be chronically ill. Blood pressure was 130/70, pulse 80 and regular with infrequent premature beats. No venous distention was noted. No rales were audible in the lungs. The heart showed cardiomegaly and an area of paradoxical pulsation inside the apical region; normal S1 and S2 with an S4 and S3 at the apex. There was no hepatosplenomegaly or peripheral

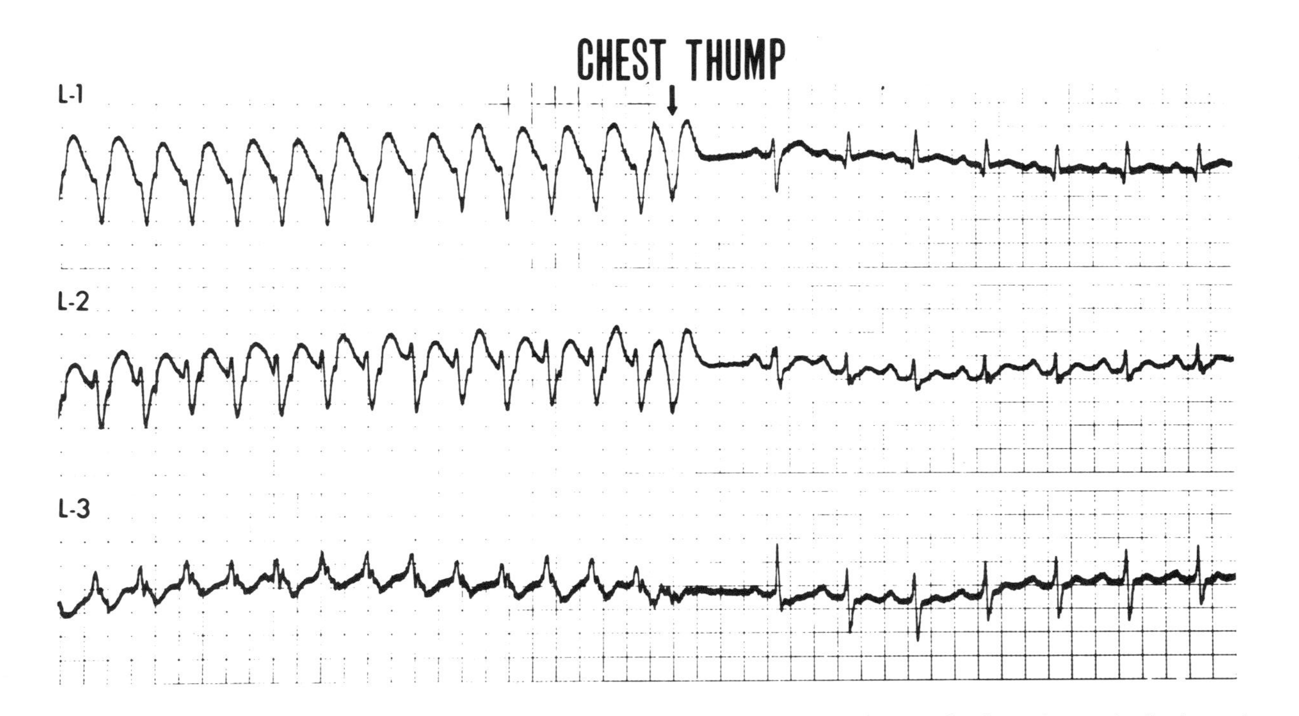

Figure 17–2. ***(Case 2).*** Demonstrates conversion of ventricular tachycardia to normal sinus rhythm after a single chest thump applied to an area of paradoxical pulsation. The chest thump induced a premature ventricular beat which was followed by a sinus beat with aberrant conduction and then resumption of sinus rhythm.

edema and the peripheral pulses were all present. The admission electrocardiogram showed normal sinus rhythm and an anterior wall myocardial infarction with elevation of the ST segments in leads V2, V3 and V4. All laboratory tests, including blood count, automated chemical profile and coagulation studies were normal. Cardiac catheterization showed normal right heart pressures with an elevated pulmonary wedge pressure of 16 mmHg. A left ventriculogram in the right oblique projection showed an anteroapical aneurysm. The left coronary artery showed complete occlusion of the anterior descending above the first septal branch and diffuse disease of the circumflex. The right coronary artery showed mild irregularities. After the study had been completed and while the left-sided catheter was in the aorta, R on T phenomenon occurred and the patient went into ventricular tachycardia (Fig. 17-3).

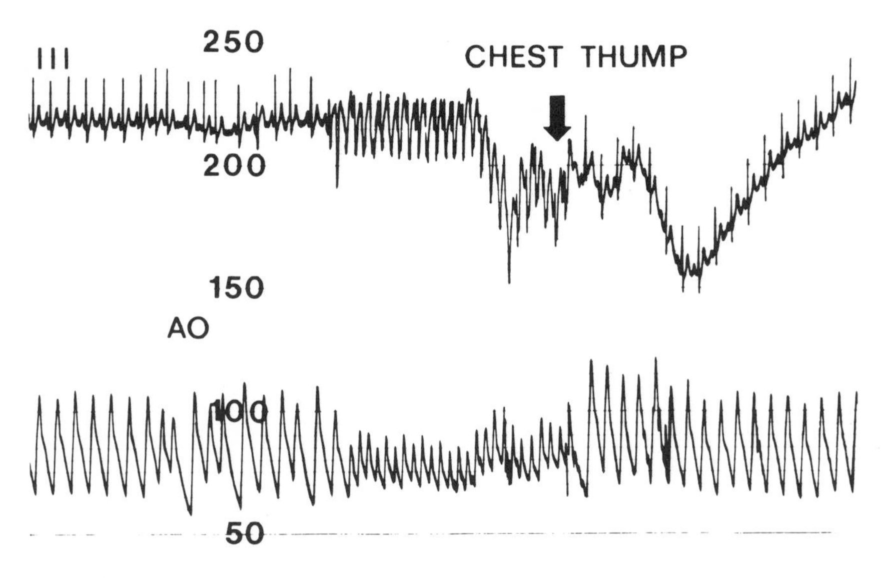

Figure 17-3. *(Case 3).* Demonstrates a patient who had just undergone coronary arteriography in whom an R on T VPC induced ventricular tachycardia. Note that a chest thump on the area of paradoxical pulsation converted the rhythm to sinus. A fall in the aortic pressure is noted while the patient was in ventricular tachycardia.

Two chest thumps, the first one to the lower sternum and the second to the area of paradoxical pulsation, converted the rhythm to sinus. Note a fall in the aortic pressure. Then he was started on a lidocaine drip but a second episode of ventricular tachycardia with a right bundle branch morphology occurred (Fig. 17-4). This episode was also abolished by a chest thump. The patient was then started on oral procainamide every

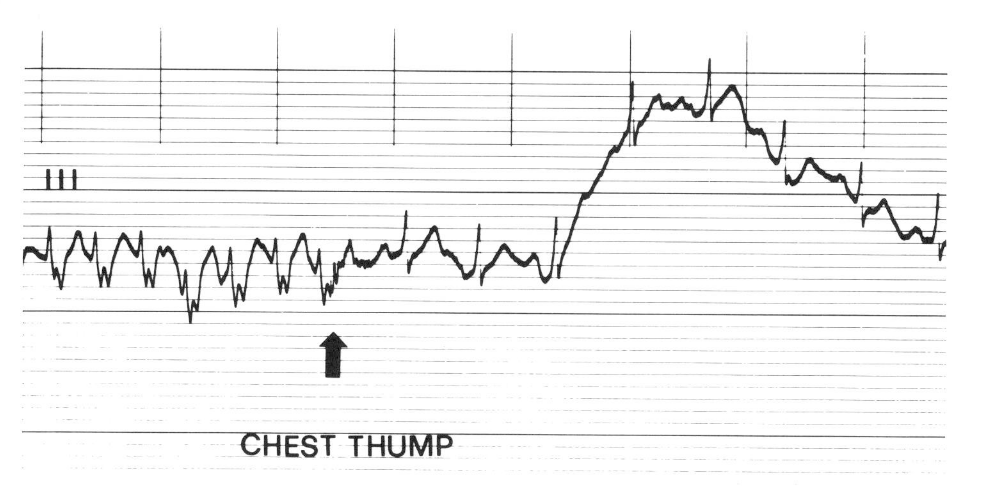

Figure 17-4. *(Case 3).* Demonstrates the same patient as on Figure 17-3 who sustained a second episode of ventricular tachycardia, this time displaying a right bundle branch block morphology. This episode was also abolished by a chest thump.

four hours and afterload reducing agents. The heart failure improved and the premature beats decreased in frequency.

An example of conversion of a run of ventricular tachycardia with a stimulus in the left ventricle is shown in Figure 17-5. This run occurred while patient was undergoing coronary arteriography. The catheter was promptly introduced into the left ventricle and one single stroke corrected the arrhythmia.

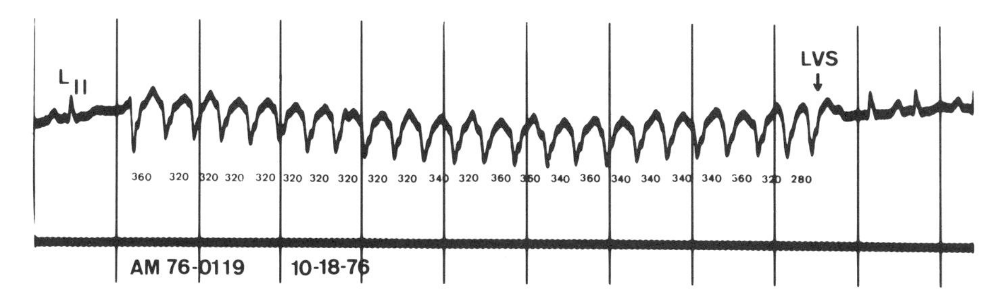

Figure 17-5. It is taken from a patient, A.M., who had undergone left ventriculography and while the catheter was in the aorta, had the sudden onset of ventricular tachycardia probably induced by a late VPC, not falling on the T wave and converted by a late ventricular stimulus produced with the angiocatheter. Note that the slightly premature beat induced by the catheter (labeled LVS) probably induced a retrograde T wave and then resumption of sinus rhythm. (Reproduced with permission from Befeler, B.: Mechanical stimulation of the heart. Its therapeutic value in tachyarrhythmias. *Chest* 73: 832–838, 1978.)

A case of supraventricular tachycardia in a patient with Lown-Ganong-Levine syndrome was interrupted by a stimulus in the right ventricle and it is shown in Figure 17-6.

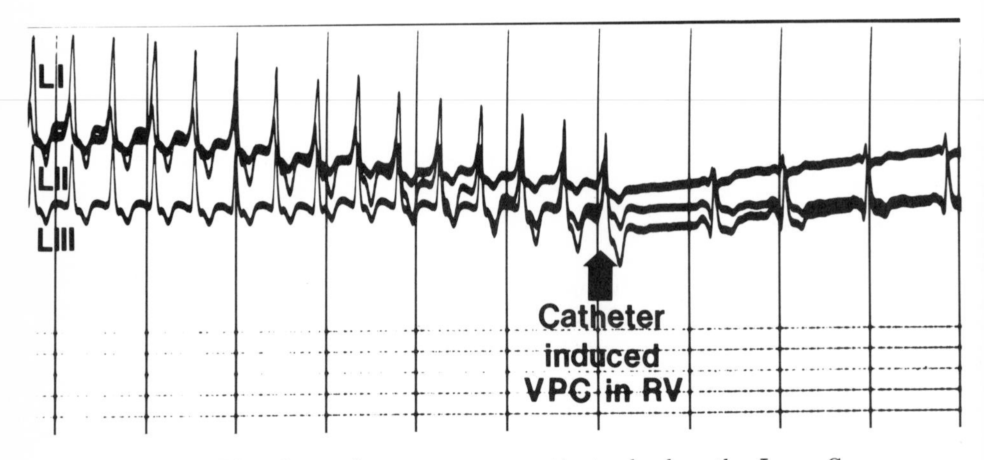

Figure 17-6. This figure demonstrates a patient who has the Lown-Ganong-Levine Syndrome and who had recurrent spontaneously occurring supraventricular tachycardia. This figure demonstrates the interruption of the supraventricular tachycardia induced by a VPC in the right ventricle with a catheter. Note the supraventricular tachycardia terminates with the VPC induced by the catheter and then resumption of sinus rhythm with a short PR interval. (Reproduced with permission from Befeler, B.: Mechanical stimulation of the heart. Its therapeutic value in tachyarrhythmias. *Chest* 73: 832–838, 1978.)

DISCUSSION

Prompt conversion of tachyarrhythmias is of great clinical relevance because they may degenerate into irreversible rhythms or because they may impair hemodynamic function. In general, various means for conversion are available which are very effective. They require various types of instruments, or this can be accomplished by pharmacologic agents. All have advantages and drawbacks. Electric cardioversion is effective and can be performed at the bedside, but requires anesthesia and the availability of the instrument. Various drugs are effective, but their onset of action varies, depending on the route of administration.

Direct mechanical stimulation can be applied promptly, at the bedside, and does not require special instrumentation. Because of its position in the chest within the rib cage, the heart is relatively inaccessible to direct mechanical stimulation. This creates the need to deliver large amounts of energy through the wall of the chest in order to effect the stimulation desired. This can be accomplished with a chest thump or with the delivery of variable amounts of energy through a catheter electrode inside the cardiac chambers,[8,9] either as a single pulse[10] or as a rapid sequence of pulses.[7] The minimal amount of mechanical energy necessary to produce a detectable cardiac effect has not been defined, although Zoll et al.[11] have stated that 0.4 to 0.7 joules is necessary. The upper limit of energy is tempered by the patient's tolerance of such stimulus, and this limit has made continuous pacing by this technique impractical.

Other applications of chest thump have been in the treatment of profound bradycardia due either to marked sinus bradycardia or sinus arrest or in cases of cardiac arrest with poorly defined or unclear electrocardiographic rhythm. This is a commonly used resuscitative maneuver during cardiac arrest.

We[5] have found that small amounts of mechanical energy delivered to the chest wall near the area of the production of the arrhythmias (i.e., a ventricular aneurysm) can interrupt a reentrant tachycardia, whereas the same amount of energy applied to the wall of the chest away from the area of paradoxical pulsation failed to interrupt such tachycardia. Similarly, if small amounts of mechanical energy can be applied to areas of the heart which either originate the ectopic impulse or make up part of a reentrant pathway, these small amounts of energy may interrupt such circuits and terminate the arrhythmia. This method requires the use of an intracardiac catheter, which makes this technique particularly suitable for use during diagnostic intracardiac studies. The use of a chest thump to deliver the energy through the wall of the chest can be reserved for the situation when intracardiac catheters are not readily available. Other types of energy have not been explored to pace or stimulate the heart, despite the tremendous technologic advances in the use of laser beams, ultrasonic energy, ultraviolet light, etc., but may find applications in the future.

Approximately 100 patients have been treated with mechanical stimulation of the heart, both external and internal. Internal stimulation was carried out by a catheter placed in the right atrium or ventricle. The site of stimulation was selected depending on convenience; that is, if a catheter was in place in the cardiac chambers it was used. If not, external stimulation was applied.

Twenty-two percent of the patients with atrial tachycardia responded to intracardiac stimulation, two-thirds to right ventricular stimulation and one-third to right atrial stimulation.

Fifty percent of the patients with junctional tachycardia responded to either right atrial or right ventricular stimulation. Forty-one percent of the patients with ventricular tachycardia responded to mechanical stimulation, approximately fifty percent to chest thump, two patients to left ventricular stimulation and the rest to right ventricular stimulation.

The mechanism by which a low-energy mechanical stimulus induces either an atrial or a ventricular premature beat and interrupts tachyarrhythmias is not completely understood. It is possible that such an extrasystole interrupts a reentrant pathway, allowing for the underlying normal pacemaker to surface. Also, it is conceivable that in situations where the tachyarrhythmia is due to repetitive firing, the extrasystole abolishes (or overdrives) the automatic focus. Both of these mechanisms appear to be operative in high-energy direct current cardioversion.[11]

It seems then that a blow to any area of the percordium may not alter the regions involved in the reentry sequence. If a blow to the area of maximal paradoxical pulsation appears to be effective, it implies that the aneurysm itself either gives rise to the ectopic impulse or makes up an important portion of the reentrant route. The depolarization of this region creates temporary local block which prevents further conduction. This mechanism of local delay may also be operative in the action of certain drugs, as suggested recently,[12] such as procaineamide which delays the coupling interval of the ventricular premature depolarization until the arrhythmia disappears. This effect is more apparent as the blood level of the drug increases.

The tachyarrhythmias treated in this study were essentially of three types, i.e., atrial, junctional, and ventricular. Atrial fibrillation was not affected by mechanical atrial stimulation, primarily because of the inability to "capture" the atria. Ventricular stimulation used early in the study in atrial fibrillation also appeared to be ineffective and was not utilized subsequently.

In our study, the timing of the mechanical stimulus was uncontrolled and was applied on an empirical basis. Further development of this technique requires the design of a device that can time the stimulus at a preset interval coupled with the QRS complex of the electrocardiogram, in a manner similar to the programmed electrical stimulation that is applied[2] for diagnostic and therapeutic purposes. The relatively low effectiveness of mechanical stimulation in converting some arrhythmias may be due to a lack of proper timing of the mechanical impulse or to the low energy developed by the stimulus in the area of reentrant pathway.

From our experience, these techniques appear to be safe. No complications were encountered in the cases reported, and no deterioration of a disturbance in rhythm was noted. No ventricular fibrillation was noted in the attempts to treat ventricular tachycardia by a chest thump. Complications such as rupture of the heart or arterial embolization from intramural thrombi were not encountered.

As a consequence of the experience gained with this study, it is recommended that patients with ventricular tachycardia should be initially treated with a chest thump. If an area of paradoxical pulsation is present, the thump should be applied to that area. This should be repeated several times. If this procedure is not successful, pharmacologic intervention may follow. For supraventricular or junctional tachycardia, if an intracardiac catheter is in place, mechanical stimulation should be attempted in each case, prior to other intervention in the atria or ventricles.

Mechanical stimulation by chest blow is advocated only as an initial intervention which carries low risk, can be performed at bedside, and can always be followed by more definitive treatment, such as direct current cardioversion or drug therapy.

REFERENCES

1. Lown, B., Amarasnagham, R., and Venman, J.: New method for termination of cardiac arrhythmias. *J.A.M.A.* **182**: 548–555, 1966.
2. Wellens, H.J.J.: Electrical stimulation of the heart in the study and treatment of tachyarrhythmias. Baltimore, University Park Press, 1971.
3. Scherlag, B.J., Lau, S.H., Helfant, R.H., et al.: His Bundle activity in man. *Circulation* **30**: 13, 1969.
4. Befeler, B.: Mechanical stimulation of the heart. Its therapeutic value in tachyarrhythmias. *Chest* **73**: 832–838, 1978.
5. Befeler, B., and Aranda, J.M.: Termination of ventricular tachycardia by a chest thump over the area of paradoxical pulsation. *Am. Heart J.* **94**: 773–775, 1977.
6. Bierfeld, J.L., Rodriguez–Viera, V., Aranda, J.M., Castellanos, A., Lazzara, R., and Befeler, B.: Termination of ventricular fibrillation by chest thump. *Angiology* (in press).
7. Pennington, J.E., Taylor, J., and Lown, B.: Chest thump for reverting ventricular tachycardia. *N. Eng. J. Med.* **283**: 1192–1195, 1970.
8. Zeft, H.J., Cobb, F.R., Waxman, M.B., et al.: Right atrial stimulation in the treatment of atrial flutter. *Ann. Intern. Med.* **70**: 447–456, 1969.
9. Zeft, J.H., and McGowan, R.L.: Termination of paroxysmal junctional tachycardia by right ventricular stimulation. *Circulation* **40**: 919–926, 1969.
10. Barold, S.S., Linhart, F.W., Samet, P., et al.: Supraventricular tachycardia initiated and terminated by a single electrical stimulus. *Am. J. Cardiol.* **24**: 37–41, 1969.
11. Zoll, P.M., Belgard, A.H., Weintraub, M.J., et al.: External mechanical cardiac stimulation. *N. Eng. J. Med.* **294**: 1274–1275, 1976.
12. Giardina, E.G.V., and Bigger, J.T., Jr.: Procaine amide against re-entrant ventricular arrhythmias. Lengthening R-V intervals of coupled ventricular premature depolarizations as an insight into the mechanism of action of procaine amide. *Circulation* **48**: 959, 1973.

18

Relevance of Phase 3 and Phase 4 Block in Clinical Electrophysiology

Mauricio B. Rosenbaum, M.D., Marcelo V. Elizari, M.D., Julio O. Lázzari, M.D., Raúl J. Levi, M.D., Gerardo J. Nau, M.D., Pablo A. Chiale, M.D., M. Susana Halpern, M.D., and Julio Przybylski, M.D.

The notion of phase 3 and phase 4 block, introduced at the beginning of the present decade,[1–7] gave rise to some confusion and controversy[8] regarding the concept itself as well as its terminology and clinical significance. The following review is merely an attempt to clarify some of these problems.

ELECTROPHYSIOLOGICAL BASIS

Figure 18-1*A* shows the intracellular recording of a normal fiber of the canine His bundle possessing strong automatic activity. Automaticity is expressed by the ascending slope during phase 4 of the action potential, commonly referred to as spontaneous diastolic depolarization (SDD)[9] or pacemaker potential.[10] Figure 18-1*B*, taken from the classic publication by Weidmann,[11] shows a similar recording from a peripheral Purkinje fiber of the bovine heart. It may be seen that when the fiber is stimulated at different times, the response is poor both in amplitude and rate of rise of phase O only during two intervals: at the end of phase 3 (during systole), and very late during phase 4 (at the end of diastole), simply

This work was supported in part by the Comisión para el Estudio Integral de la Enfermedad de Chagas and the Fundación de Investigaciones Cardiológicas Einthoven.

because the rate of rise of the action potential is voltage-dependent.[11] Since conduction velocity depends (among other factors) on the rate of rise of phase O, it is theoretically possible and has actually been verified by Singer et al.[9] that conduction in a fascicle composed of Purkinje fibers may be slow or cause block both prematurely, during phase 3 and late, during the final part of phase 4 (Fig. 18-1*C*). It is then reasonable that the two clinical varieties of block occurring under these different circumstances were called by us "phase 3 block" and "phase 4 block", respectively.[1–7]

Figure 18-2*A* illustrates schematically that in addition to the classic relative refractory period (RRP) at the end of systole, another refractory period (RP) may exist at the end of diastole. In a *normal* fiber or fascicle, an impulse falling prematurely on the first RP will be abnormally conducted. A familiar example is the aberrant ventricular conduction of premature supraventricular beats (upper panel in Fig. 18-3), which is thus a "physiologic" or "functional" form of phase 3 or systolic block. On the contrary, a late impulse falling—always in a normal fiber—on the second and eventual RP is generally conducted in a normal fashion. In other words, the second RP is, normally, just a potential possibility and so far as we know, there is no evidence whatsoever of the existence of an

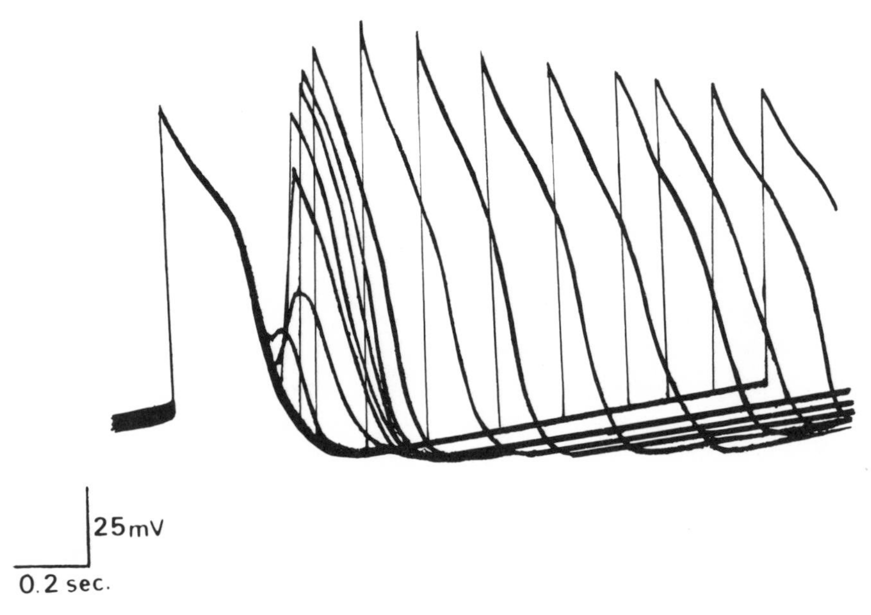

Figure 18-1. *A*, Intracellular recording of a normal fiber from the His bundle of the canine heart.

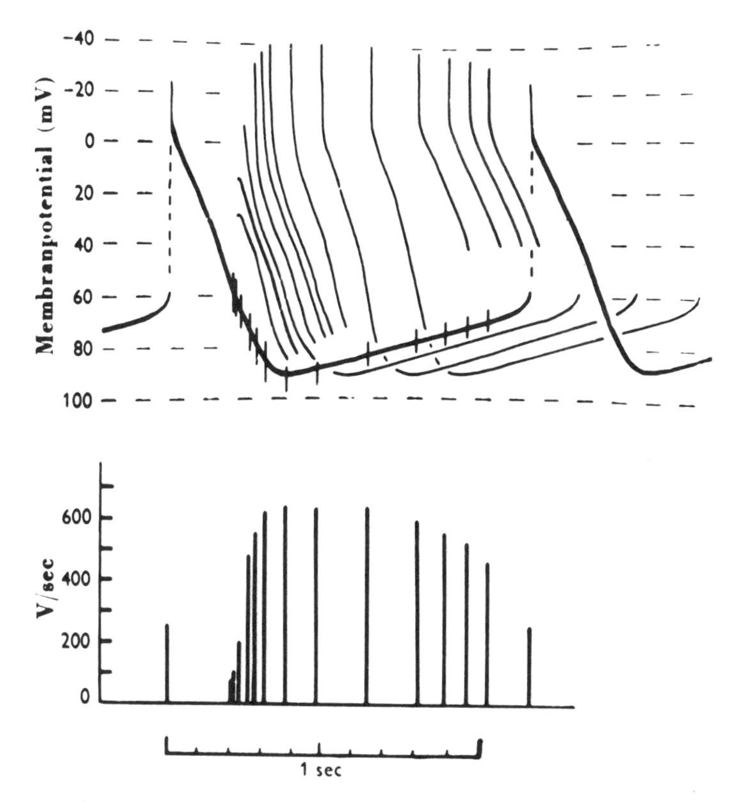

Figure 18-1. *(Continued).* *B*, Intracellular recording from a peripheral Purkinje fiber of the bovine heart. (Reproduced with permission from Weidmann, S.: Effect of cardiac membrane potential on the rapid availability of the sodium carrying system. *J. Physiol. (Lond.)* **127**: 213, 1955.) In both *A* and *B* the fiber was stimulated at different intervals. The lower panel in *B* shows the upstroke velocity in volts/sec.

aberrant conduction of late impulses as an equivalent to the aberrant conduction of premature beats. This is probably due to the fact that when a fiber is stimulated late in diastole, the reduction in the rate of rise of the action potential is compensated by a greater proximity to the threshold potential (implying greater excitability), in such a way that conduction velocity tends to be preserved (Fig. 18-2*A*). This phenomenon does not occur during phase 3 because the threshold potential has not yet reached the horizontal stable level of full diastole. Therefore, under normal conditions, there is only a systolic refractory period, and the late or diastolic refractory period is more a theoretical possibility than a real fact. However, in a pathological condition this possibility may turn into reality, giving rise to phase 4 block.

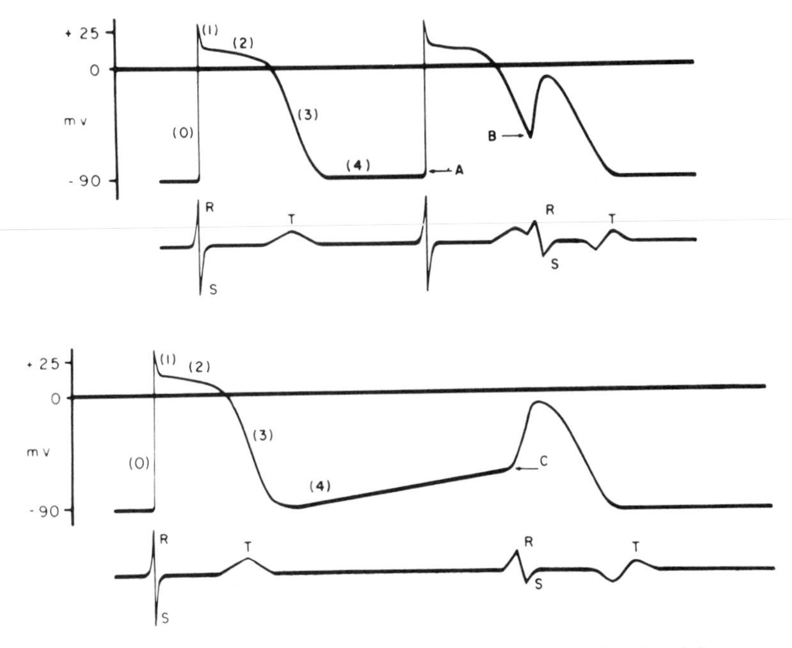

Figure 18–1. *(Continued). C*, Demonstrates that conduction in a fascicle composed of Purkinje fibers may cause block (as shown in the simultaneous electrogram) both prematurely and during the final part of phase 4. (Reproduced with permission from Singer, D.H., et al.: Interrelationship between automaticity and conduction in cardiac Purkinje fibers. *Circ. Res.* **21**: 537, 1967.)

In order for a real phase 3 block to occur, there must be abnormal prolongation of the action potential and/or the refractory period and, in addition, the involved fascicle must be stimulated at a relatively rapid rate. For this reason, this type of block is commonly referred to us as "tachycardia-dependent" (Figure 18-3, middle panel). The concurrence of phase 4 block requires an enhancement or at least the presence of a pacemaker potential, a shift of the threshold potential toward zero (Fig. 18-2*B*) and a certain degree of hypopolarization. Hypopolarization is probably the most important single factor, because there is evidence that a moderate degree of hypolarization causes secondarily an enhancement of spontaneous diastolic depolarization and a shift of the threshold potential.[12] For the phase 4 block to be uncovered, the heart rate must be sufficiently slow and consequently, this kind of block is frequently designated as "bradycardia-dependent" (Fig. 18-3, bottom panel). A depression of a membrane responsiveness (DMR) caused by antiarrhythmic drugs may contribute to widen the extension of the phase 3 and phase 4 block ranges (Fig. 18-2*C*).

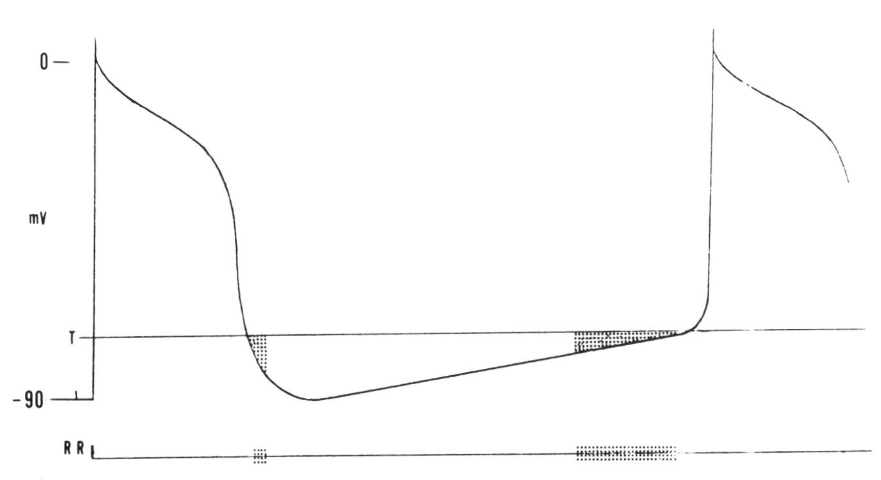

Figure 18–2. *A*, Schematic drawing indicating that, in addition to the classical relative refractory period at the end of systole (during phase 3), a second refractory period may exist at the end of diastole (during phase 4). In accordance with the facts shown in Figure 18-1, Line T corresponds to the threshold potential, which is normally the "ceiling" of the pacemaker potential.

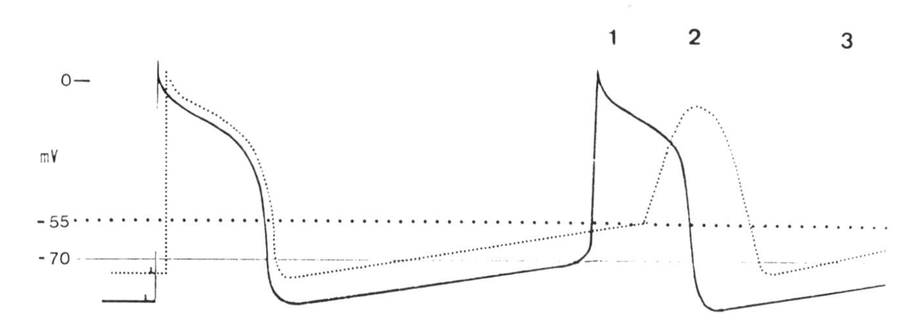

Figure 18–2. *(Continued). B*, A shift of the threshold potential (in the present drawing from −70 to −55 mV) and a certain degree of hypopolarization (seen at the beginning of the two superimposed action potentials) are required for the spontaneous diastolic depolarization to carry the membrane potential to the low levels at which slow conduction will occur (action potential 2). In the normal fiber, firing and normal conduction will occur (action potential 1) when spontaneous diastolic depolarization reaches the level of the normal threshold potential.

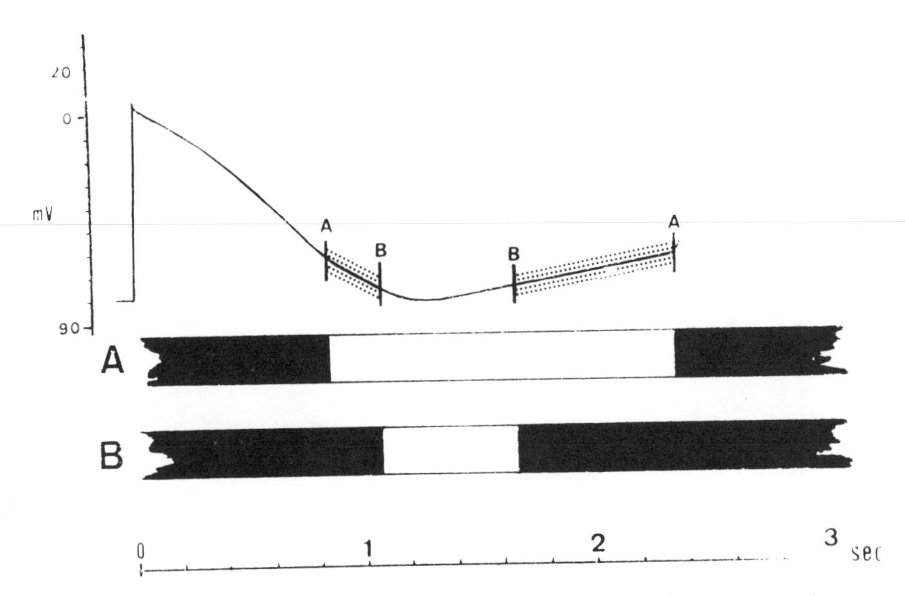

Figure 18-2. *(Continued). C,* A moderate depression of membrane responsiveness is assumed to act preponderantly at levels AB and BA of the membrane potential, thus extending the duration of the two refractory periods (represented by the black bars).

In summary, phase 3 block can be either physiologic, when an impulse is excessively premature, or pathologic, when the action potential and/or the refractory period are abnormally prolonged (Fig. 18-3, panels A and B). When the prolongation of the refractory period is very small, it may be difficult to distinguish a physiologic phase 3 block or aberrant conduction of premature beats from the pathologic phase 3 block indicating the slightest degree of a conduction disturbance. It is likely that some cases conventionally considered to indicate physiologic aberrant conduction may already represent the beginning of a pathologic phase 3 block. In contradistinction to phase 3 block, phase 4 block is always abnormal and is related to the presence of spontaneous diastolic depolarization (enhanced or not), a shift of the threshold potential toward zero (implying a decrease in excitability), and a slight or moderate hypolarization. A depression of membrane responsiveness may favor both forms of block or cause by itself a total or partial conduction block which may be rate-independent. On the contrary, phase 3 and phase 4 block are essentially and always rate-dependent.

Figure 18-4 shows the intracellular recordings from two experiments in which phase 4 block was provoked by slight mechanical injury to the right bundle branch in an in vitro preparation of the canine conducting

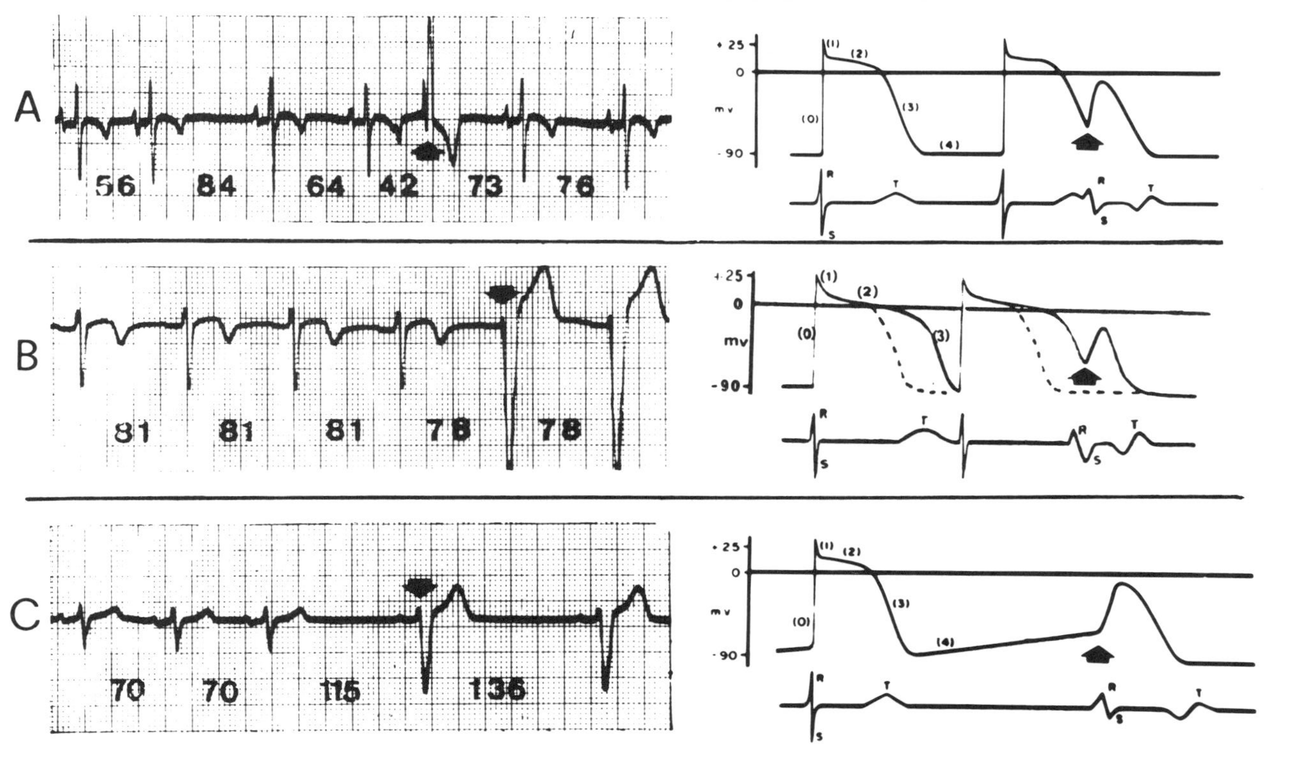

Figure 18–3. The fifth beat in panel *A* is a premature atrial beat with aberrant ventricular conduction or "physiological" phase 3 right bundle branch block. Panel *B* shows an example of "pathological" phase 3 or tachycardia-dependent left bundle branch block. Panel *C* shows an example of phase 4 or bradycardia-dependent left bundle branch block. In the three panels, the recorded lead was V1. Intervals in hundredths of a second. The right section of each panel indicates the underlying corresponding electrophysiological mechanism. (Modified from Singer, D.H., et al.: Interrelationship between automaticity and conduction in cardiac Purkinje fibers. *Circ. Res.* **21**: 537, 1967.)

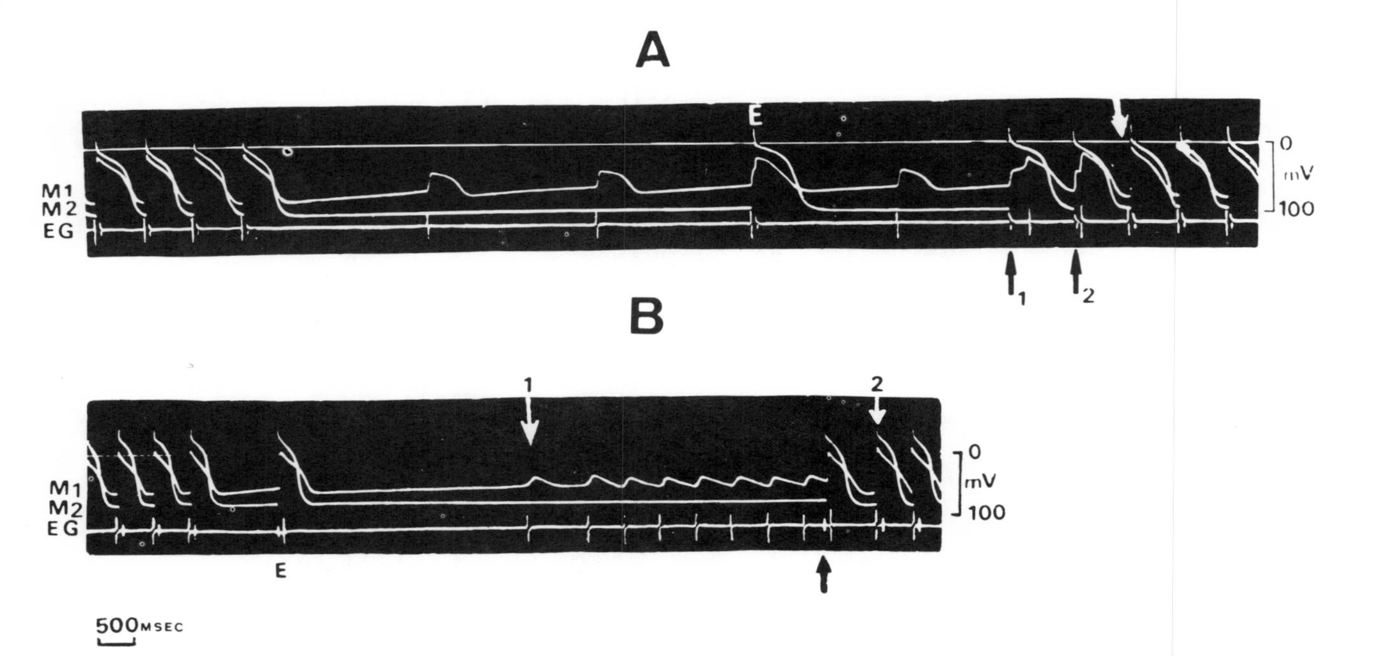

Figure 18–4. Two experiments in which phase 4 block was induced in the right bundle branch by mechanical injury, in an in vitro preparation of the canine conducting system.[13] A microelectrode (M1) was impaled in the injured segment and its recording verifies that the phase 4 block was related to a moderate hypopolarization (compare with the recording of microelectrode M2 impaled in a noninjured segment), causing secondarily an enhancement of the pacemaker potential and a shift of the threshold potential toward zero. (See text for further details.)

system.[12] It may be seen that the phase 4 block was related to a small degree of hypopolarization which caused secondary enhancement of the pacemaker potential. The shift of the threshold potential can be inferred from the fact that escapes did not occur when the SDD displaced the membrane potential beyond −70 or −60 mV. Note that the blocked anterograde impulses show some degree of penetration in the injured region, without being able to provoke its full discharge. On the other hand, a retrograde impulse is able to penetrate and fully discharge and reset the injured segment, favoring thus the resumption of conduction.

PHASE 3 AND PHASE 4 BLOCK IN INTERMITTENT BUNDLE BRANCH BLOCK

Figure 18-5 illustrates diagrammatically the sequence of conduction changes occurring when a conducting fascicle is injured transiently.[7,13] Initially, there is an apparently total and rate-independent interruption of conduction, but in a few minutes the typical ranges of systolic and diastolic block appear, separated by an intermediate normal conduction range which is narrow at the beginning, but which in a few more minutes opens itself progressively, pushing the phase 3 and phase 4 block ranges towards the left and right, respectively, until a complete normalization of conduction is reached.

The similarity between these experimental observations and the clinical cases of intermittent bundle branch block is striking. An intermittent bundle branch block may resemble any one of the stages 1 to 4 of Figure 18-5. Moreover, a single patient may—if studied repeatedly for weeks, months or years—swing back and forth from one stage to the other, probably in relation to small changes occurring in the injured region responsible for the conduction disturbance (Fig. 18-6). This phenomenon, which is nearly constant in the *chronic* cases of intermittent bundle branch block has been described under the name of Troilo effect or accordion effect,[1] which has no relation whatsoever to the so-called "concertina effect"[14] seen in patients with the Wolff-Parkinson-White syndrome. The accordion effect can be demonstrated equally well either when a single case is studied at different times (Fig. 18-6) or when a sufficiently large number of cases are compared to each other (Fig. 18-7). It can thus be seen that the two refractory periods or phase 3 and phase 4 block seem to change, to a greater or lesser extent, the intermediate normal conduction range. According to experimental studies[12,13] it may be assumed that a narrowly closed accordion indicates a greater degree of fascicular injury, and that a widely open accordion corresponds to a much milder degree of injury. When the accordions are graphically depicted as in Figures 18-6 and 18-7, it is clear that there are

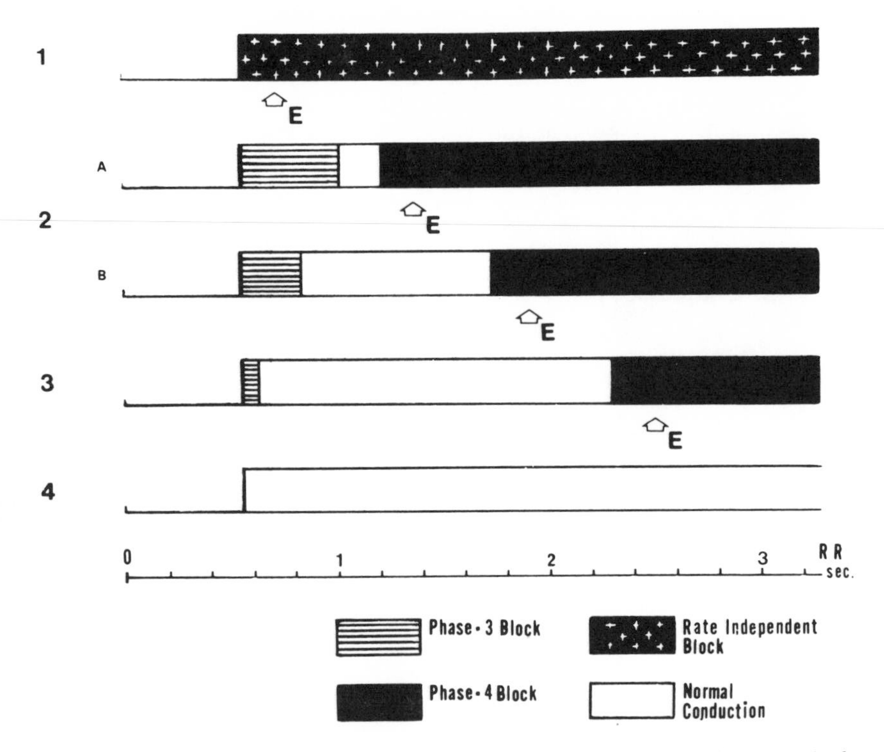

Figure 18–5. See text for description. Arrows labeled *E* correspond to ventricular escapes arising from the injured fascicle.

two rates or critical diastolic intervals separating (on of them) the phase 3 block range from the normal conduction range, and the other, the normal conduction range from the phase 4 block range. To demarcate the boundaries and extension of the two refractory periods, systolic and diastolic, it is imperative that each patient be studied at different rates and, above all, that sufficiently long R-R intervals be obtained. The latter is eloquently demonstrated by the case illustrated in Figure 18-8, which at the same time shows how the phase 3 and phase 4 bundle branch block should be "chased". The duration of the systolic refractory period or phase 3 block range was somewhere between 1480 and 1600 msec, and it is quite clear that, if pauses of the latter magnitude were not obtained, the phase 3 block would not have been documented and the erroneous conclusion could have been reached that the bundle branch block was permanent. On the other hand, the manifest beginning of the diastolic RP or phase 4 block range was between 2049 and 2450 msec, and it is again obvious that without pauses of the latter length, the phase 4 block would remain silent or concealed.

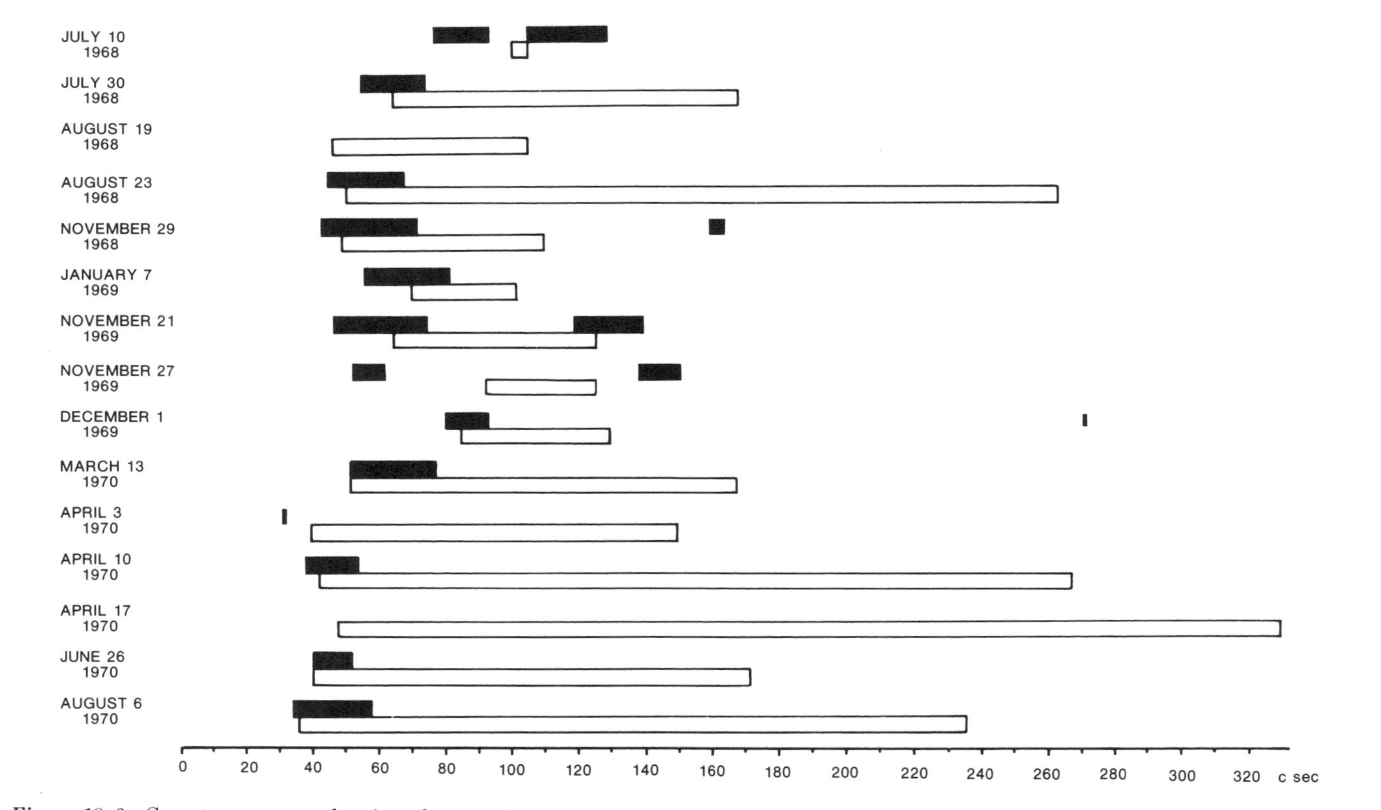

Figure 18–6. Spontaneous conduction changes in a case of intermittent LBBB during a follow-up of more than two years, during which repeated studies were performed. Black bars to the left: phase 3 block range, or systolic refractory period; black bars to the right: phase 4 block range, or diastolic refractory period; white bars: normal conduction range.

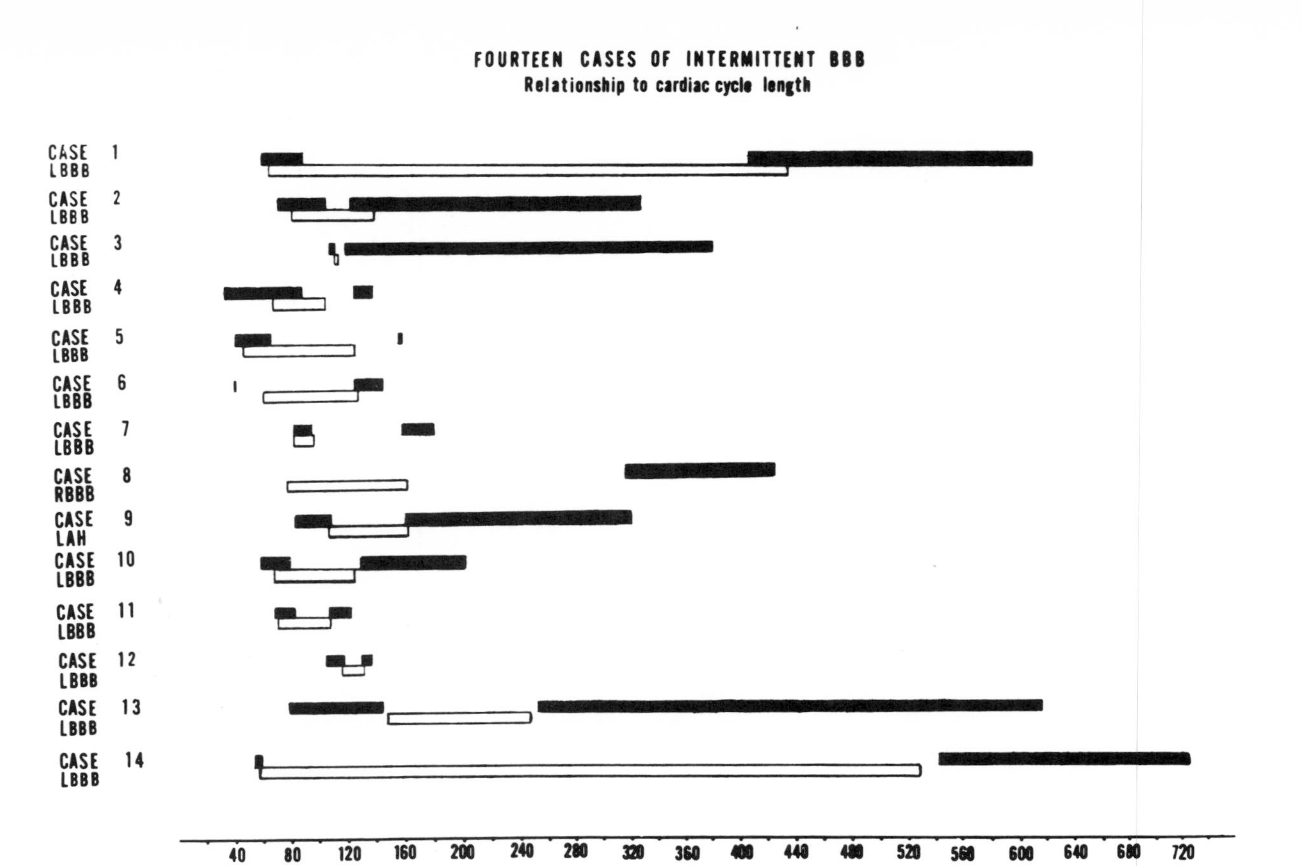

Figure 18–7. Boundaries and extension of the phase 3 and phase 4 block ranges (black bars), representing the systolic and diastolic refractory period respectively, in 14 different cases of intermittent bundle branch block. The accordion effect is clearly apparent

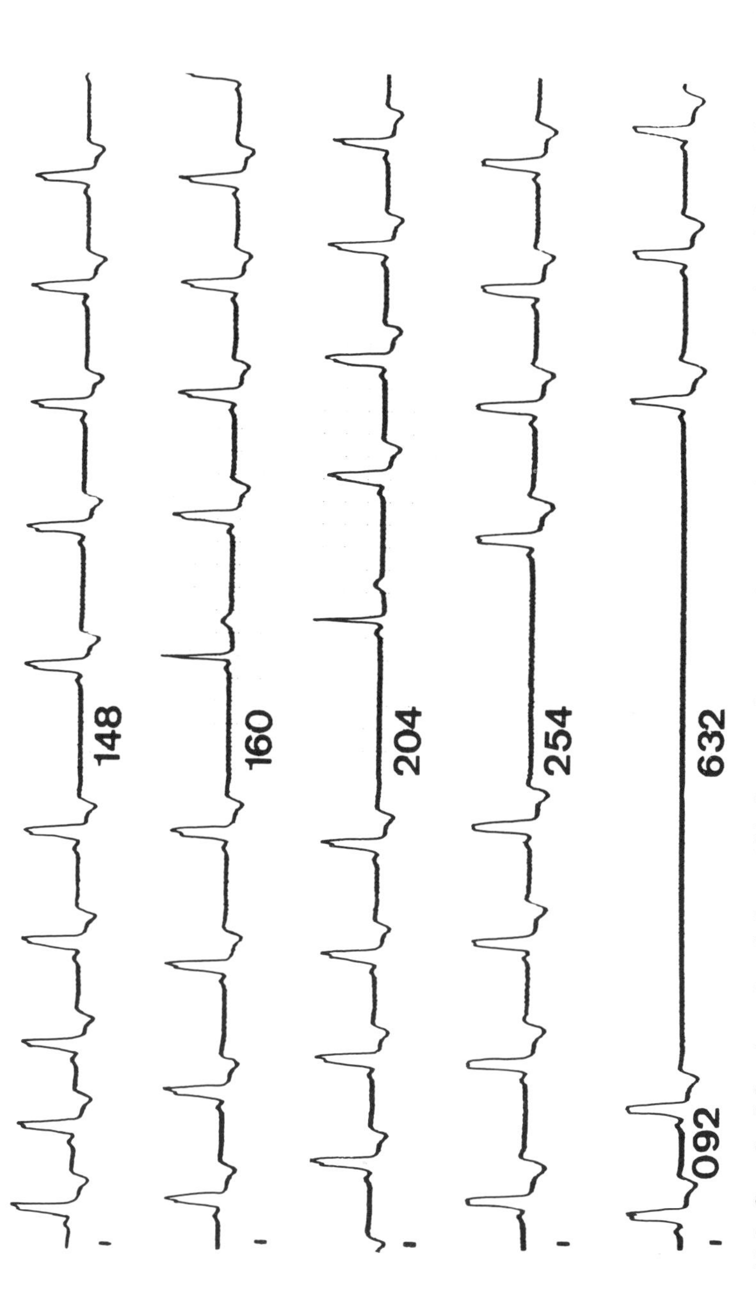

Figure 18–8. Search of the phase 3 and phase 4 block ranges in a case of apparently permanent left bundle branch block, in which the systolic refractory period was enormously long (around 1500 msec). The five discontinuous strips were ordered according to an increasing degree of effectiveness of the vagal stimulation (carotid sinus massage) in provoking longer and longer diastolic pauses. Normally conducted beats are seen only twice, terminating the long pauses in the second and third strip. All the other beats show a typical "complete" left bundle branch block pattern. Intervals are in hundredths of seconds. See text for further description.

Figure 18-9 shows the study of a patient in whom phase 3 and phase 4 bundle branch block had been readily documented at common cardiac rates previously and in whom conduction had apparently been normalized. However, when pauses as long as 6710 msec were provoked (not without difficulty), the existence of phase 4 block was still demonstrated. This case, which is far from being exceptional in our material, suggests that it may be difficult or impossible to determine whether phase 4 block exists. A good example is the phase 4 left bundle branch block occurring in some patients with an acute diaphragmatic infarction which can only be documented in the very late beats or at the very slow rate due to the AV block caused by the same infarct.[15] Difficult as it is to uncover phase 4 bundle branch block when the accordion is wide open as in the case of Figure 18-9, it may be equally hard or laborious to study cases in which the accordion is narrow, with a tight normal conduction range, particularly when the latter is displaced to the left. In such cases, if the appropriate heart rates are not induced, it may be erroneously concluded that the bundle branch block is stable or rate-independent. Or if the small normal conduction hiatus is uncovered, the wrong diagnosis of supernormal conduction may be entertained. In some of these cases, the persistence of a pattern of incomplete bundle branch block during the intermediate hiatus is another indication of a greater degree of fascicular injury and suggests that the tissue is significantly hypopolarized.

Figure 18-10 illustrates another interesting phenomenon. In a case of chronic left anterior hemiblock numerous degrees of hemiblock were recorded in relation to changes in cycle length. The degree of hemiblock was thus shown to increase toward the left and much more slowly and gradually to the right within the phase 4 block range. The latter is particularly revealing because it suggests that the late or diastolic refractory period rises gradually to a maximum in a fashion highly compatible with a gradual rising slope of the pacemaker potential.

A WORD ON METHODOLOGY

Intermittent bundle branch block constitutes the original model by which phase 3 and phase 4 block as well as their mutual relationship was initially demonstrated [1–7] However, in general, intermittent bundle branch block has been poorly studied. This is in part due to the fact that its physiologic importance may not have a direct clinical application because in essence it is a matter of methodology.

The study of permanent or intermittent bundle branch block is usually performed by recording a His bundle electrogram while stimulating the atria at rapid rates or by the extrastimulus method. And this is clearly insufficient. In order to study most cases of phase 3 bundle branch block,

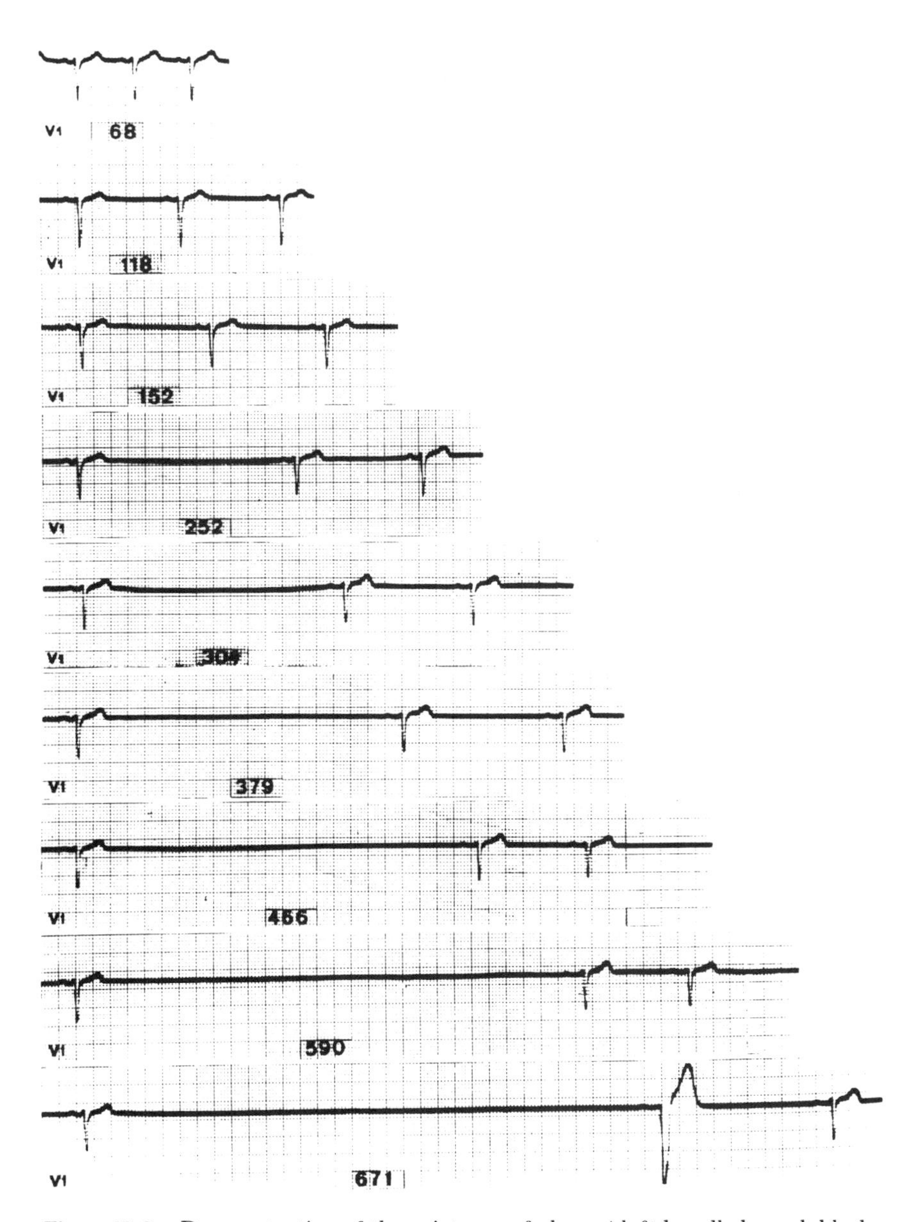

Figure 18-9. Demonstration of the existence of phase 4 left bundle branch block, only after extremely long diastolic intervals, in a patient in whom conduction was apparently normal or normalized. See text for further description. Intervals in hundredths of seconds. The different strips were ordered according to increasing length of diastolic pauses, provoked by vagal stimulation.

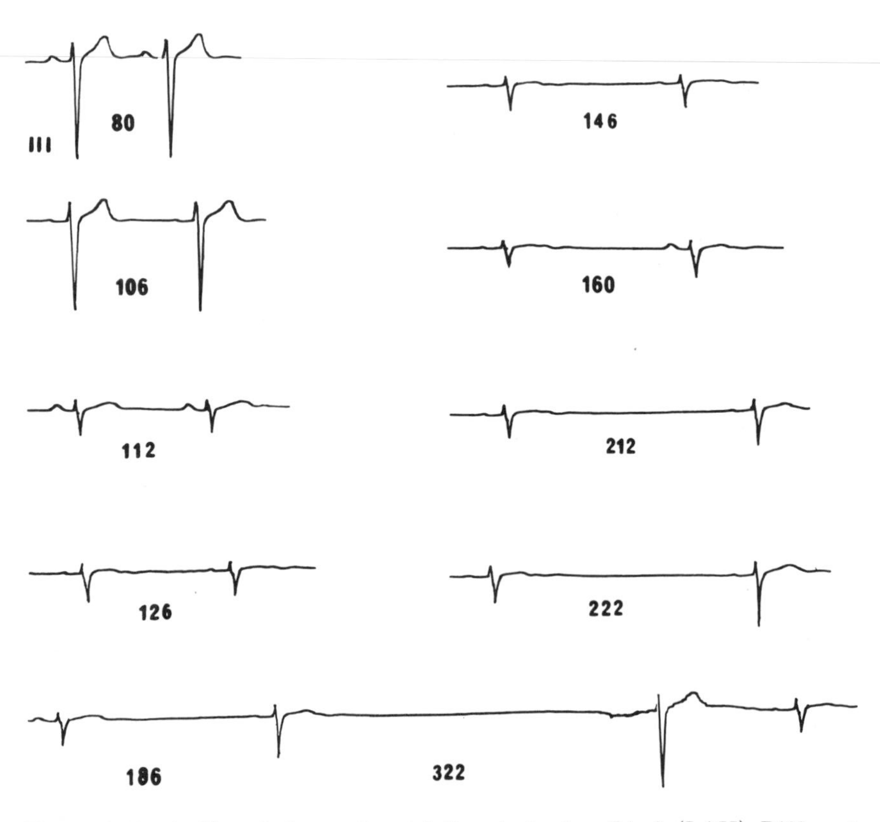

Figure 18-10. *A*, Chronic intermittent left anterior hemiblock (LAH). Different strips were ordered according to increasing degree of diastolic intervals provoked by a vagal stimulation. As the R-R interval increases, there is first a decrease in the degree of LAH (the S wave becomes smaller and smaller), and then again a progressive increase in the degree of the LAH (the S wave becomes deeper and deeper). Intervals in hundredths of seconds.

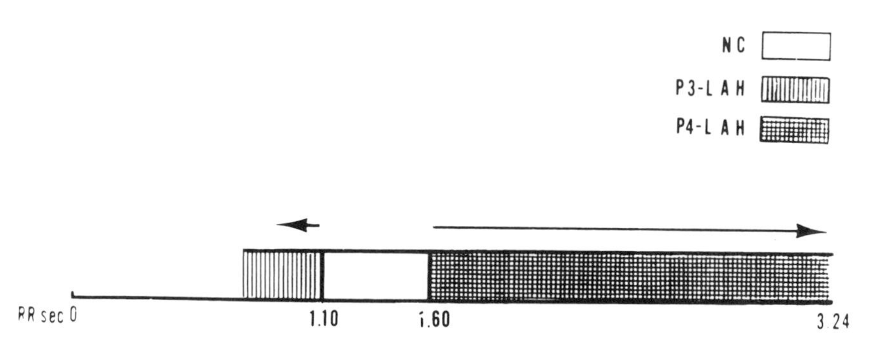

Figure 18-10. *(Continued).* *B*, Diagrammatic representation, showing the phase 3 and phase 4 LAH ranges, and the normal conduction range. The arrows indicate the direction and lapse of time during which the LAH increases in degree.

electrical stimulation at rapid rates is unnecessary or useless simply because, when the phase 3 block range lasts 1000 msec or more (which is quite common), what is needed is to slow down and not to increase the heart rate. The requirement is even more drastic if phase 4 bundle branch block is to be identified, because the only sensible approach—with all its limitations—is to provoke sufficiently long pauses by way of vagal stimulation. It is only so that phase 4 bundle branch block can be demonstrated and that the study of a patient can be truly completed regarding the functional integrity of the His intraventricular conduction system. To say that a patient has (or has not) bundle branch block at normal rates is to tell very little indeed. Unless we prepare ourselves to study routinely all cases of bundle branch block (BBB) at both rapid and slow rates, we will never be able to learn the natural history of BBB, the way in which BBB commences, the duration of the stage of intermittent BBB (which may last for years), and when or how stages of permanent anterograde or bidirectional BBB are reached, if ever. It is natural that, if in the presence of any stable or intermittent BBB the physiology of the diseased fascicle is practically unknown, not much can be expected from the attempts to correlate this almost elementary electrocardiographic finding with histological studies of the conduction system. In our laboratory, approximately 25 percent of the cases of BBB can be shown to be intermittent and to exhibit phase 3 and/or phase 4 BBB.[7] Such incidence is several times greater in left BBB than in right BBB.

FURTHER APPLICATIONS OF THE PHASE 3 AND PHASE 4 BLOCK CONCEPT

The same mechanisms underlying the occurrence of intermittent BBB can be shown to operate, some times decisively, in most cases of paroxysmal atrioventricular block (PAVB)[12,16,17] in some forms of ventricular parasystole,[18] and in many cases of pre-excitation.[18–21] Another valuable extension of the concept of phase 3 and phase 4 block was the development of a clinical model to study the effects of antiarrhythmic drugs on "diseased Purkinje fibers of the human heart".[7,22,23] All these topics have been extensively discussed in the above quoted publications.

Terminology

The term "phase 3 block" implies the existence of a refractory period abnormally prolonged at the end of the systole. The name "phase 4 block" indicates the presence of an abnormal RP at the end of diastole. There is a generalized tendency to designate these two forms of block as "tachycardia- and bradycardia-dependent", respectively. However, we believe this term has the following disadvantages: (1) It applies well to intermittent bundle branch block, but rather poorly to the phase 3 and phase 4 block occurring in paroxysmal atrioventricular block. (2) A phase 3 bundle branch block is tachycardia-dependent only relatively, occurring when the rate increases and disappearing when it decreases. However, when the phase 3 block range is greatly prolonged, lasting not uncommonly between 1000 and 1500 msec, the phase 3 block can only be uncovered by slowing the rate below 60 or 40 beats per minute, as in the case shown in Figure 18-8, in which pauses longer than 1500 msec were needed. It does not seem realistic or entirely correct to describe this phenomenon as "tachycardia-dependent". (3) Similar considerations apply to some cases of phase 4 bundle branch block. When the phase 4 block range is shifted to the left (commonly a manifestation of acute fascicular injury), it can be documented at normal or rapid cardiac rates, sometimes beyond 100 beats per minute. It is again not totally correct to call bradycardia-dependent the block occurring at this heart rate. (4) In phase 4 paroxysmal AV block, the AV block is provoked by a slowing of the sinus rate, but is not corrected by an increase of rate.[12,16] The block is thus bradycardia-dependent ragarding its initiation, but not its form of termination. And there is a different form of paroxysmal AV block related to supernormal conduction[24] which is authentically bradycardia-dependent regarding both initiation and termination, and which is however a variety of phase 3 block. Several other inconsistencies can be traced, but to summarize, the main drawback of this nomenclature is the fact that the same terms are often used to designate pathogenic processes which are completely different. Let us now consider some of the advantages and disadvantages of the terms "phase 3" and "phase 4" block.

The term phase 4 block does not appear to raise many doubts. Whether or not acceptance is given to its relation with the presence of spontaneous diastolic dipolarization there is not question that phase 4 block occurs really during phase 4 or electrical diastole of the action potential. On the other hand, when we first suggested the term phase 3 block together with phase 4 block,[1–7] it was because this approach seemed to us a simple and pragmatic way to distinguish and at the same time interconnect these two basic mechanisms of block (as they are indeed interconnected in clinical practice), without ignoring that the former could be partially incorrect. Although it is true that in phase 3 block most of the impulses fall on phase 3 of the action potential, this may not be so in two circumstances: (a) extremely premature isolated impulses may actually fall on phase 2, but this is unlikely to occur at a stable rapid rate; (b) in the presence of hypopolarization (or under the effect of antiarrhythmic drugs), the refractory period is prolonged beyond the end of the action potential, and this may cause tachycardia-dependent block with impulses actually falling beyond phase 3 of the action potential. The term "postrepolarization refractoriness"[25] applied to the latter phenomenon can also be considered to be unsatisfactory because it does not set apart or distinguish the classical or systolic refractory period from the late or diastolic refractory period, which may also be a "postrepolarization refractoriness". Phase 3 and phase 4 block have also been called "systolic" and "diastolic" block, respectively.[18] The latter terminology appears to be simple and descriptive and at the same time conveys some pathogenic meaning, without entering into basic details not yet well elucidated.

REFERENCES

1. Garcia, H., and Rosenbaum, M.B.: El "efecto fuelle" en los bloqueos intermitentes de rama. *Rev. Argentina de Cardiologia* **40**: 75, 1972.
2. Elizari, M.V., Lázzari, J.O., and Rosenbaum, M.B.: Phase 3 and phase 4 intermittent left anterior hemiblock. Report of first case in the literature. *Chest* **62**: 673, 1972.
3. Rosenbaum, M.B., Elizari, M.V., Lázzari, J.O., et al.: The physiological basis of intermittent bundle branch block. In Dreyfus, L.S., and Likoff, W. (eds.): *Second Symposium on Cardiac Arrhythmias*. New York, Grune & Stratton, 1973, p. 349.
4. Rosenbaum, M.B., Elizari, M.V., Lázzari, J.O., et al.: The mechanism of intermittent bundle branch block. Relationships to prolonged recovery, hypopolarization and spontaneous diastolic depolarization. *Chest* **63**: 666, 1973.
5. Elizari, M.V., Lázzari, J.O., and Rosenbaum, M.B.: Phase 3 and phase 4 intermittent bundle branch block occurring spontaneously in a dog. Correlation with histological study of the conducting system. *Eur. J. Cardiol.* **1**: 95, 1973.

6. Rosenbaum, M.B, and Elizari, M.V.: Mechanism of intermittent bundle branch block and paroxysmal atrioventricular block. *Postgrad. Med.* **53**: 87, 1973.
7. Rosenbaum, M.B., Elizari, M.V., Chiale, P.A., et al.: Relationships between increased automaticity and depressed conduction in the main intraventricular conducting fascicles of the human and canine heart. *Circulation* **49**: 818, 1974.
8. El-Sheriff, N., Scherlag, B.J., Lázzara, R., and Samet, P.: Pathophysiology of tachycardia and bradycardia-dependent block in the canine proximal His-Purkinje system after acute myocardial ischemia. *Am. J. Cardiol.* **33**: 529, 1974.
9. Singer, D.H., Lazzara, R., and Hoffman, B.F., Interrelationship between automaticity and conduction in cardiac Purkinje fibers. *Circ. Res.* **21**: 537, 1967.
10. Noble, D.: *The Initiation of the Heart Beat.* Oxford, Clarendon Press, 1975.
11. Weidmann, S.: Effect of cardiac membrane potential on the rapid availability of the sodium carrying system. *J. Physiol. (Lond.)* **127**: 213, 1955.
12. Elizari, M.V., Novakosky, A., Quinteiro, R., et al.: The experimental evidence for the role of phase 3 and phase 4 block in the genesis of A-V conduction disturbances. In Wellens, H.J., Lie, K.I., and Janse (eds.): *The Conduction System of the Heart.* Leiden, H.E., Stenfert Kroese, B.V., 1976, p. 360.
13. Elizari, M.V., Nau, G.J., Levi, R.J., et al.: Experimental production of rate dependent bundle branch block in the canine heart. *Circ. Res.* **34**: 730, 1974.
14. Ohnell, R.F.: Pre-excitation, a cardiac abnormality. *Acta Med. Scand.* **152. (Suppl.)**: 74, 1944.
15. Lie, K.I., Wellens, H.J., Schuilenburg, R.M., and Durrer, D.: Mechanism and significance of widened QRS complexes during complete AV block in acute myocardial infarction. *Am. J. Cardiol.* **33**: 833, 1974.
16. Rosenbaum, M.B., Elizari, M.V., Levi, R.J., and Nau, G.J.: Paroxysmal atrioventricular block related to hypopolarization and spontaneous diastolic depolarization. *Chest* **63**: 678, 1973.
17. Corrado, G., Levi, R.J., Nau, G.J., and Rosenbaum, M.B.: Paroxysmal atrioventricular block related to phase 4 bilateral bundle branch block. *Am. J. Cardiol.* **33**: 553, 1974.
18. Rosenbaum, M.B., Lázzari, J.O., and Elizari, M.V., The role of phase 3 and phase 4 block in clinical electrocardiography. In Wellens, H.J., Lie, K.I. and Janse (eds.): *The Conduction System of the Heart.* Leiden, H.E. Stenfert Kroese B.V., 1976, p. 126.
19. Przybylski, J., Chiale, P.A., Quinteiro, R.A., et al.: The occurrence of phase 4 block in the anomalous bundle of patients with Wolff-Parkinson-White syndrome. *Eur. J. Cardiol.* **3**: 267, 1975.
20. Chiale, P.A., Przybylski, J., Halpern, M.S., et al.: Comparative effects of ajmaline on intermittent bundle branch block and the Wolff-Parkinson-White syndrome. *Am. J. Cardiol.* **39**: 651, 1977.
21. Przybylski, J., Chiale, P.A., Halpern, M.S. et al.: Existence of automaticity in anomalous bundle of Wolff-Parkinson-White syndrome. *Br. Heart J.* **40**: 672, 1978.

22. Rosenbaum, M.B.: A new clinical and experimental model for studying the effects of antiarrhythmic drugs upon automaticity and conduction. *Acta Cardiol.* **Suppl. 18**: 289, 1974.
23. Chiale, P.A., Levi, R.J., Halpern, M.S., et al.: Efecto de diferentes drogas antiarritmicas sobre un caso de bloqueo de rama intermitente. *Medicina (Buenos Aires)* **35**: 1, 1975.
24. Levi, R.J., Elizari, M.V., Lázzari, J.O., et al.: Las diferentes variedades de bloqueo AV paroxistico. *Rev. Lat. de Cardiol.,* in press.
25. Lazzara, R., El-Sheriff, N., and Scherlag, B.J.: Disorders of cellular electrophysiology produced by ischemia of the canine His bundle. *Circ. Res.* **36**: 444, 1975.

19

Electronic Pacemakers: Recent Advances

Michael D. Klein, M.D., and Paul A. Levine, M.D.

As the pace of modern life has quickened, the human heart has not always kept pace. Whether from disease or senescence, the heart may falter, failing to initiate or propel its impulse efficiently. Heart block, excessive tachycardias, and alternating bradycardia and tachycardia all reflect electrical dysfunction of the heart which may require electronic pacemaker therapy.

In less than one quarter of a century, pacemaker systems have gone through several generations of improvement which have rendered them smaller, more durable, and more versatile. As is always the case, however, their worth and safety depend upon the quality control maintained during their manufacture, the quality control used during their insertion, and the surveillance control exercised during their operating lives. The present communication will review certain advances in pacemaker design and is based upon our experience at Boston University Medical Center with more than 250 pacemaker insertions over the past four years.

PULSE GENERATOR SIZE

Advances in microelectronics and battery technology have resulted in a substantial reduction in pacemaker size and weight. The current generation of pulse generators average about 50 to 60 grams, which represents about a two-fold reduction in weight from their counterparts we were using just three years ago. Better cosmetic features are an obvious advantage of the shrinking pacemaker size. This is especially important in the cachectic patient with advanced heart disease in whom the fashioning of a subcutaneous pouch for pacemaker installation free of erosion and local difficulties can be an arduous task.

BATTERY TYPE

The lithium cell has replaced the mercury-zinc cell as the preferred energy source for most implantable pacemakers. While pacemakers employing different types of lithium batteries are available from various manufacturers, the widest experience has been compiled with the lithium iodide cell. Lithium iodide batteries have certain potential advantages over batteries using other lithium salts, such as silver chromate, cupric sulfide, thionyl chloride. The lithium iodide cell contains no liquid electrolyte. It does not require a separator material to keep the lithium anode from contacting the iodine-poly-2-vinylpyridine cathode; total volume of the cell remains essentially constant during discharge; no gas is produced by chemical reactions and no gas, therefore, is emitted by the cell.

One feature of lithium iodide cells which differs between manufacturers involves the shielding of the iodine cathode from the stainless steel encapsulating case. The Catalyst Research Corporation (800 series) of batteries is constructed with a centrally located cathode current collector and a lithium envelope which surrounds and contains the iodine depolarizer material. A second barrier of fluorocarbon plastic surrounds the lithium envelope. Thus, two barriers, the lithium and fluorocarbon, separate the iodine depolarizer material from the stainless steel casing, preventing corrosion and potential foreshortening of battery life. In the Wilson-Greatbatch 755 lithium iodide cells, iodine depolarizer is poured directly into the stainless steel case and may result in surface corrosion. Whether the surface corrosion can result in corrosion of deeper levels and shortening of battery life remains controversial.

Comparative features of lithium cells are depicted in Table 19-1. Projected life time for all of these cells is between seven to ten years. As yet, however, there has been only a limited experience with lithium cells in continuous human use for more than five years. Thus, the actual longevity of these batteries in humans has yet to be established.

PROGRAMMABILITY

Heart disease or dysfunction, of whatever sort, is rarely a static problem. Change and variability is the rule, often mandating change and readjustment of medication. With some models of cardiac pacemakers, heretofore, it has been possible to alter their rate of discharge and energy output subsequent to permanent implantation. Altered pacemaker parameters are achieved noninvasively by delivering a small electromagnetic pulse transcutaneously to the implanted pacemaker. A reduction in pacemaker rate and amplitude of discharge provides certain potential advantages: conservation of battery life; decrease in cardiac work in

Table 19-1. Cell Comparisons

	802/23 (CRC)	702E (CRC/WG)	752 (WG)	755 (WG)	Li-210 (SAFT)	LSA 900-6 (Mallory)	Lithium-Thionyl Chloride
Anode	Lithium	Lithium	Lithium	Lithium	Lithium	Lithium	Lithium
Cathode	Iodine	Iodine	Iodine	Iodine	Silver Chromate	Lead Iodide	Thionyl Chloride
Volts/Cell O.C.	2.8	2.8	2.8	2.8	3.5	5.7	3.6
Weight (g)	34	80	27	33	9.04 ± .15	4.0	13
Size (mm)	23 × 13.5 × 45.1	32 × 14 × 45	33 × 9 × 40	33 × 9 × 40	21 ± .05 × 9.06 ± 0.16	12 dia × 4.4 long	14.3 dia × 50 long
Volume (cm³)	11.8	31	9.5	9.5	3.14	10.1	8
Energy vs. Vol. (Watt hr/cm³)	.41	.28	.395				
Energy vs. Wt (WH/g)	.140	.109	.138	.79	—	.40	.915
Capacity (Ah)	2.3	3.5	1.5	.227	—	.100	.113
Self-Discharge	0.19 AH/10 yrs.	10%/10 yrs.	10%/10 yrs.	3.0	.6	.9	2.0
				10%/10 yrs.	—	—	—

patients with severe angina pectoris. An increase in pacemaker rate and amplitude of discharge provides certain other potential advantages: overdriving of refractory tachyarrhythmias which may be rate-dependent at their inception; leaway in stimulating a myocardium whose threshold may be elevated further during the course of a chronic or acute intermittent illness.

Within the past year further advances in technology have ushered in the era of multi-parameter programmability. At least two systems, the Pacesetter Programalith and the Medtronic Spectrax, allow the physician to alter noninvasively a wide range of parameters subsequent to pulse generator installation. Additionally, the Programalith can be interrogated to verify that it is operating according to specifications and assess the status of the battery and electrode. In Table 19-2, the programmable features and additional interrogatable characteristics of the Programalith system are listed. The energy delivered by the pacemaker can be modulated by modifying either the output voltage or pulse width so as to maximize battery life and meet changing myocardial threshold requirements. The Pacemaker's demand rate and excape interval (hysteresis) can be adjusted, if required, for setting optimal work loads for the heart and for optimum suppression of dysrhythmias. Rate adjustments between 45–110/min can be made in 12 increments. Hysteresis can be added from a 0–600 msec longer escape interval than demand interval, which in certain patients will preserve synchronous atrioventricular conduction and help optimize cardiac output over a wider range of heart rates. Additionally, the pulse generator can be interrogated and respond with its working parameters: battery impedance, battery current and stimulation impedance. These last three items provide information on the status of the lithium power cell and the integrity of the electrode. Finally, all the above-mentioned data are automatically printed out for incorporation into patient records.

Totally programmability may be a scientific marvel, but is the complexity and additional cost of such pacemaker systems worthwhile? With

Table 19-2. Programalith Pacemaker

I. Programmable and Interrogatable Items:
- A. Discharge rate
- B. Output voltage
- C. Refractory period
- D. Pulse width
- E. Hysteresis
- F. Sensitivity

II. Interrogatable Items:
- A. Battery impedance
- B. Lead impedance
- C. Battery current drain

additional complexity comes the increased likelihood of system malfunction. Cost becomes a consideration when the specific clinical problem for which the pacemaker is to be used does not require such extensive pulse generator modulation.

Arguments in favor of total programmable pacemaker systems center around the increasing life expectancy of these devices and, conceivably, the patients they serve. Lithium power cells may give a pacemaker and its electrode a potential working life of ten of more years. Specifications for optimal myocardial pacing may change by virtue of disease or senescence during this time interval requiring a change of a nonprogrammable unit even if functioning normally. Multi-parameter programmability allows the pacemaker to be fine tuned to the changing needs of the patient. Although provisional data on multi-parameter programmable pacemakers do not point toward a greater random failure rate than in standard nonprogrammable units, the likelihood of some electronic malfunction or electrode dysfunction will be increased over this prolonged life span. In addition, further experience with programmable pacemakers may obviate the need for special design units required to extend the working range of standard pacemakers.

The following case illustrates the use of a programmable pacemaker. A 64-year-old male was eight years post mitral valve replacement (Beall Valve). He had right bundle branch block, left posterior hemiblock, periods of rapid ventricular tachycardia, chronic atrial fibrillation with episodic ventricular bradycardia (< 30/min) and tachycardia (> 110/min). His medications included digoxin, furosemide and procainamide. For several reasons, a Programalith pacemaker was selected for control of the periodic high grade A-V block: (1) The interrelationship between ambient heart rate of the rapid ventricular tachycardia was unclear. Ventricular irritability arose when the ventricular response rate to atrial fibrillation decreased to below 60; but ventricular tachycardia was also triggered from faster ventricular response rates. Therefore, a rate adjustable pacemaker was utilized. (2) With right bundle branch block, left posterior hemiblock and multiformed ventricular premature beats prevalent, it was thought advisable to have an adjustable sensitivity lest sensing failure occur at the permanent electrode site and paced beats in the T-wave of the sinus of extrasystolic beats induce repetitive ventricular responses. (3) Should sensing failure nonetheless occur, pacing with the minimal effective energy level would minimize the likelihood of pacer-induced ventricular fibrillation.

During the first few weeks after pacemaker insertion, ventricular tachycardia and cardiac arrest recurred requiring defibrillation. Cardiorenal failure ensued with eventual digoxin and procainamide intoxication. Digoxin was withheld and procainamide discontinued. As cardiac and renal function improved, digoxin was restarted and low dose propranolol initiated for suppression of ventricular irritability. Because of persistent 5-8 beat salvoes of ventricular tachycardia at a rate of 160, the pacemaker was progressively programmed upward in rate with better containment of the ventricular arrhythmias.

ELECTRODES

Enhanced life expectancy of pulse generators has spurred efforts to design and fabricate more durable electrodes. One of the more innovative devices is the tined electrode first introduced by Medtronic but now manufactured by others as well. It is equipped with four symmetrically placed, short (2.5 mm), flexible silicone rubber tines positioned at a 45° angle to the lead shaft, 3.1 mm proximal to the tip electrode. The tip is comprised of platinum-iridium rather than elgiloy as in the older electrodes and is an annular ring with a surface area of 8mm^2.[1]

The tined electrode was designed to minimize four problems experienced with previous electrode models:

1. Dislodgement
2. Perforation
3. Sensing Failure
4. Exit Block

Securing of the electrode tip in the webbing of the right ventricle should be easier, as the tines are caught amongst the crevices in the trabeculae. Flexibility and short length of the tines should reduce problems of myocardial perforation associated with older model flange-tipped electrodes with their rigid shoulders. Exit block and sensing failure should be obviated, as the tined electrode tip is snug against the right ventricular endocardium.

Early experience with the Medtronic 6961 (Unipolar) and 6962 (Bipolar) electrode leads has been most favorable. A series comparing 50 consecutive patients receiving the bipolar tined lead with 48 patients receiving the older flange-tip electrode showed mean stimulation threshold to be 32 percent less in volts and 28 percent less in milliamps with the tined electrode.[2] R-wave sensitivities were comparable in both groups. Though mean lead impedance was under 600 Ohms with both types of electrode, it was 13 percent lower with the tined electrode. In this report series, dislodgement was not observed with the tined electrodes, whereas it did occur with 21 percent of the flange-tipped electrodes, requiring lead re-manipulation or replacement. (However, we have a 0.75 percent (1/250) dislodgement rate with the older flange-tip electrode and none out of 50 tined electrodes, but this difference is not statisically significant.)

While we believe that stability of the electrode to be largely a function of implantation technique, we have found the tined electrode to offer about a 10 percent reduction in stimulation threshold requirements as compared to a variety of older leads. The tined electrode has proven especially helpful in agitated patients and in patients with large right ventricles, either with or without tricuspid insufficiency.

The Cardiac Pacemakers, Inc. (CPI) porous electrode represents a different approach to the problems of electrode dislodgement, sensing failure and exit block.[3] The cathode electrode tip consists of a meshwork of 25 μm platinum fibers occupying 10 percent of the electrode volume. The remaining 90 percent of electrode volume is occupied by blood, cellular and fibrinous components, together with some fluid, which penetrate the platinum mesh. Thus, in principle, the electrode should form a secure, low-resistance bond with the right ventricular endocardium, lowering both pacing and sensing thresholds. Diameter of the platinum fibers is comparable to the size of cardiac cells and calculated to minimize the foreign body reaction to electrode tip emplacement. In animal studies, porous electrodes have been observed to have thinner fibrotic capsules around the electrode tip than have solid electrodes.[4]

Porous electrodes may also reduce polarization impedance, a measure of the efficiency in converting electronic current to a depolarizing ionic current at the metallic surface area contacting NaCl electrolyte. Both the outside and the inside of the platinum wire mesh contact the electrolyte with a total surface area of about 50 mm^2, despite an outside surface area of only 7.5 mm^2. The fraction of pacemaker energy dissipated as polarization impedance has been estimated as only 12 percent with a 1 msec duration depolarization spike in a porous electrode.[4] With the larger surface area for sensing, it has been estimated that R-wave attenuation with the porous electrode is only about 6 percent, whereas for solid electrodes it is about 13 percent.

PHYSICIAN

With any pacemaker system, the final common pathway to the heart is the implanting physician. Advances in electrode and pulse generator design will doubtless have some bearing upon problems of dislodgement, perforation, pacing and sensing failure. It is the physician, not the engineer, however, who exerts quality control over the installation of the pacemaker system. The advantages of a qualified, careful, experienced, interested doctor doing the work are dramatic. In our own institution, for example, one cardiologist (PAL) has performed or personally supervised the last 150 pacemaker insertions. The problem of electrode dislodgement is rare, only one in 15 cases for an incidence of 0.75 percent.

Electrode perforation during insertion has been seen in only four of 150 cases, and quickly remedied by withdrawal of the electrode tip and repositioning it on the endocardium; and the problem of exit block has occurred in only three pacemakers in this group.

REFERENCES

1. Lathrop, T.J.: Synopsis of clinical report on the models 6961/6962 tined leads. *Medtronic News*, Sept. 1978, p. 6.
2. Holmes, D.R., Jr., Nissen, R.G., Maloney, J.D., et al.: Transvenous tined electrode systems: an approach to acute dislodgement. *Mayo Clin. Proc.* **54**: 219, 1979.
3. Amundson, D., McArthur, W., and Mosharrafa, M.: The porous endocardial electrode. *Pace* **2**: 40, 1979.
4. Amundson, D.C.: Characteristics of the CPI porous tip electrode. *Impulse* **14**: 7, 1979.

20

Clinical Implications of Chronic Conduction System Disease

Dietmar Gann, M.D., and Philip Samet, M.D.

INTRAVENTRICULAR CONDUCTION DEFECTS

Sclerodegenerative disease of the conduction system (Lenègre's disease-Lev's disease) is probably the most common cause of chronic atrioventricular (AV) block and intraventricular conduction defects (IVCD). Lenègre described sclerosing degenerative changes of the bundle branches and main His bundle of unknown etiology, not associated with any known pathological condition.[1] Lev postulated that fibrosis and calcification of the left side of the cardiac skeleton secondarily impinged on the conduction system and produced atrioventricular block.[2-4]

A multitude of other conditions can result in chronic conduction problems—hypertension, aortic valve disease, coronary artery disease, myocarditis, congenital heart disease, endocarditis, rheumatic heart disease, and more.[2,5-12]

Rosenbaum et al.[13,14] introduced the concept of electrocardiographically diagnosed fascicular blocks. The intraventricular conduction system consists of three fascicles—right bundle, left anterior superior fascicle of the left bundle, and left posterior inferior fascicle of the left bundle. Various patterns on the electrocardiogram are recognized as being unifascicular (right bundle branch block [RBBB], left anterior hemiblock [LAH], and left posterior hemiblock [LPH]); bifascicular (left bundle branch block [LBBB] or combinations of RBBB with LAH or LPH); and trifascicular (alternating LBBB and RBBB, or RBBB with alternating LAH and LPH if incomplete or complete heart block, if all three fascicles are blocked). The concept of fascicular blocks is clinically very useful, but well-defined anatomical correlates have not been identified.[15]

A pattern of bifascicular disease (especially RBBB and LAH) often precedes the development of complete heart block.[16,17] Various clinical follow-up studies have estimated the risk of developing complete heart block with bifascicular disease at anywhere from 0 to 21 percent.[18,19] These widely varied results demonstrated our inability to predict from the surface electrocardiogram when an intraventricular conduction defect would progress to complete heart block.

After the introduction of His bundle recording into clinical practice in 1969,[20] it was hoped that this tool would make possible more accurate predictions of impending complete heart block. His bundle recording made it possible to subdivide the PR segment of the surface electrocardiogram into three time intervals:[21] PA—from the beginning of the P wave to the beginning of the low right atrial electrogram (normal 25–45 msec); AH—from the onset of the low right atrial electrogram to the beginning of the His spike (normal 50–120 msec); and HV—from the onset of the His potential to the beginning of the QRS complex (normal 35–55 msec). The PA time reflects intra-atrial conduction, AH time the conduction through the AV node, and HV time the conduction through the His-Purkinje system. Lengthening of the His spike to more than 20 msec indicates conduction delay in the main His bundle.

His bundle studies in patients with intraventricular conduction defects and various patterns of fascicular disease have shown that, despite similarities in the surface electrocardiograms, there were differences in conduction intervals, especially the HV times. The HV time remains normal as long as one fascicle conducts without delay. However, HV times were prolonged in up to 30 percent of patients with LAH, 40 percent of patients with LPH, 32 percent of patients with RBBB, 72 percent of patients with RBBB + LAH, 79 percent of patients with LBBB and 87 percent of patients with RBBB and LPH.[22,23] Therefore, a substantial number of patients with mono- or bifascicular disease have additional disease in the remaining fascicles or the main His bundle that is not detectable from the surface electrocardiogram. There is suggestive evidence in the literature that a markedly prolonged HV interval (> 70 msec) may be associated with an increased risk of sudden death or development of high-degree AV block.[24–28] Others, however, differ with these findings.[22,29–31] Possible explanations for the differences in our opinion may be the variability of symptoms, age and cardiac disease in the populations studied.

Management of Patients with Intraventricular Conduction Defects (Table 20–1)

How do the results of these studies affect our present-day approach to patients with intraventricular conduction defects, especially those pa-

Table 20-1. Approach to Symptomatic Patients With Bifascicular Blocks (LBBB, RBBB + LAH, RBBB + LPH)

Patients with syncope and/or recurrent dizziness undergo medical evaluation, including neurological workup. If no cause for symptoms is found, proceed with 24-hour continuous electrocardiographic monitoring.

Documented second- or third-degree A-V block → Permanent pacemaker

Symptoms during recording unexplained by findings on avionics → Look for other causes

No symptoms during recording
No second- or third-degree AV block
→ His bundle study

His bundle study → Prolonged HV interval 50–55 msec → Permanent pacemaker

His bundle study → Normal HV time → Observe
Look for other causes

tients with so-called bifascicular disease? There is a general consensus that *asymptomatic* patients with intraventricular conduction defects do not require any conduction studies. In order to glean the few with markedly prolonged HV times who might profit from prophylactic pacing, a large number of patients would need to be studied, an unacceptable approach today, when medical economics and cost-effectiveness of a procedure are taken into consideration.

In the elderly population, intraventricular conduction defects in the cardiogram and episodes of dizziness and/or syncope are relatively common problems, which may occur in tandem. Symptoms of such patients could possibly be related to intermittent high-degree or complete AV block. It is not uncommon for a patient with bifascicular disease to exhibit transient complete heart block and then persistent 1:1 AV conduction which lasts for days or weeks. Therefore, the finding of 1:1 conduction even during prolonged monitoring does not rule out the possibility of intermittent AV block. If a thorough medical evaluation including neurological work-up and 24-hour monitoring does not establish a diagnosis for the dizzy episodes or syncopal attacks in patients with intraventricular conduction defects, we proceed to His bundle recording. A normal HV time makes intermittent AV block as a cause of the symptoms an unlikely possibility and we do not recommend pacing for these patients. However, it is our opinion that a prolonged HV time in those patients with unexplained dizziness or syncope establishes the need for permanent pacing.

Our experience over the last ten years, and similar reports from other institutions, justifies this approach.[24,28] Studies of patients with bifascicular block, transient complete heart block or Mobitz type II second-degree AV block reveal that a very high percentage exhibited prolonged HV times during 1:1 antegrade conduction.[24, 32–34] These findings support the concept that a prolonged HV is almost a necessary prerequisite for the development of complete heart block. A total of 20 patients from our institution with RBBB, LAH and syncopal episodes were found to have normal HV times. None of these patients was permanently paced, and only one developed subsequent complete heart block. However, this occurred after the patient had an acute myocardial infarction. Similar results were obtained by Altschuler et al.[24] In 16 patients with various intraventricular conduction defects accompanied by syncope or dizziness who had normal HV times, there was no sudden death and no development of AV block over a mean period of 22 months. In contrast to this, of 11 similar patients with prolonged HV times who were not paced in spite of symptoms, three died suddenly and another three progressed to high-degree AV block requiring permanent pacing.

ATRIOVENTRICULAR BLOCK

Based on the PR interval in the surface electrocardiogram AV blocks have been divided into several groups:

a. *First degree*—PR interval is longer than 0.20 seconds
b. *Second-degree Wenckebach or Mobitz type I*—PR interval progressively increases until a P-wave is blocked (Fig. 20-1)
c. *Second degree Mobitz type II*—constant PR interval with abrupt cessation of P-wave conduction (Fig. 20-2)
d. *High degree*—only occasional P-waves are conducted
e. *Complete*—no P-waves are conducted

First- and second-degree AV block have been described in the atrium, AV node, His bundle, bundle branches and Purkinje network. Third-degree AV block occurs in all these locations except the atrium.[35] His bundle recording allows the division of AV blocks into *supraHis*, *intra-His* and *infraHis*. There is some evidence in the literature that location of the block has prognostic implications.[36–38] A supraHis block generally occurring in the AV node (and less often in the atrium) is considered relatively benign.[36] The escape pacemaker in supraHis blocks usually originates above the bifurcation of the His bundle, is fairly reliable, faster than 40/min, and responds in some degree to exercise and atropine.[37,38] In contrast, intra- and infraHis blocks often result in Stokes-Adams attacks or sudden death. The escape pacemakers are unreliable, with rates often below 40/min, and respond poorly to any stimulation.

From the surface electrocardiogram and clinical picture it is often possible to determine the site of the block with reasonable accuracy. In a minority of patients exact determination of the site of block cannot be made; if therapeutic decisions are to be based on knowledge of the site of the block, conduction studies are necessary.

SupraHis blocks are usually located within the AV node. The AH interval is prolonged (> 120 msec). This block is commonly associated with digitalis intoxication, inferior wall myocardial infarction and congenital heart block. At times it is seen in young healthy athletes, due to excessive vagotonia. Most first-degree AV blocks occur in the AV node. Second-degree supraHis block is almost always of the Wenckebach type. Mobitz II block in the AV node has been described, but the validity of the interpretation of these studies has been questioned.[39] The QRS complex of the escape pacemaker is narrow, if no additional bundle branch defects exist.

IntraHis blocks are less common, occurring in 14 to 17 percent of patients with chronic complete heart block,[37,40] predominantly elderly females. The QRS complex is narrow if no additional bundle branch

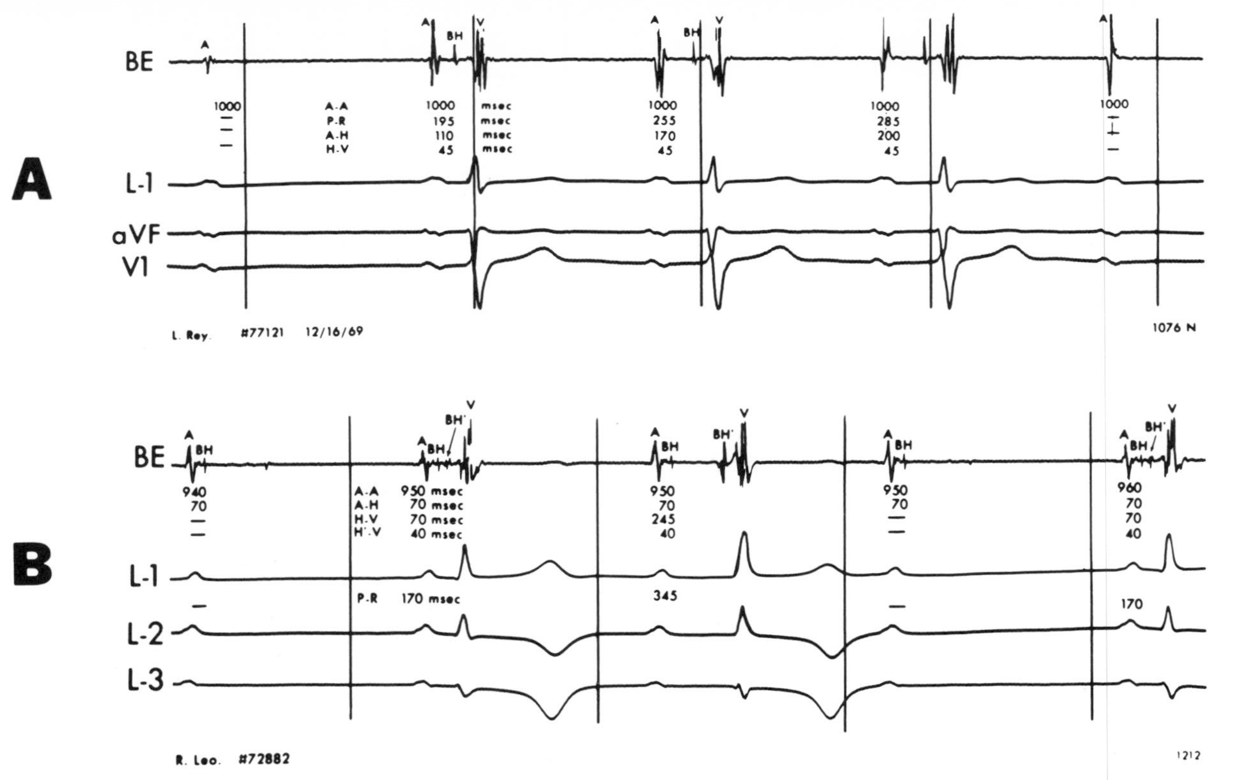

Figure 20–1. Two patients with Mobitz type I atrioventricular block. *A*, Progressive PR prolongation due to delayed AH conduction. Blocked P-wave is not followed by a BH spike and is therefore blocked in the AV node. *B*, Progressive PR prolongation due to delayed intraHis conduction ($BH\text{-}BH^1$). Blocked P-wave is followed by a BH spike but not a BH^1 spike. BE = Bipolar electrode recording His bundle activity.

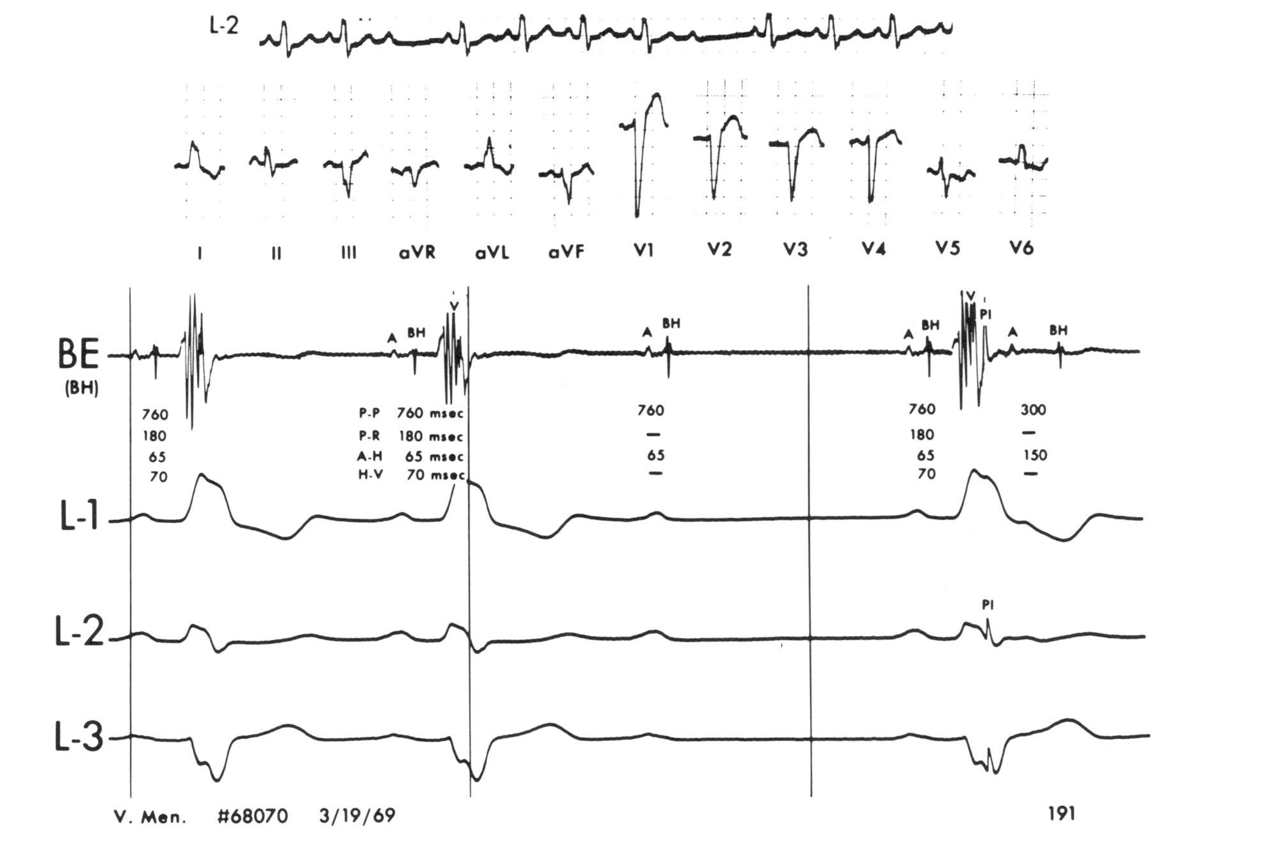

Figure 20–2. Mobitz type II block. Rhythm strip L-2 shows normal sinus rhythm, normal PR interval and intermittently nonconducted P-wave. Regular electrocardiogram demonstrates left bundle branch block. His bundle recording (BE) demonstrates a constant HV prolongation of 70 msec on all conducted P-waves. P-waves are blocked distal to the His bundle spike (BH).

blocks exist. Second-degree AV block can be of the Mobitz I or Mobitz II type. The criteria for main His bundle diseases are a wide His bundle deflection (≥ 25 msec), split His potentials or a prolonged HV time in a patient with a narrow QRS complex. Generally, prolongation of the His bundle conduction time without block cannot be suspected or diagnosed from the surface electrocardiogram and can only be established by His bundle studies. The prognosis of intraHis blocks is probably no different from that of infraHis blocks.

InfraHis blocks are commonly associated with sclerodegenerative disease of acute anterior wall myocardial infarction. The QRS complex is wide (≥ 12 sec). The HV time is either prolonged or block occurs distal to the His deflection. Second-degree AV block is usually of the Mobitz II type and on rare occasions Mobitz I type. The escape pacemaker is located either in the bundle branches or in the Purkinje system, hence the escape rate is low and the pacemaker is unreliable.

Management of Patients with AV Block (Table 20–2)

Patients with first-degree AV block require no therapy. The approach to patients with second- and third-degree AV block depends on their symptoms. All *symptomatic* patients with syncope, dizziness, congestive heart failure or low cardiac output are candidates for permanent cardiac pacing if the symptoms are thought to be related to the bradycardic rhythm. No conduction studies are needed for these patients. On the other hand, treatment of *asymptomatic* patients with second- and third-degree AV block has to be individualized. In general, we recommend permanent pacing for patients with heart rates persistently below 40/min, since they rarely remain asymptomatic for any length of time. In all other asymptomatic patients with second- and third-degree AV block, we attempt to base our decision for or against pacing on the site of the AV block. Patients with block localized to intraHis or infraHis sites are paced permanently. They have an increased risk of Stokes-Adams attacks or sudden death. Patients with second- and third-degree block localized to a supraHis site are followed clinically and not paced.

In selected patients, localization of the block can be made from the surface electrocardiogram. Demonstration of typical Mobitz II block indicates disease of the intraHis or infraHis system, regardless of QRS duration, and we recommend permanent pacing without conduction studies. In patients with narrow QRS, Mobitz type I or complete heart block and heart rates persistently above 50/min the block is most commonly supraHis, usually in the AV node. No pacing is needed for this group of patients as long as they are asymptomatic. In asymptomatic patients with second- and third-degree AV block, heart rates between

40–50/min and narrow or wide QRS, we cannot predict from the surface electrocardiogram with reasonable certainty where the block is located. These patients undergo electrophysiological studies. If supraHis block is demonstrated we elect to observe the patients. Patients with intraHis or infraHis block are permanently paced.

Table 20.2. Approach to Patients With Atrioventricular Block

First-degree AV block		No therapy
Second- and third-degree AV block		
	—if symptomatic from bradycardic rhythm ...	Permanent pacing
	—if heart rate remains persistently below 40 per minute ...	Permanent pacing
	—if there is demonstration of Mobitz type II block (usually intraHis or infraHis) ...	Permanent pacing
	—if heart rate is persistently above 50 per minute (block usually supraHis) ...	Observe
	—if asymptomatic with heart rates from 40–50 per minute regardless of QRS width ...	Conduction study
	∨	
	∨	
	—if block is intraHis or infraHis ...	Permanent pacing
	—if block is supraHis ...	Observe

Pseudo-Second-Degree AV Block (Figure 20-3)

In a rare patient, His bundle extrasystoles may simulate an ECG pattern of Mobitz type I or Mobitz type II block.[41–43] His bundle extrasystoles may exhibit antegrade block and may not produce a QRS complex. Retrogradely, however, they penetrate the AV node and collide with the subsequent normal P-wave, producing intermittent block of the P-wave or PR prolongation. An exact diagnosis can only be established with His bundle recordings. One may suspect His bundle extrasystole if the pattern of the blocked P-waves is not persistent, if both Mobitz II and Mobitz I patterns are seen on one tracing and at other times

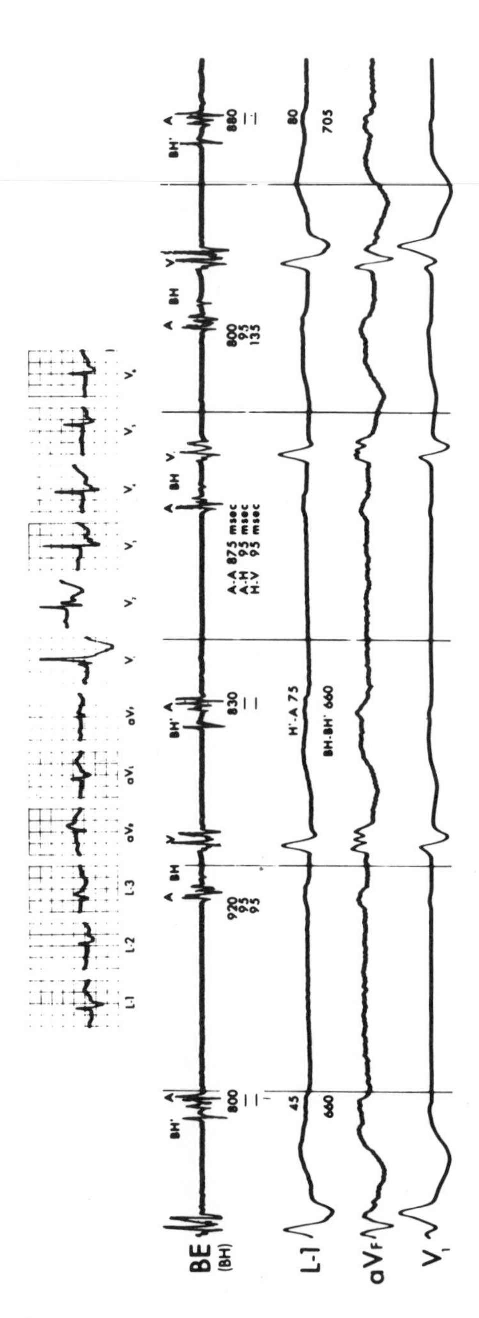

Figure 20–3. Pseudo-AV block due to His bundle premature beats. Intermittently, P-waves are not conducted because premature His beats interfere with their conduction through the AV node. The premature His beats cannot be seen on a regular cardiogram because they are blocked antegradely and therefore produce no QRS complex.

premature ventricular or junctional beats are seen. Therapy for these pseudoblocks is antiarrhythmic medication.[44] They may, however, be an indication of a diseased His-Purkinje system. The HV time is prolonged in many such patients.[45,46]

SINUS NODE DYSFUNCTION

The sick sinus syndrome is related to primary default of impulse formation in the sinus node, delay or block of conduction across the sinoatrial junction, or both. It encompasses sinus bradycardia, sinoatrial block, sinus arrest and the tachycardia-bradycardia syndrome.[47–50] Dizziness, syncope, weakness and, less often, congestive heart failure are the major symptoms associated with a diseased sinus node.[51,52] Sinus node disorders are estimated to account for 50 percent of permanent pacemakers implanted.[53]

Evaluation of Patients with Suspected Sinus Node Disease (Table 20-3)

Twenty-four hour monitoring is probably the most useful test in the initial evaluation of patients with suspected sick sinus syndrome. A normal sinus rhythm on a routine electrocardiogram does not exclude the possibility of a diseased sinus node. Electrocardiographic manifestations as well as symptoms are often intermittent. Recording of long pauses (> 2–2.5 sec) in a symptomatic patient is an indication for permanent pacing (Fig. 20-4). Recording of regular rhythm without bradycardia during episodes of dizziness or syncope excludes the diagnosis of sick sinus syndrome as the cause of this patient's symptoms. During prolonged electrocardiographic recording, the response of the sinus node to exercise and medications such as atropine and isoproterenol can also be evaluated. The response of the sinus node to carotid sinus massage is not necessarily a useful indication of the functional state of the sinus node. A prolonged episode of sinus arrest following carotid sinus massage is in our experience a nonspecific response. This is found in many elderly patients, and of course depends often on the intensity of the massage applied. Patients with the tachycardia-bradycardia syndrome may be symptomatic because of rapid supraventricular tachycardias, and not bradycardia. This can clearly be documented during continuous monitoring. If the rate during the bradycardic episode is not below 45 to 50/min, the only therapy necessary may be antiarrhythmic medication.

Electrophysiological Evaluation

Not infrequently, however, we encounter elderly patients with intermittent episodes of dizziness or syncope who show only sinus bradycardia

Table 20.3. Approach to Patients With the Sick Sinus Syndrome

I. Persistent sinus bradycardia <40/min (except in healthy athletes), regardless of symptoms.	>	Permanent pacing
II. Intermittent periods of sinus arrest or sinoatrial block >2.5–3 seconds, regardless of symptoms.	>	Permanent pacing

Symptomatic patients (dizziness or syncope) with only sinus bradycardia above 40/min on routine electrocardiogram undergo 24-hour monitoring and complete medical and neurological evaluation.

V

I. Symptoms during monitoring:		
A. Correlate with asystolic periods.	>	Permanent pacing
B. Rhythm remains normal or shows only moderate sinus bradycardia.	>	Look for other causes
C. Symptoms related to supraventricular or ventricular tachycardia.	>	Antiarrhythmics
II. No symptoms during monitoring:		
A. Substantial abnormalities are recorded (intermittent sinus bradycardia <40/min or periods of sinus arrest around 1.5–2 sec); therapy is individualized.	>	Permanent pacing—further monitoring—electrophysiological evaluation
B. Either normal sinus rhythm or moderate sinus bradycardia is recorded and no other cause for symptoms is found.	>	Electrophysiological evaluation* V V if normal → V → observe if abnormal → V → permanent pacing

*See text for details.

or short (1–1.5 sec) periods of asystole during monitoring and who remain asymptomatic during the monitoring period. Therefore, we have some suggestive evidence of a malfunctioning sinus node, but not enough evidence to make definite therapeutic recommendations. Electrophysiological study may be helpful in these situations.

The most useful and consistent test in the evaluation of the sinus node at our disposal is the corrected sinus node recovery time before and after the administration of atropine. The sinus node recovery time is the interval from the last paced beat to the first spontaneous sinus beat after one or two minutes of atrial pacing at rates varying from 100 to 150/min. The corrected sinus node recovery time is derived by deducting the prepacing sinus cycle length from the sinus node recovery time. The upper limit of normal in our laboratory for the corrected sinus node recovery time is 525 msec[54] (Fig. 20-5).

The overall accuracy of an abnormal corrected sinus node recovery time in predicting serious sinus node disease requiring pacemaker therapy was 92 percent for patients with sinus bradycardia and dizziness and 100

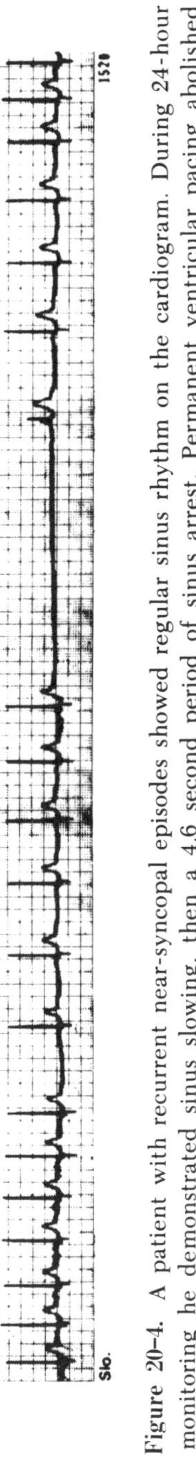

Figure 20-4. A patient with recurrent near-syncopal episodes showed regular sinus rhythm on the cardiogram. During 24-hour monitoring he demonstrated sinus slowing, then a 4.6 second period of sinus arrest. Permanent ventricular pacing abolished all symptoms.

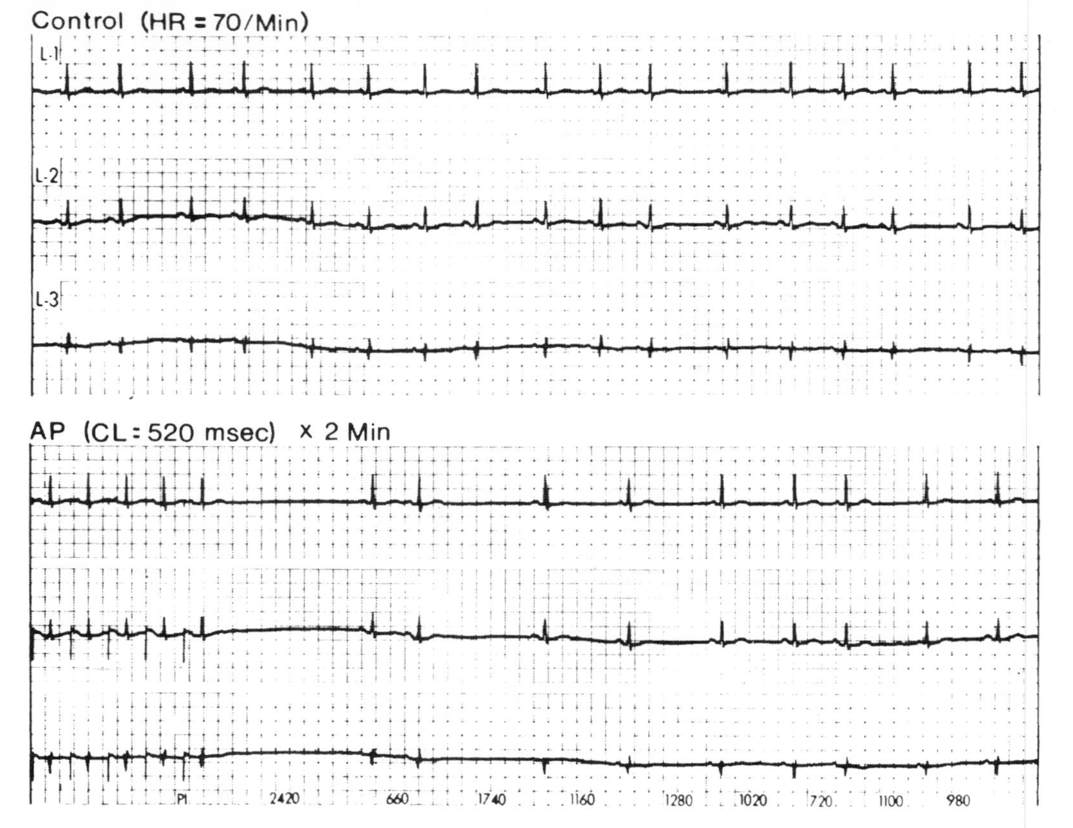

Figure 20–5. Recording of the sinus node recovery time. The control tracing with leads 1, 2 and 3 demonstrates normal sinus rhythm with sinus arrhythmia. Average heart rate is 70/min (cycle length 860 msec). The second tracing is recorded at the termination of atrial pacing (AP). The atrium is paced for 2 minutes at a cycle length of 520 msec, then pacing is abruptly stopped. The first sinus beat escapes only after 2420 msec. Deducting the 860 msec cycle length during control rhythm from

percent for patients with sinus bradycardia and syncope.[55] However, of 56 patients with sinus bradycardia and nonspecific findings on 24-hour monitoring who later proved to have definite sick sinus syndrome, only 37 (66%) had an abnormal sinus node recovery time.[55] Therefore, the test is very specific, but not very sensitive. Additional useful information can be obtained in individual patients by measuring the sinoatrial conduction time[56] or evaluating the first ten beats after cessation of atrial pacing.[57] Obtaining the intrinsic heart rate after paralysis of the sympathetic and parasympathetic system with propranolol and atropine is a new approach which needs further clinical evaluation.[58]

If syncopal attacks and dizzy spells remain unexplained after a thorough medical work-up including neurological evaluation, 24-hour monitoring and electrophysiological testing, permanent pacing is not indicated, and it is generally safe just to observe the patient. There will still be some patients who will subsequently demonstrate clearly diseased sinus nodes. However, patients with sinus node disease very rarely die or suffer irreversible damage during recurrent symptomatic episodes,[58,59] and approximately 50 percent of patients with unexplained syncope or dizziness have no recurrent symptoms at all. Therefore, it is justifiable to wait until a clear relationship between symptoms and bradycardia can be established before deciding to pace the patient permanently.

REFERENCES

1. Lenègre, J.: Les lesions du systeme de His-Tawara dans les blocs auriculo-ventriculairies d'un degre. *Cardiologia* **46**: 261–267, 1965.
2. Lev, M., and Bharati, S.: Atrioventricular and intraventricular conduction disease. *Arch. Intern. Med.* **135**: 405–410, 1975.
3. Lev, M.: Anatomic basis for atrioventricular block. *Am. J. Med.* **37**: 742–748, 1964.
4. Lev, M.: The pathology of complete atrioventricular block. *Prog. Cardiovasc. Dis.* **6**: 317–326, 1964.
5. Davies, M.I.: *Pathology of Conducting Tissue of the Heart.* New York, Appleton-Century-Crofts, 1971.
6. Rossi, L.: *Histopathologic Features of Cardiac Arrhythmias.* Milan, Casa Editrice Ambrosiana, 1969.
7. Knieriem, J.H., and Effert S.: Morphologische Befunde beim kompletten Herzblock. *Klin. Wochenschr.* **44**: 349–360, 1966.
8. Harper, J.R., Harley, A., Jackel, D.B., et al.: Coronary artery disease and major conduction disturbances: A pathological study designed to correlate abnormalities with electrocardiogram. *Am. Heart. J.* **77**: 411–422, 1969.
9. Lev, M., Kinare, S.G., and Pick, A.: The pathogenesis of atrioventricular block in coronary disease. *Circulation* **42**: 409–425, 1970.
10. James, T.N.: The coronary circulation and conduction system in acute myocardial infarction. *Prog. Cardiovasc. Dis.* **10**: 410–449, 1968.

11. Lev, M.: The pathology of atrioventricular block. *Cardiovasc. Clin.* **4**: 159–186, 1972.
12. Hunt, D., Lie, J.T., Vohra, J., et al.: Histopathology of heart block complicating acute myocardial infarction. *Circulation* **48**: 1252–1261, 1973.
13. Rosenbaum, M.B., Elizari, M.V., and Lazzari, J.O.: The hemiblocs. Oldsmar, *Tampa Tracings*, 1970.
14. Rosenbaum, M.B., Elizari, M.V., Lazzari, J.O., et al.: Intraventricular trifascicular blocks. Review of the literature and classification. *Am. Heart J.* **78**: 450–459, 1969.
15. Definitions of terms related to cardiac rhythm. World Health Organization ISFC Task Force. *Eur. J. Cardiol.* **8**: 127–144, 1978.
16. Lasser, R.P., Haft, J.I., and Friedberg, C.K.: Relationship of right bundle branch block and marked left axis deviation (with left parietal or periinfarction block) to complete heart block and syncope. *Circulation* **37**: 429–437, 1968.
17. Scanlon, R.J., Pryor, R., and Blount, S.G.: Right bundle branch block associated with left superior or inferior intraventricular block. Clinical setting, prognosis and relation to complete heart block. *Circulation* **42**: 1123–1133, 1970.
18. Watt, T.B., and Pruitt, R.D.: Character, cause and consequence of combined left axis deviation and right bundle branch block in human electrocardiograms. *Am. Heart. J.* **77**: 460–465, 1969.
19. Narula, O.S., Sherlag, B.J., Samet, P., et al.: Atrioventricular block. Localization and classification by His bundle recording. *Am. J. Med.* **50**: 146–165, 1971.
20. Scherlag, B.J., Lau, S.H., Helfant, R.H., et al.: Catheter technique for recording His bundle activity in man. *Circulation* **39**: 13, 1969.
21. Narula, O.S., Cohen, L.S., Samet, P., et al.: Localization of A-V conduction defects in man by recording of the His bundle electrogram. *Am. J. Cardiol.* **25**: 228–235, 1970.
22. Denes, P., Dhingra, R.C., Wu, D., et al.: H-V interval in patients with bifascicular block (right bundle branch block and left anterior hemiblock): clinical, electrocardiographic and electrophysiologic correlations. *Am. J. Cardiol.* **35**: 23–29, 1975.
23. Narula, O.S.: Intraventricular conduction defects. In Narula, O.S. (ed.): *His Bundle Electrocardiography and Clinical Electrophysiology.* Philadelphia, F.A. Davis Co., 1975, p. 177.
24. Narula, O.S., Gann, D., and Samet, P.: Prognostic value of HV intervals. In Narula, O.S. (ed.): *His Bundle Electrocardiography and Clinical Electrophysiology.* Philadelphia, F.A. Davis Co., 1975, p. 437.
25. Scheinman, M.M., Peters, R.W., Modin, G., et al.: Prognostic value of infranodal conduction time in patients with chronic bundle branch block. *Circulation* **56**: 240–244, 1977.
26. Gupta, P.K., Lichstein, E., Chadda, K.D., et al.: Follow-up studies in patients with right bundle branch block and left anterior hemiblock. Significance of H-V interval. *J. Electrocardiol.* **10**: 221–224, 1977.

27. Altschuler, H., Fisher, J.D., and Furman, S.: Prolonged H-V interval: preventable early mortality in symptomatic patients with documented heart block (abstract). *Clin. Res.* **25**: 203A, 1977.
28. Altschuler, H., Fisher, J.D., and Furman, S.: Significance of isolated HV interval prolongation in symptomatic patients without documented heart block. *Am. Heart J.* **97**: 19–26, 1979.
29. Dhingra, R.C., Denes, P., Wu, D., et al.: Chronic right bundle branch block and left posterior hemiblock. Clinical, electrophysiologic and prognostic observations. *Am. J. Cardiol.* **36**: 867, 1975.
30. Dhingra, R.C., Denes, P.,Wu, D., et al.: Prospective observations in patients with chronic bundle branch block and marked H-V prolongation. *Circulation* **53**: 600–604, 1976.
31. McAnulty, J.H., Rahimtoola, S.H., Murphy, E.D., et al.: A prospective study of sudden death in "high risk" bundle branch block. *N. Eng. J. Med.* **299**: 209–216, 1978.
32. Vera, Z., Mason, D.T., Fletcher, R.D., et al.: Prolonged His-Q interval in chronic bifascicular block. Relation to impending complete heart block. *Circulation* **53**: 46–55, 1976.
33. Gupta, P.K., Lichstein, E., and Chadda, K.D.: Intraventricular conduction time (H-V interval) during antegrade conduction in patients with heart block. *Am. J. Cardiol.* **32**: 27–31, 1973.
34. Scheinman, M., Weiss, A., and Kunkel, F.: His bundle recordings in patients with bundle branch block and transient neurologic symptoms. *Circulation* **48**: 322–330, 1973.
35. Narula, O.S., Runge, M., and Samet, P.: Second-degree Wenckebach type AV block due to block within the atrium. *Br. Heart. J.* **34**: 1127–1136, 1972.
36. Rosen, K.M., Gunnar, R.M., and Rahimtoola, S.H.: Site and type of second-degree A-V block. *Chest* **61**: 99–100, 1972.
37. Rosen, K.M., Dhingra, R.C., Loeb, H.S., et al.: Chronic heart block in adults. Clinical and electrophysiological observations. *Arch. Intern. Med.* **131**: 663–672, 1973.
38. Dhingra, R.C., Denes, P., Wu, D., et al: The significance of second-degree atrioventricular block and bundle branch block: observations regarding site and type of block. *Circulation* **49**: 638–646, 1974.
39. Narula, O.S.: Wenckebach type I and II atrioventricular block (revisited). *Cardiovasc. Clin.* **6**: 137–167, 1974.
40. Narula, O.S., Scherlag, B.J., Javier, R.P., et al.: Analysis of the A-V conduction defect in complete heart block utilizing His bundle electrograms. *Circulation* **41**: 437–448, 1970.
41. Narula, O.S.: Conduction disorders in the A-V transmission system. In Dreifus, L.S., and Likoss, W. (eds.): *Cardiac Arrhythmias.* 25th Annual Hahnemann Symposium. New York, Grune & Stratton, 1973, p. 259.
42. Eugster, G.S., Godfrey, C.C., Braumell, H.L., et al.: Pseudo A-V block associated with AH and HV conduction defects. *Am. Heart J.* **85**: 789–796, 1973.

43. Cannom, D.S., Gallagher, J.J., Goldreyer, B.N., et al.: Concealed bundle of His extrasystoles simulating non-conducted atrial premature beats. *Am. Heart J.* **83**: 777–779, 1972.
44. Rosen, K.M., Rahimtoola, S.H., and Gunnar, R.M.: Pseudo A-V block secondary to premature nonpropagated His bundle depolarization: documentation by His bundle electrocardiography. *Circulation* **42**: 367–373, 1970.
45. Narula, O.S.: Current concepts of atrioventricular block. In Narula, O.S. (ed.): *His Bundle Electrocardiography and Clinical Electrophysiology.* Philadelphia, F.A. Davis Co., 1975, p. 139.
46. Grolleau, R., Peuch, P., Latour, H., et al.: Les dépolarisations hisiennes ectopiques non propagées. *Arch. Mal. Coeur* **65**: 1069–1080, 1972.
47. Imperial, E.S., Carballo, R., and Zimmerman, H.A.: Disturbance of rate, rhythm and conduction in acute myocardial infarction: A statistical study of 153 cases. *Am. J. Cardiol.* **5**: 24–29, 1960.
48. Ferrer, M.I.: The sick sinus syndrome. *Circulation* **47**: 635–641, 1973.
49. Reiffel, J.A., Bigger, J.T., Cramer, M., et al.: Ability of Holter electrocardiographic recording and atrial stimulation to detect sinus nodal dysfunction in symptomatic and asymptomatic patients with sinus bradycardia. *Am. J. Cardiol.* **40**: 189–194, 1977.
50. Ferrer, M.I.: The sick sinus syndrome in atrial disease. *J.A.M.A.* **206**: 645–646, 1968.
51. Bower, P.J.: Sick sinus syndrome. *Arch. Intern. Med.* **138**: 133–137, 1978.
52. Kaplan, B.M.: The tachycardia-bradycardia syndrome. *Med. Clin. N. Am.* **60**: 81–89, 1976.
53. Kaplan, B.M.: Sick sinus syndrome (editorial). *Arch. Intern. Med.* **138**: 28, 1978.
54. Narula, O.S., Samet, P., and Javier, R.P.: Significance of the sinus-node recovery time. *Circulation* **45**: 140–158, 1972.
55. Gann, D., Tolentino, A., and Samet, P.: Electrophysiological evaluation of elderly patients with sinus bradycardia. A long-term followup study. *Ann. Intern. Med.* **90**: 24–29, 1979.
56. Strauss, H.C., Bigger, J.T., Jr., Saroff, A.L., and Giardina, E.G.V.: Electrophysiologic evaluation of sinus node function in patients with sinus node dysfunction. *Circulation* **53**: 763–776, 1976.
57. Benditt, D.G., Strauss, H.C., Scheinman, M.M., et al.: Analysis of secondary pauses following termination of rapid atrial pacing in man. *Circulation* **54**: 436–441, 1976.
58. Jordan, J.L., Yamaguchi, I., and Mandel, W.J.: Studies on the mechanism of sinus node dysfunction in the sick sinus syndrome. *Circulation* **57**: 217–223, 1978.
59. Gann, D., Rahman, E., and Samet, P.: Electrophysiological evaluation in patients with unexplained syncope. Follow-up study. Submitted for publication.

21

Atrioventricular Sequential Demand Pacing for Treatment of Arrhythmias

B. V. Berkovits, F.A.C.C.

Electrical stimulation of the heart is now a therapeutic choice for disorders of impulse generation and transmission in the cardiac conduction system. Pacemaker stimuli may be applied in the atria, in the ventricles or in both chambers. Ventricular stimulation has been the method chiefly used to sustain heart action in patients with asystole of various forms.

However, current indications for pacemaker therapy make it important that for both hemodynamic and electrophysiologic reasons, the proper sequence of atrial and ventricular depolarizations be preserved. Proper AV synchrony provides regularized ventricular filling and increased cardiac output,[1–3] reduces oxygen need of the heart,[4] and affords protection against some arrhythmias[5,6] and against retrograde conduction.[7–9]

As early as 1916, Gesell[10] wrote that "auricular systole increased ventricular output about 50% over that maintained by venous pressure alone." After the advent of artificial pacing in the early 1960's, there was increased interest in understanding the hemodynamic role of atrial contraction. A number of studies,[1,11–14] were reported strengthening and amplifying such reports as Gesell's. It has been shown that atrial contribution with proper AV timing may, in patients with failing heart, increase cardiac output up to 30 percent.[2,3]

APPLICATIONS

In patients with acute myocardial infarction, DeSanctis[3] has reported increased cardiac output with AV sequential pacing compared to ventricular pacing (Fig. 21-1).

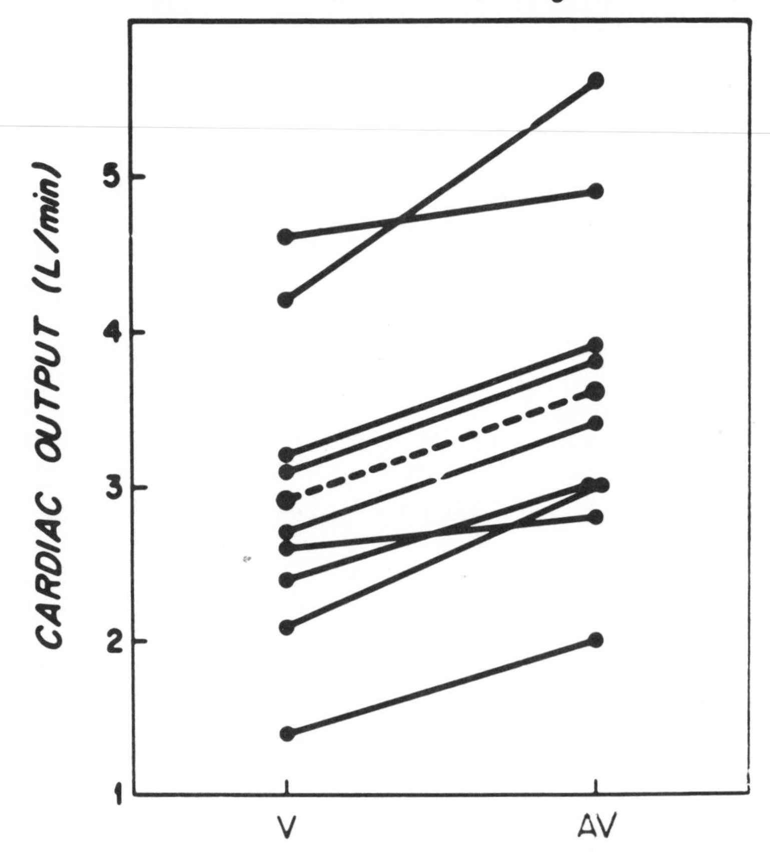

Figure 21-1. Increase of cardiac output with AV sequential pacing. (Courtesy of Dr. Roman DeSanctis)

Sharma and co-workers[4] found that when stimulating at the same heart rate the myocardial oxygen consumption was about 15 percent higher with ventricular pacing than with atrial pacing.

Irregular filling of the ventricles caused by atrioventricular dissociation can result in beat-to-beat variations of arterial blood pressure (Fig. 21-2 *A*).

These variations in arterial pressure and the cannon waves caused by atrial contraction against closed AV valves are sometimes observed by the patient as palpitations. This so-called "pacemaker syndrome" is eliminated by sequential pacing (Fig. 21-2 *B*). Alicandri et al.[15] reported

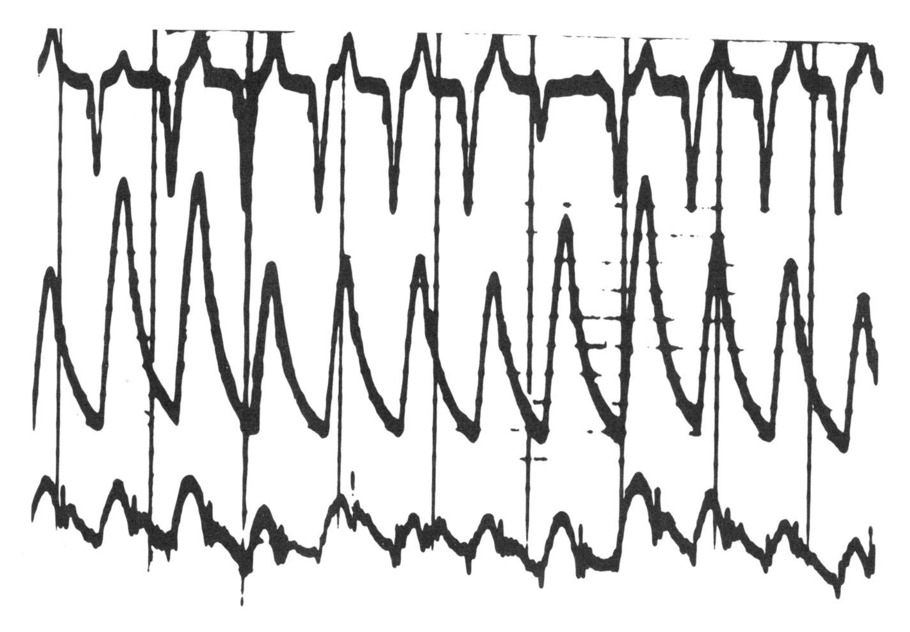

Figure 21-2. Pressure tracings: *A*, ventricular pacing.

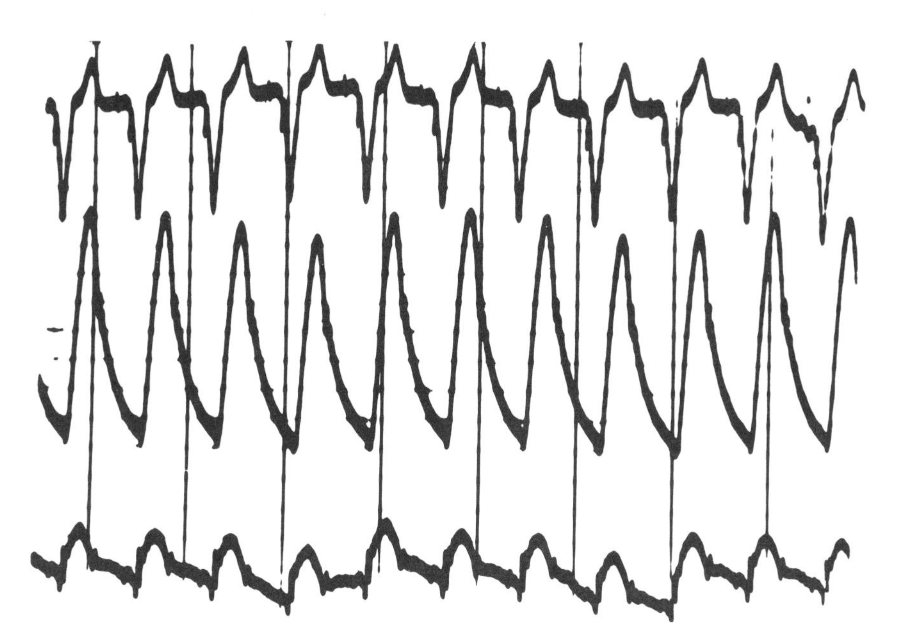

Figure 21-2. *(Continued). B,* sequential pacing. (Courtesy of Dr. Victor Parsonnet)

on three patients in whom significant postural hypotension occurred, sometimes resulting in syncope, when atrial-ventricular dissociation was induced by ventricular pacing. They suggested that this complication may have been accentuated by a reflex from the sudden atrial distention that occurs during AV dissociation.

Atrial pacing can be used to preserve AV synchrony when electrophysiologic studies assure that AV conduction is intact. This provides the benefit of AV synchrony and normal ventricular depolarization but affords no protection if an AV block develops later.

METHODOLOGY

The AV sequential demand (bifocal) pacemaker has been developed to combine the benefits of atrial, ventricular, and sequential pacing without their limitations. It automatically adapts to the patient's needs. It may be totally dormant, stimulate only the atria, or stimulate both the atria and ventricles with a preset sequence. Technically, the AV sequential demand pacemaker consists of two demand units, (Fig. 21-3): a conventional QRS-inhibited ventricular demand pacemaker and a QRS-inhibited atrial demand pacemaker. Both of these units are in a single package sharing the battery and the QRS detecting circuit. They act in synchrony and provide QRS-inhibited AV sequential stimulation.

Figure 21-4 illustrates how the AV sequential demand pacemaker operates under various clinical conditions.

It is to be emphasized that intrinsic atrial activity has no effect on the operation of the pulse generator. Sensing is done only in the ventricle, thus avoiding the difficulties found in the past with systems requiring atrial sensing.

Figure 21-5 shows ECG tracings from a patient with an AV sequential demand pacemaker, illustrating clearly the various modes of operation of this pacemaker as it adapts to variations in the patient's spontaneous rhythm.

AV sequential pacing has been successfully used for treatment of bradycardia-related heart failure with or without AV block, sick sinus syndrome, bradytachyarrhythmias, some reentry tachycardias, and to suppress by overdrive pacing ectopic activity or tachycardia in either chamber.

In patients with heart failure brought on by bradycardia, the sequential pacer improves cardiac output not only by increasing heart rate but also by maintaining proper AV synchrony. Nager and Kappenberger[16] reported in many patients disappointing long-term hemodynamic results with ventricular pacemaker therapy. They state that prevention of AV dissociation by use of atrial-triggered or bifocal pacing could improve

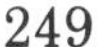

DEMAND PACEMAKER

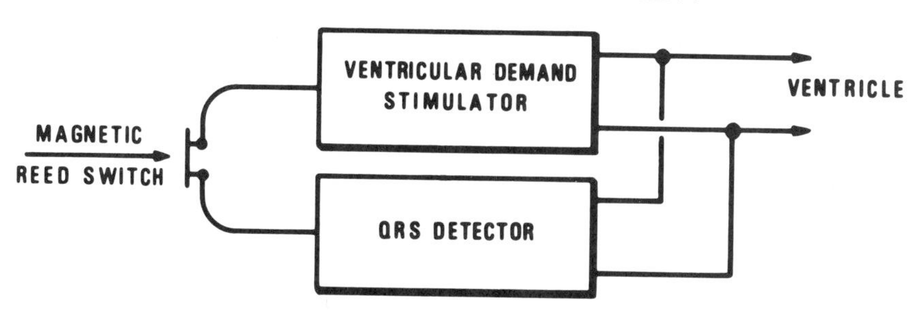

BIFOCAL DEMAND PACEMAKER

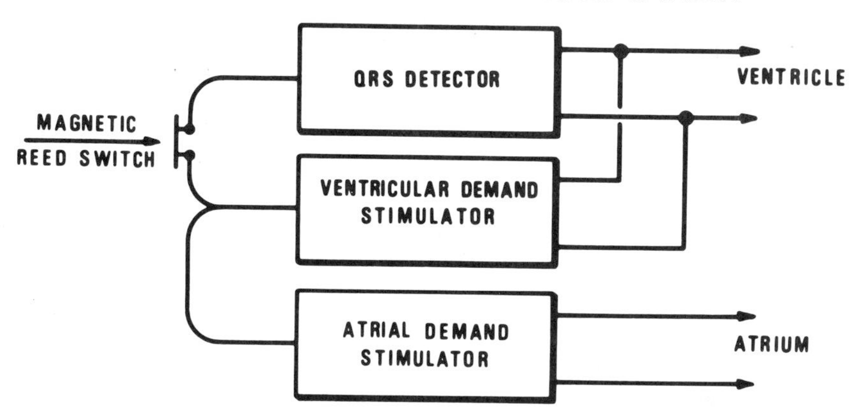

Figure 21-3. Block diagram of demand and AV sequential demand (bifocal) pacemakers.

hemodynamics for these patients. They predict that these modalities will certainly be the first choice for pacing patients with heart failure in the future.

OTHER APPLICATIONS

While the original indication for use of the AV sequential demand pacemaker was the need to improve cardiac output, today this modality is also used for the treatment of various arrhythmias. One estimate[17] is that 40 percent of present pacemaker implantations are for sick sinus syndrome. Moss and Davis[18] wrote that management of such patients is a "formidable therapeutic challenge" and Bower[19] reported that "drug therapy alone has been uniformly unsuccessful." Fields et al.[7] reported on successful treatment of sick sinus syndrome by AV sequential pacing in

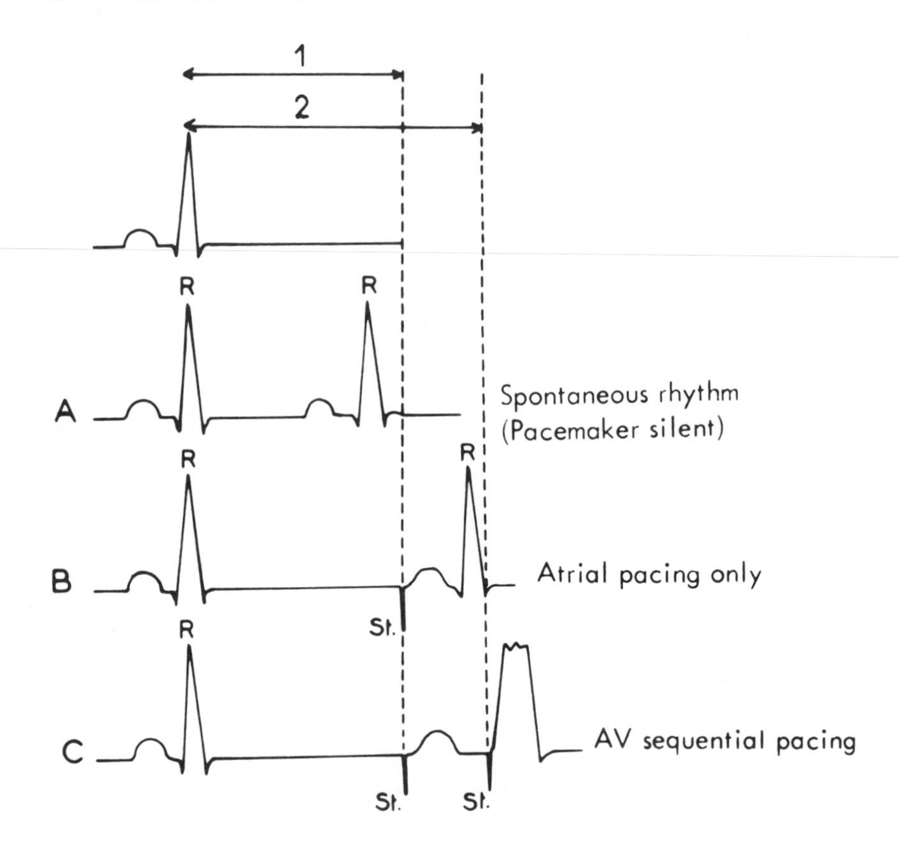

Figure 21-4. Modes of operation of the AV sequential demand pacemaker.

A. When the patient's spontaneous R to R interval is shorter than the atrial escape interval of the pulse generator both atrial and ventricular outputs are inhibited by the sensed ventricular depolarization, and the unit produces no stimuli (inhibited mode).

B. When the R to R interval exceeds the pulse generator atrial escape interval, an atrial output pulse is emitted. If the patient's PR interval is shorter than the pulse generator AV sequential interval, the conducted R-wave will inhibit the generator's ventricular stimulus and only the atria will have been stimulated.

C. After an atrial output pulse, if the patient's PR interval exceeds the pulse generator AV sequential interval, a ventricular output pulse will also be emitted (AV sequential pacing mode). (Courtesy of Dr. S. Levy)

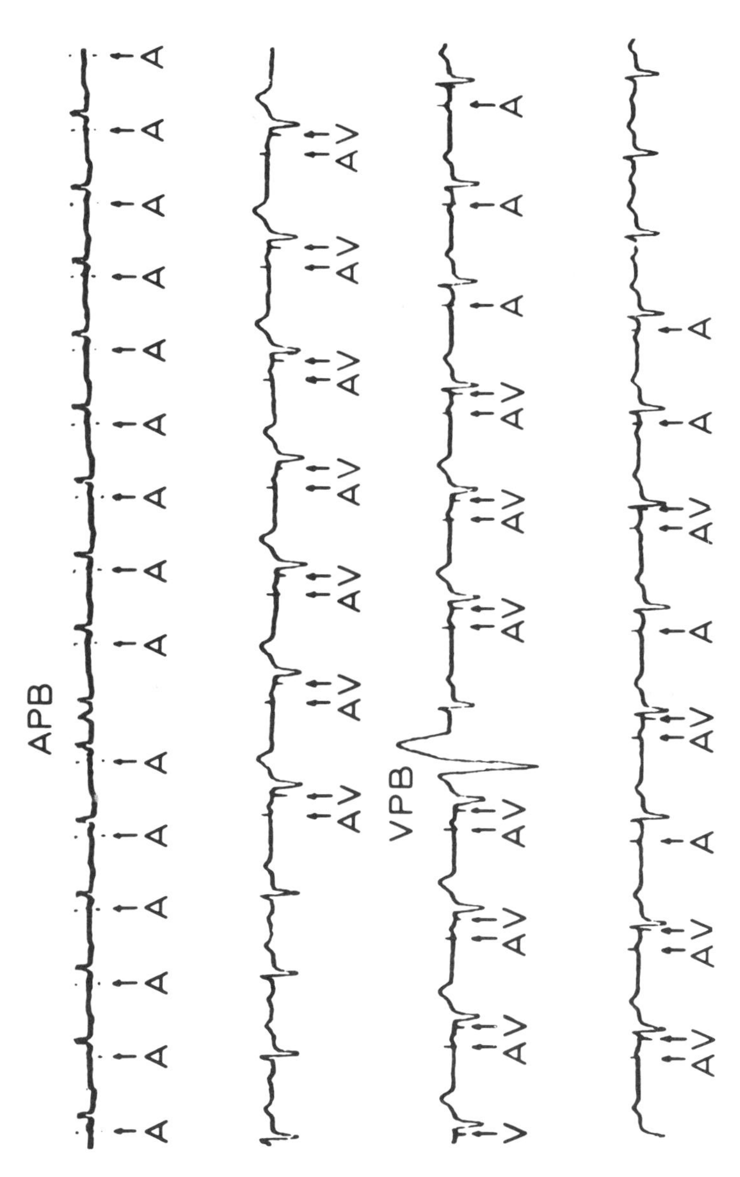

Figure 21-5. ECG tracings with AV sequential demand pacemaker.

42 patients. In some of these patients with brady-tachyarrhythmias, antiarrhythmic drugs have been progressively discontinued two to three months after implantation. The atrial stimulation not only protected against the bradycardia but also suppresses the episodes of tachycardia. Since sick sinus syndrome patients are especially sensitive to atrial contribution to ventricular filling,[20] the AV sequential demand pacer fills a major need in therapy for this group of patients. Radford and Julian[21] wrote that for sick sinus syndrome "the theoretically ideal method of pacing is with a sequential atrioventricular demand system."

Bifocal pacing facilitates the treatment of some tachyarrhythmias by suppressing both atrial and ventricular ectopic foci, by entering and blocking the reentry loop, by improving the hemodynamic function and by protecting against prolongation of the PR interval.

Experimental studies[22] found that reversed sequence (VA activation) causes greater reduction of blood pressure and cardiac output than random atrial activation (AV dissociation) or atrial flutter-fibrillation. Witz[9] observed retrograde stimulation occurring during ventricular pacing and found that reestablishing AV synchrony by AV sequential demand pacing appreciably improved hemodynamics. He found that this was particularly true for patients with myocardial infarction accompanied by left ventricular insufficiency, and states that for such patients the restoration of AV synchrony is necessary and should "perhaps finally improve the prognosis." Retrograde conduction was reported by Rost et al.[8] to occur in 90 percent of a group of pacer patients with intact AV conduction and in one-third of a group with AV block. In their reported experience bifocal stimulation prevented the retrograde activation of the atria.

For overdrive suppression of tachyarrhythmias, sequential pacing is more effective than ventricular pacing because at these high pacing rates the benefits of atrial contribution to cardiac output are especially significant and conduction at the AV junction is less reliable.

For temporary pacing following cardiac surgery, Curtis et al.[23] prefer atrial or AV sequential demand over ventricular pacing because of the significantly increased cardiac output. This preference was also expressed in two other reports.[24,25]

Equipment

Figure 21-7 shows a 6-pole catheter for temporary transvenous pacing. It provides two distal electrodes for ventricular stimulation and four proximal electrodes for atrial stimulation. The use of this catheter was first described by Castellanos et al.[26] They chose an appropriate vein in the upper torso and placed the ventricular electrodes in the accustomed

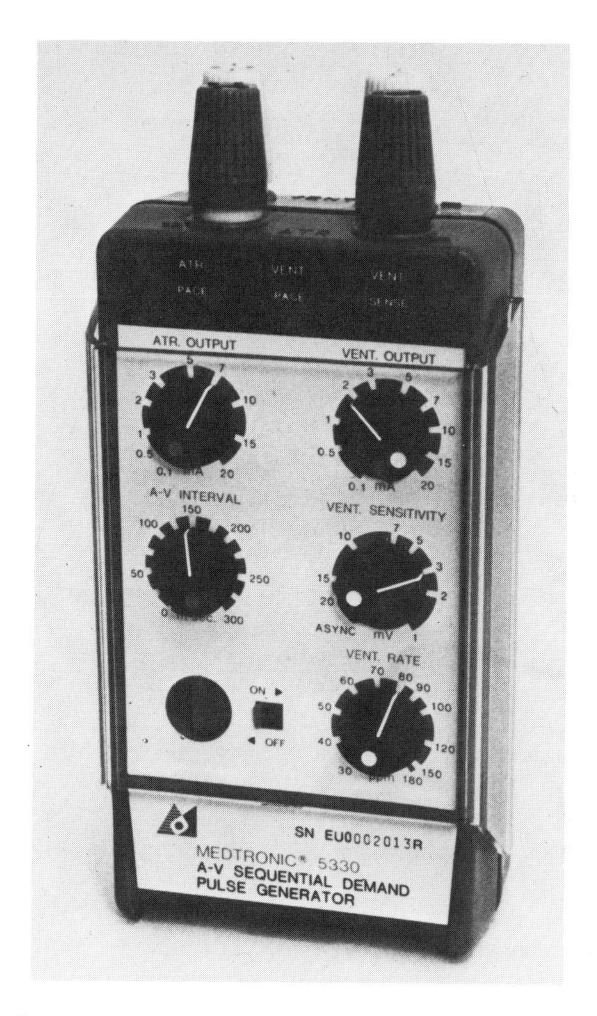

Figure 21-6. External AV sequential demand pacemaker used for temporary pacing.

manner under fluoroscopic control. To assure proper placement of the distal electrodes in the right ventricle, they made sure that the ventricular stimulation threshold was less than 1 mA and a bipolar intraventricular electrogram of more than 6 mV was measured. Then they tested the four proximal electrodes for atrial stimulation threshold and chose that pair with the lowest threshold.

Figure 21-9 shows an implantable, non-invasively programmable sequential pacemaker (Medtronic, Inc., Model 5992) with its external pro-

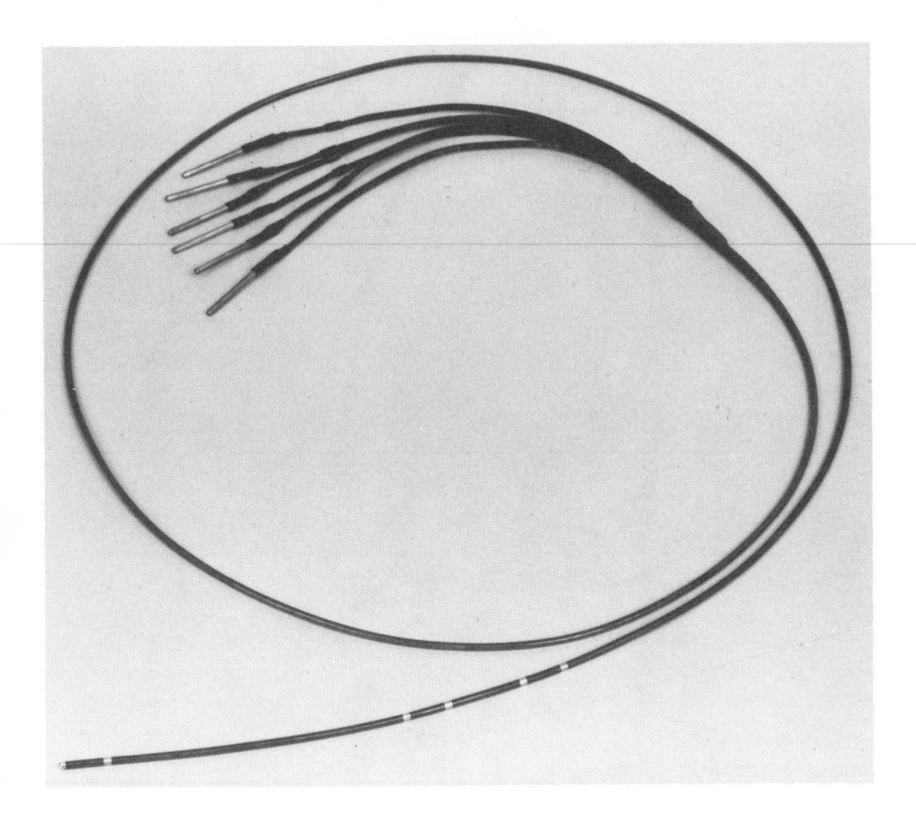

Figure 21-7. Hexapolar catheter for use in temporary AV sequential demand pacing. (Made by USCI, Model 004178)

grammer (Medtronic, Inc., Model 9600). The parameters of this unit are noninvasively selected after implantation to accomodate the patient's condition.

A number of myocardial and endocardial electrodes are now available for permanent sequential pacing. For transvenous pacing, two bipolar leads are used, one placed in the right ventricular apex, the other in the right atrial appendage or in the coronary sinus. One of the J-leads is shown in Figure 27-10.

The use of J-leads has been described by Zucker et al.[27] The atrial J-lead is introduced with its stiffening stylet until the tip lies in the distal right atrium just above the inferior vena cava. The stylet is withdrawn and a little manipulation will cause the J-curve to reset itself with the tip pointing cephalad. The lead is next pulled upward, with the tip of the J anterior and slightly to the left, until it enters and becomes lodged in the atrial appendage, and the J-loop has begun to straighten out slightly. Proper positioning of the lead is confirmed by the swaying of the tip from

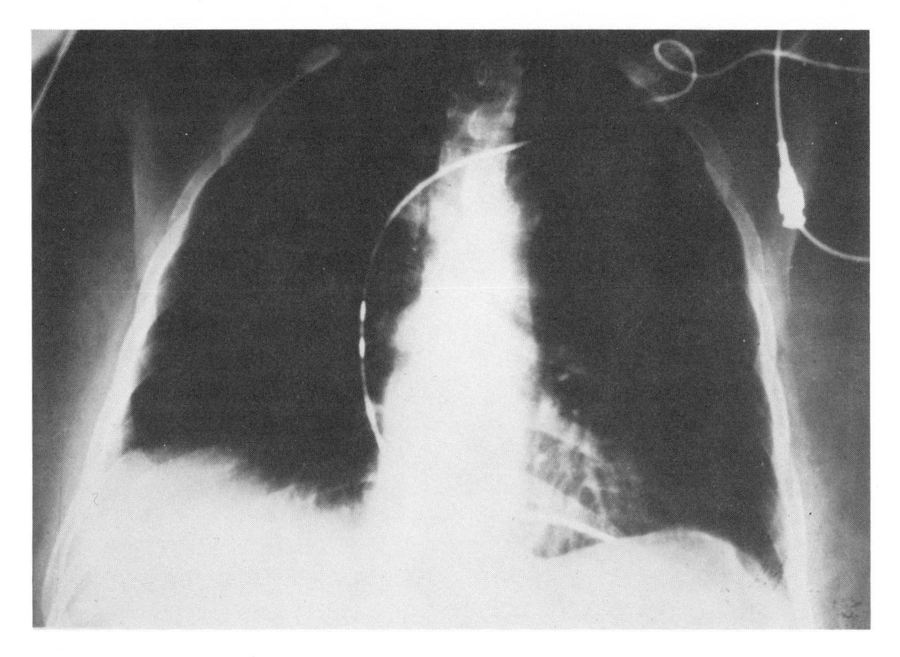

Figure 21–8. Anteroposterior x-ray view showing the sextapolar catheter properly positioned in the heart to achieve sequential atrioventricular pacing.

side to side with each atrial contraction (Fig. 21-11). In the case of no spontaneous atrial activity, movement can be produced by stimulation of the atria through the electrode.

Excitation thresholds are then measured. Acute thresholds in the atrial appendage are found to be higher than in the ventricle; usually they are from 1.5 to 2.0 milliamperes.

When pacer implantation is completed, posteroanterior and lateral chest x-rays are made to confirm the proper anatomical position; these should show the tips to be far anterior (Fig. 21-12).

In general the results with atrial J-electrodes have been better than anticipated. One report[7] of 49 permanent implants with atrial J-leads states that only three early and one late repositionings were necessary. In another set of 12 patients[28] no complications were reported with the atrial electrodes. With these J-electrodes, there will surely be increased use of the new smaller, lighter, lithium-powered, noninvasively programmable sequential pacemakers.

SUMMARY

Pacing therapy has undergone marked changes during its relatively brief existence; electrical pacemakers have become a common and accepted method of therapy for many bradyarrhythmias. Management of sick sinus syndrome and tachydysrhythmias by pacing has increased in recent times and may be expected to continue to grow in the future.

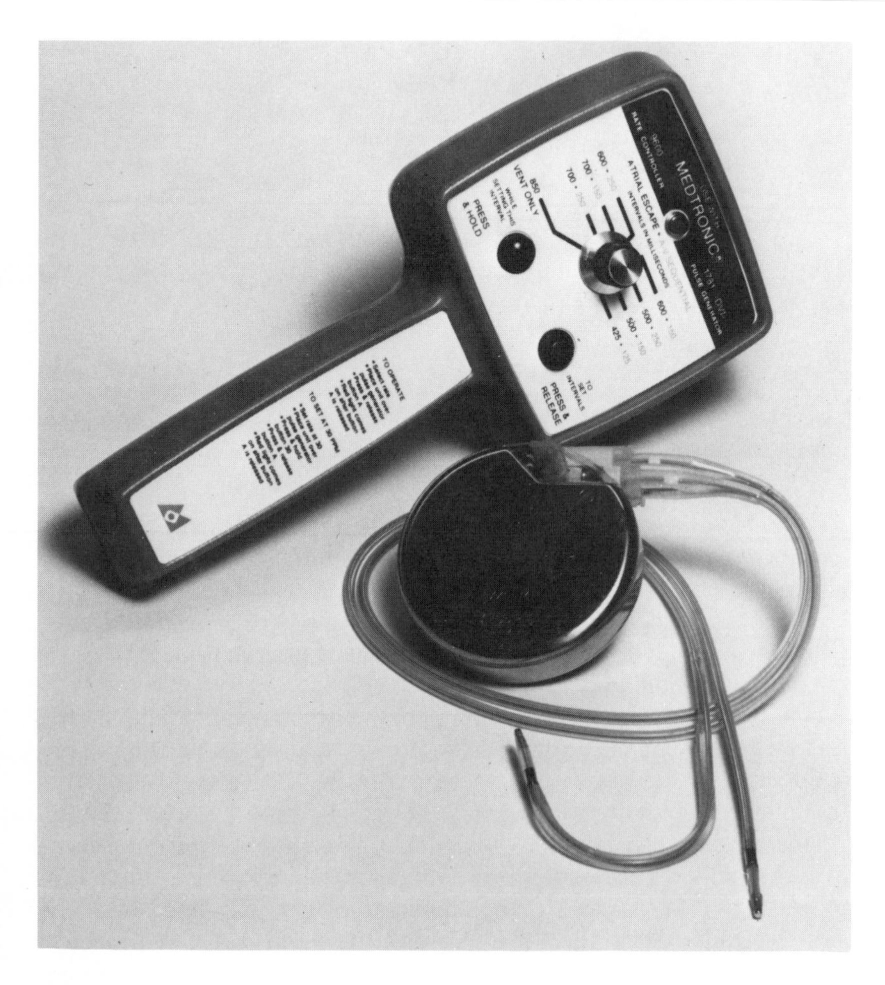

Figure 21–9. Implantable bifocal pacemaker with programmer.

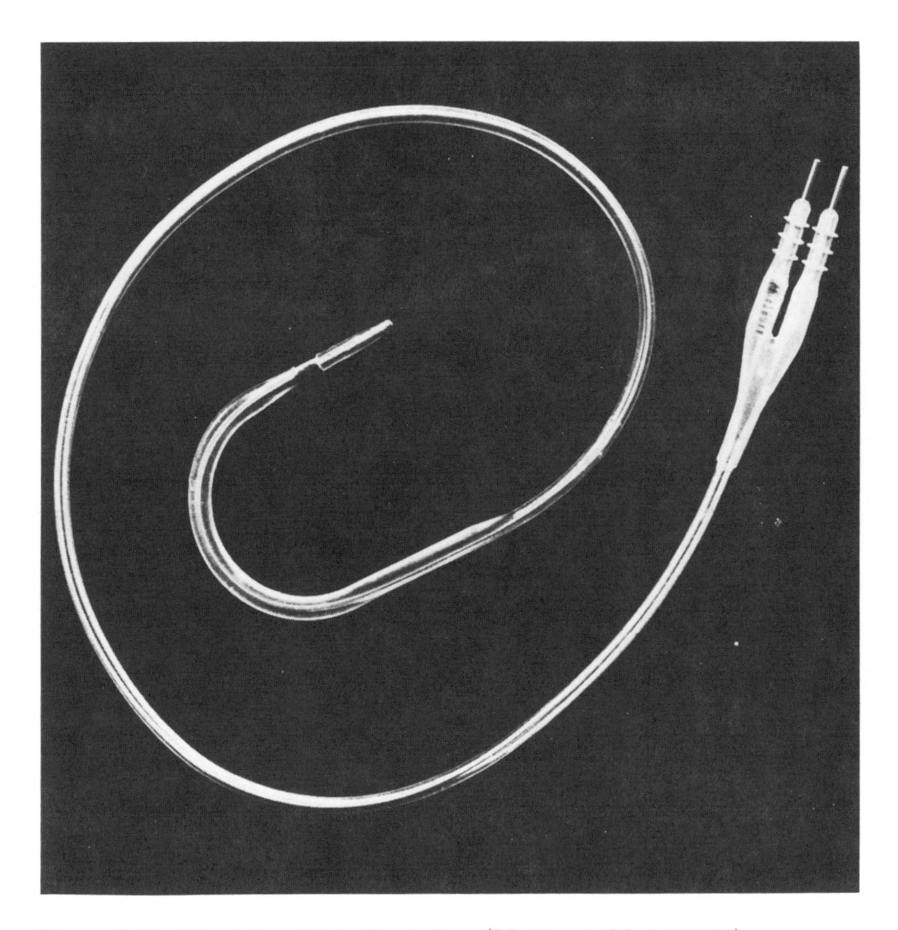

Figure 21-10. J-lead for atrial stimulation. (Medtronic Model 6994)

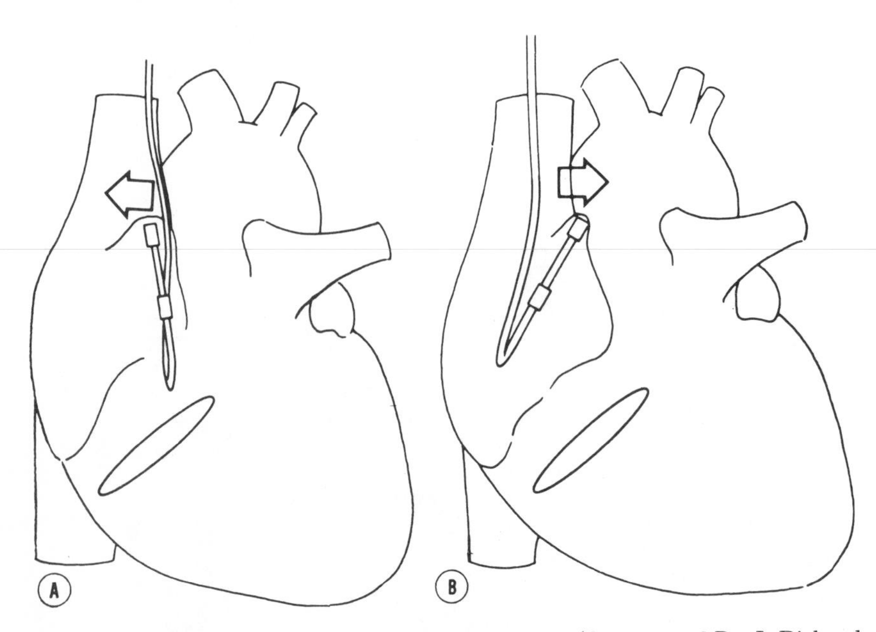

Figure 21-11. Diagram of J-electrode tip movement. (Courtesy of Dr. I. Richard Zucker)

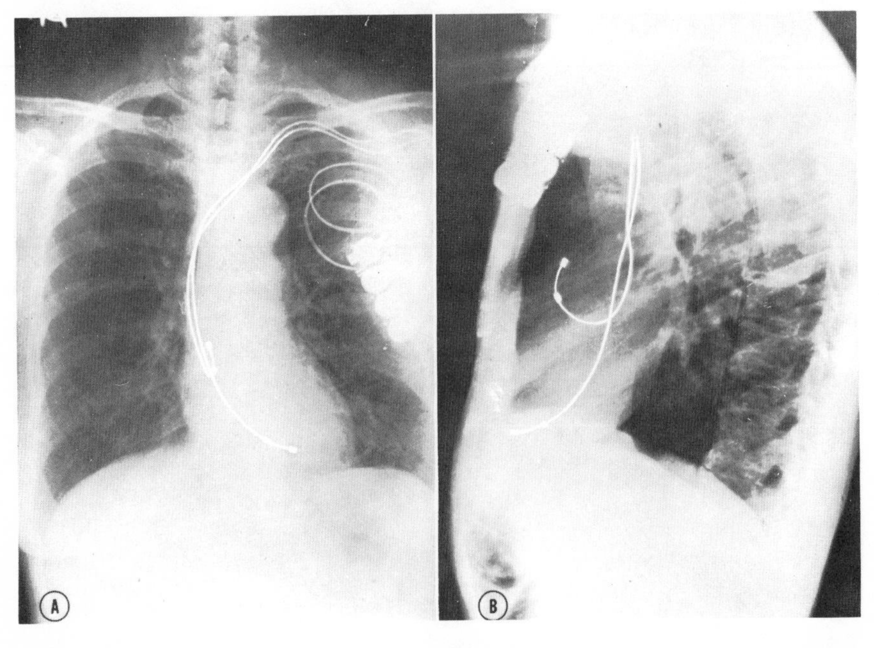

Figure 21-12. Posteroanterior (*A*) and lateral (*B*) x-rays of the chest of a patient with a transvenously implanted AV sequential demand pacemaker. (The films have been retouched for illustrative clarity.) (Courtesy of Dr. I. Richard Zucker)

REFERENCES

1. Gilmore, J.P., Sarnoff, S.J., Mitchell, J.H., and Linden, R.J.: Synchronicity of ventricular contraction: Observations comparing hemodynamic effects of atrial and ventricular pacing. *Br. Heart J.* **25**: 299–307, 1963.
2. Samet, P., Castillo, C., and Bernstein, W.H.: Hemodynamic sequelae of atrial, ventricular, and sequential atrioventricular pacing in cardiac patients. *Am. Heart J.* **72**: 725–729, 1966.
3. DeSanctis, R.W.: Diagnostic and Therapeutic Uses of Atrial Pacing (Lecture). American Heart Association, 43rd Scientific Sessions, Atlantic City, N.J., November 13, 1970. Published as Audio-Visual Aid EM-529 by American Heart Association.
4. Sharma, G.V.R., Kumar, R., Molokhia, F., et al.: Oxygen cost of atrial and ventricular pacing in the intact conscious dog, III-58. Supplement III (Abstracts) to *Circulation* **41, 42**: 285, 1970.
5. Heiman, D.F., and Helwig, J., Jr.: Suppression of ventricular arrhythmias by transvenous intracardiac pacing. *J.A.M.A.* **195**: 172–175, 1966.
6. Zipes, D.P., Festoff, B., Schaal, S.F., et al.: Treatment of ventricular arrhythmia by permanent atrial pacemaker and cardiac sympathectomy. *Ann. Intern. Med.* **68**: 591–597, 1968.
7. Fields, J., Berkovits, B.V., and Matloff, J.M.: Surgical experience with temporary and permanent A-V sequential demand pacing. *J. Thorac. Cardiovasc. Surg.* **66**: 865–877, 1973.
8. Rost, W., Gattenhohner, W., Schneider, K.W., and Stegmann, N.: Untersuchungen zum hemodynamischen Effekt der Ventrikularen, Atrialen und bifokalen Stimulation. *Intensivmedizin* **11**: 72–78, 1973.
9. Witz, F.: Le Role Hemodynamique de la Systole Auriculaire Gauche dans L'infarctus du Myocarde au Stade Aigu. Thesis for the M.D. degree. Facultes A et B de Medecine, Universite de Nancy 1, 1974.
10. Gesell, R.A.: Cardiodynamics in heart block as affected by auricular systole, auricular fibrillation and stimulation of the vagus nerve. *Am. J. Physiol.* **40**: 267–313, 1916.
11. Sarnoff, S.J.: Certain aspects of the role of catecholamines in circulatory regulation. *Am. J. Cardiol.* **5**: 579–588, 1960.
12. Linden, R.J., and Mitchell, J.H.: Relation between left ventricular diastolic pressure and myocardial segment length and observations on the contribution of atrial systole. *Circ. Res.* **8**: 1092–1099, 1960.
13. Sarnoff, S.J., and Mitchell, J.H.: The regulation of the performance of the heart. *Am. J. Med.* **30**: 747–771, 1961.
14. Mitchell, J.H., Gilmore, J.P., and Sarnoff, S.J.: The transport function of the atrium, factors influencing the relation between mean left atrial pressure and left ventricular end diastolic pressure. *Am. J. Cardiol.* **9**: 237–247, 1962.
15. Alicandri, C., Fouad, F.M., Tarazi, R.C., et al.: Three cases of hypotension and syncope with ventricular pacing: possible role of atrial reflexes. *Am. J. Cardiol.* **42**: 137–142, 1978.
16. Nager, F., and Kappenberger, L.: Hemodynamik nach Schrittermacherimplantation. *Internist* **18**: 14–20, 1977

17. News item: Sick sinus syndrome label for many cardiac problems. *J.A.M.A.* **239**: 597, 1978.
18. Moss, A.J., and Davis, J.: Brady-tachy syndrome. *Prog. Cardiovasc. Dis.* **16**: 439–454, 1974.
19. Bower, P.J.: Sick sinus syndrome. *Arch. Intern. Med.* **138**: 133–137, 1978.
20. Sowton, E.: Haemodynamic aspects of cardiac stimulation (Abstract). IVth International Symposium on Cardiac Pacing. Gröningen/the Netherlands, April 1973.
21. Radford, D.J., and Julian, D.G.: Sick sinus syndrome: Experience of a cardiac pacemaker clinic. *Br. Med. J.* 3: 504–407, 1974.
22. Ogawa, S., Dreifus, L.S., Shenoy, P.N., Brockman, S.K., and Berkovits, B.V.: Hemodynamic consequences of atrioventricular and ventriculoatrial pacing. *Pace* **1**: 8–15, 1978.
23. Curtis, J.J., Maloney, J.D., Barnhorst, D.A., et al.: A critical look at temporary ventricular pacing following cardiac surgery. *Surgery* **82**: 888–893, 1977.
24. Wisheart, J.D., Wright, J.E.C., Rosenfeldt, F.L., and Ross, J.K.: Atrial and ventricular pacing after open heart surgery. *Thorax* **28**: 9–14, 1973.
25. Hartzler, G.O., Maloney, J.D., Curtis, J.J., and Barnhorst, D.A.: Hemodynamic benefits of atrioventricular sequential pacing after cardiac surgery. *Am. J. Cardiol.* **40**: 232–236, 1977.
26. Castellanos, A., Berkovits, B.V., Castillo, C.A., and Befeler, B.: Sextapolar catheter electrode for temporary sequential atrioventricular pacing. *Cardiovasc. Res.* 8: 712–714, 1974.
27. Zucker, I.R., Parsonnet, V., and Gilbert, L.: A method of permanent transvenous implantation of an atrial electrode. *Am. Heart J.* **85**: 195–198, 1973.
28. Levy, S., Jausseran, J.M., Boyer, C.: La stimulation "sequentielle" auriculo-ventriculaire par stimulateur "bifocal" implantable. *Arch. Mal. Coeur* **69**: 1285–1292, 1976.

22

Anatomic Basis of Pre-excitation

Lino Rossi, M.D.

The Wolff-Parkinson-White (WPW) syndrome[1] was described in 1930 as an association of left bundle branch block, short PR interval, and tendency to paroxysmal tachycardia. In 1932 Holzmann and Scherf[2] suggested that this pattern was due to pre-excitation of the ventricles via an anomalous atrioventricular (AV) connection with the impulse circumventing or short-circuiting the AV junction. A large body of literature followed these publications.

In 1970, Durrer and co-workers[3] defined pre-excitation as a conduction in which the ventricular muscle is activated earlier than would be expected had the impulse reached the ventricles via the normal AV conducting system.

Much interest has existed for the underlying anomalous bundles: Kent's,[4] Mahaim's,[5] and James'[6] types.

ELECTROCARDIOGRAPHIC FEATURES

Classic electrocardiographic signs of WPW syndrome are a short PR interval with a widened QRS complex, which starts with a "delta" wave, a fusion complex resulting from summation of two impulses reaching the ventricle separately (through an anomalous AV pathway and the conducting system, respectively). A current classification[7] subdivides WPW syndrome into type A and type B, with left-sided pre-excitation in type A, right-sided (or AV junctional) in type B. Other criteria have been proposed for surface electrocardiographic nomenclature.[8]

Lown, Ganong and Levine (LGL) syndrome[9] is a form of pre-excitation also known as syndrome of short PR interval with normal QRS (and rapid heart action); this is currently explained by the presence of atrial fibers of James[6] joining the AV junctional tissue below the AV node, beyond which the ventricular activation would proceed normally.

Ventricular pre-excitation would go unnoticed in many cases if it were not for the frequent occurrence of tachycardias (supraventricular atrial fibrillation and flutter) which utilize a reentry pathway for the impulse, via the AV system and accessory pathway. The pre-excitation features may become manifest during antegrade or retrograde conduction.

Specialized procedures such as programmed stimulation, catheter recording, body-surface and epicardial potential mapping are available for study of these patients. They have opened the way to successful surgery of life-threatening, intractable tachyarrhythmias.[10]

In the past other mechanisms have been invoked to explain pre-excitation such as the presence of an inflammatory hyperexcitation focus,[11] close vicinity of atrial and ventricular myocardium,[12] particularly in those cases of WPW syndrome in which anomalous AV pathways were not demonstrated by histological studies. These, as well as other sixty-odd alternative mechanisms,[13] have now been superceded by the anomalous pathway explanation.

ANATOMIC-PHYSIOLOGIC CONSIDERATIONS

When faced with apparent anatomoclinical discrepancy in the WPW syndrome, at least four phenomena should be taken into account: (a) impedance mismatch,[14] which in tiny atrial accessory fascicles anastomosed with the ventricular mass may establish unidirectional (antegrade) block and prevent pre-excitation while allowing for re-entrant tachydysrhythmias ("concealed WPW"); (b) electrotonic conduction, that might allow pre-excitation to be propagated from atrial to contiguous ventricular fibers, without demonstrable anatomic anastomosis (incomplete accessory AV bundles); (c) synchronized sinoventricular conduction,[15] by a shift of pacemaking in the vicinity of James' bypass fibers;[6] (d) Anatomofunctional duality in the AV junction.[16]

HISTOPATHOLOGICAL STUDIES

This presentation of the anatomy of pre-excitation is based upon histological examination of six hearts from cases of WPW syndrome, and of four specimens of anomalous AV communications without pre-excitation. Observations and discussions pertain to hearts free from gross malformations (in which several types of AV aberrant pathways can be found), though dealing with microscopic abnormalities essentially congenital in nature. A low medial tricuspid insertion has been seen in one case of WPW syndrome, reminiscent of Ebstein's anomaly,[17] which is frequently associated with the syndrome.

The histological procedure for examination of the conducting system was the usual one; both AV rims, with the adjacent atrial and ventricular walls, were entirely cut in series (every 150) perpendicularly to the plane of the annuli.[18]

After the basic studies of Oehnell,[19] and particularly of Lev and co-workers,[20] further clinicopathological investigations were carried out.[21–27] These six cases studied were of type A WPW syndrome (one of intermediate type), and five showed a left-sided AV accessory bundle; in one, a canine heart, the bundle was on the right side. Two other cases (intermittent WPW of uncertain type, and type B, respectively) were seen[28–29] in which no direct AV accessory connections were found, but only connections between the His bundle and the ventricles and the atria and His bundle.

A septoseptal accessory connection in a postinfarction WPW (type B) syndrome was also seen,[30] in contrast to five of the seven cases of Becker and co-workers[31] which showed extremely thin AV Kent's type direct bundles.

In the Lown Ganong Levine syndrome, Brachenmacher's conclusions[23,32] seem to favor, but not to confirm, the importance of James' bypass fibers.[6]

In both WPW and LGL syndrome, with tachyarrhythmias, there is functional evidence of one or more aberrant AV conducting "short-circuits" which fit anatomically inferred pathways. The fact that anatomy does not always imply function, is borne out by the finding of one or more anomalous AV tracts in hearts of pre-excitation free subjects; in turn, in pre-excited hearts AV bypasses other than those electrophysiologically inferred can be found. In one of our cases, even the surgical disruption of the AV accessory bundle with correction of WPW syndrome did not elicit any pre-exciting function; in another, an electrically silent, AV bypass was discovered by histological studies.

Therefore, morphology does not always seem to account satisfactorily for electrophysiological diagnoses supporting the existence and function of unique or multiple AV anomalous pathways in individual cases. A gap still seems to separate the demonstration of abnormal AV pathways by electrophysiological means from anatomic findings.

The present treatment of the anatomic basis of pre-excitation will, then, be founded on the all-important evidence of anomalous AV pathways. The classification of the bundles will be reviewed, since terms such as Kent, Mahaim and James fibers have been under some criticism and change,[33] and difficulties are likely to arise in coping with the use of old and new nomenclature. The newer classification[33] also falls short of satisfying all anatomic and functional facts.

The modified terminology of Anderson et al. (Table 22-1)[33] separates the various AV abnormal bundles to avoid misinterpretation of the AV short-circuit. Thus "accessory AV connections" are pathways completely outside the delay-producing junctional area (former Kent[4] and/or Paladino[34] bundles). The "nodoventricular accessory connections" defined tracts connecting the AV node directly with the ventricular myocardium (formerly a variety of Mahaim[5] fibers). The "atriofascicular bypass" tracts (former James[6] fibers) described atrial fibers anastomosing with the penetrating bundle and the "fasciculoventricular connections" are those connecting the distal parts of the junctional area directly with the ventricular myocardium (formerly another variety of Mahaim fibers). The "intranodal bypass tracts" have a rather theoretical relevance to pre-excitation, and refer to fibers within the AV node, which avoid the delay within the node (former "overlay fibers"[35]).

In some of our cases and in general the term "fasciculoventricular fibers" is quite vague to indicate "Mahaim fibers" anastomosing the root or the middle course of the bundle branches with the ventricular septum; pathophysiological implications may be different from case to case, according to the location of the upper end of the abnormal fascicle. Moreover, conducting system-mediated anomalous AV connections should be distinguished from those which are direct, and completely outside the conducting system itself. Table 22-1 illustrates the proposed histological classification of anomalous AV pathways[36] which complement that of Anderson and co-workers.[33] Some overlapping of nomenclature is unavoidable, but the present scheme outlines the location of the bundles and translates old terms into new ones.

KENT BUNDLES OR DIRECT ACCESSORY AV CONNECTIONS

These bundles are formed outside the conduction system (Figs. 22-1 to 22-5). The original Kent[4] description does not support his published evidence,[37] the eponym of Kent bundles can be retained for both historical and practical reasons[38] (Fig. 22-2). The name of "Paladino's bundle" has sometimes been used to indicate a right atrial bundle parallel to the junctional tissue, that joins the fibrous ring of the medial tricuspid leaflet and has been seen to anastomose with the conducting system or in the upper ventricular septum. However, in Paladino's original articles[34] there is only a hint at possible anastomoses of some atrial fascicles, normally joining the AV rings, with the ventricular muscle, but no illustrations or precise descriptions of these anastomoses were reported.

Table 22-1. Histological Classification of Anomalous AV Pathways

DIRECT ATRIOVENTRICULAR BYPASS OUTSIDE THE CONDUCTING SYSTEM or *Accessory connections*	KENT BUNDLES or *Accessory atrioventricular muscle bundles:* *(i) septal, (ii) parietal—specialized—* *(iii) parietal—nonspecialized—*		
MEDIATE ATRIOVENTRICULAR BYPASS THROUGH THE CONDUCTING SYSTEM	INLET ATRIO-HISIAN JUNCTION or Bypass *tracts*	→ JAMES FIBERS or	*Atriofascicular fibers—specialized or not—*
	↓ *Intranodal (alternate) pathways—specialized—*		
	OUTLET CONDUCTING SYSTEM—VENTRICLE JUNCTION	NODOVENTRICULAR UPPER MAHAIM FIBERS and/or *accessory nodoventricular muscle bundles:* *(i) Overlay—specialized or transitional—* *(ii) Deep—specialized—*	
		Fasciculo—ventricular connections—specialized or HISIO-VENTRICULAR MIDDLE MAHAIM FIBERS	
		BIFURCATION—VENTRICULAR LOWER MAHAIM FIBERS	
		BUNDLE BRANCH(ES)-VENTRICULAR LOWERMOST MAHAIM FIBERS	

CAPITALS: traditional classification, complemented by Rossi.[38]
Italics: new classification (Anderson et al.[33]).

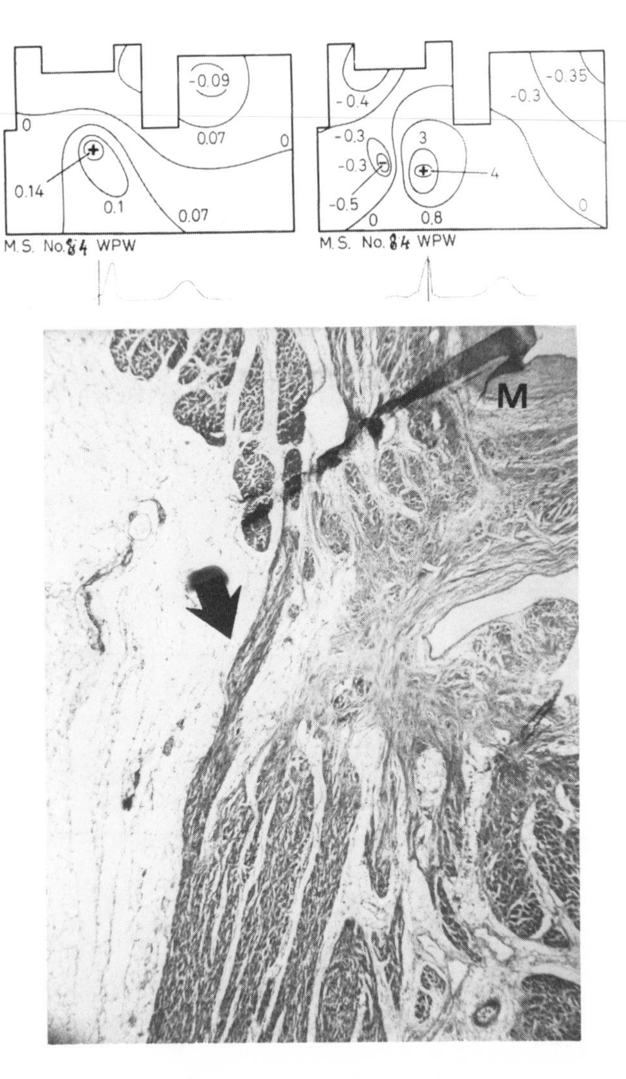

Figure 22-1. WPW syndrome (type A): left-sided ventricular pre-excitation showed by surface-body equipotential maps (related to the instant of time barred in the ECG tracings), from a left direct accessory A.V. bundle of Kent (K), astride the mitral (m) annulus, on the subepicardial side. (Hematoxylin-eosin; × 25.)

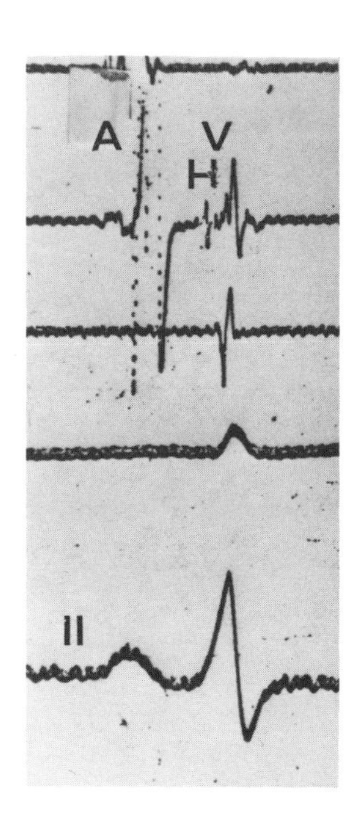

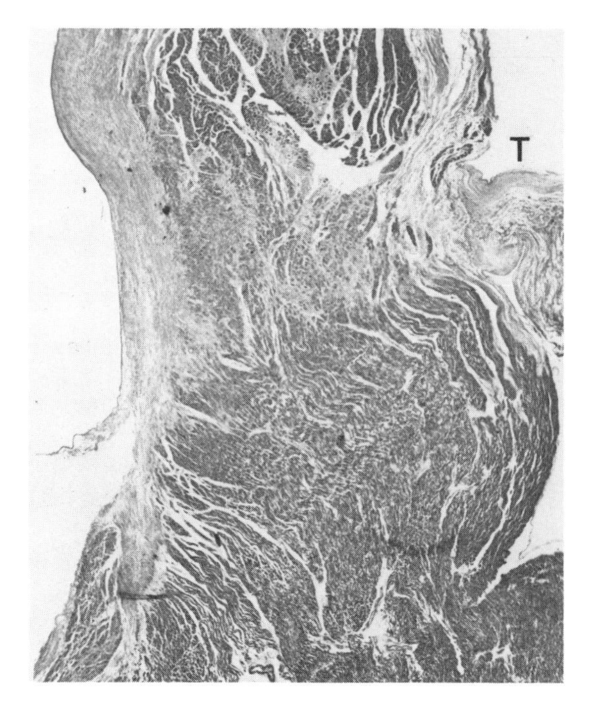

Figure 22–2. WPW syndrome (type A and B): His bundle recording of ventricular pre-excitation (HV time of −50 msec.), from a thick A.V. septoseptal accessory bundle (T= tricuspid). (Hematoxylin-eosin; × 15.)

The majority of cases studied histologically of WPW syndrome exhibited Kent's accessory bundles, and their correlation with the syndrome and arrhythmias is generally recognized.[37] It is only doubtful whether direct AV accessory connection of this type exists in normal hearts; although circus movement supraventricular tachyarrhythmias without pre-excitation do exist.[36]

Kent bundles consist of ordinary myocardium probably arising from "ring tissue",[39] and may explain the occasional finding of specialized P-cell-like elements.[25] Kent bundles, even when their size is rather conspicuous (about 1 mm thick) are not seen without thorough histological studies. They either run in the fatty subepicardial tissue mounted, or through the AV ring, to bridge the atrium with the homologous ventricle; their direction can be oblique or direct to the plane of the AV ring, and their length may vary. Septoseptal accessory connections seem to be mostly related with defective formation of the central fibrous body and/or the adjacent segments of the AV annuli. These myocardial AV bridges can be either limited to very thin fascicles or build up a conspicuous septoseptal anastomosing bundle.

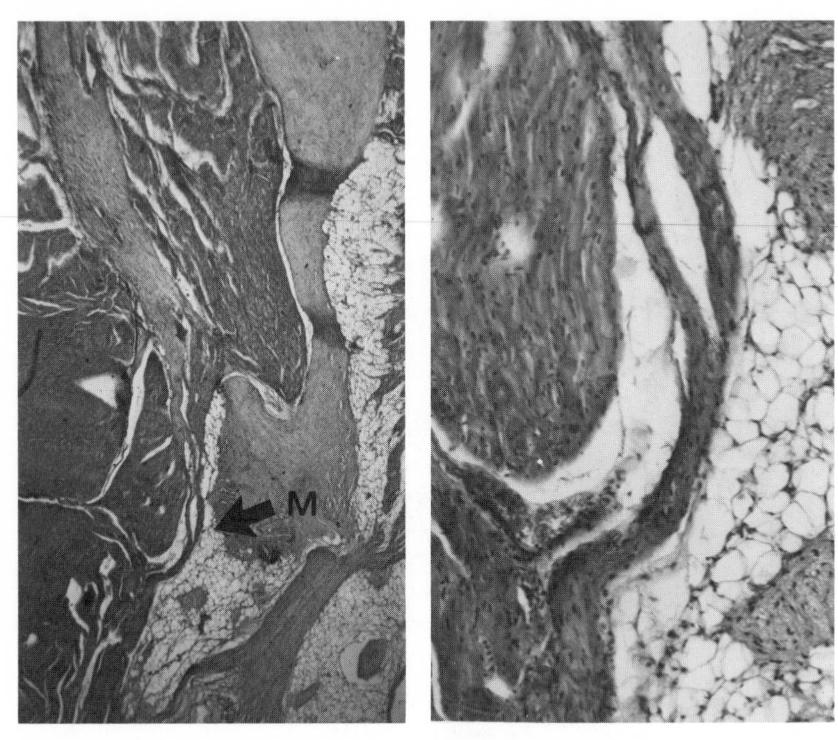

Figure 22–3. Fasciculoventricular (lower Mahaim) A.V. bundle (M) anastomosing the right side of the Hisian branching portion with the myocardium of the ventricular septum (a detail on the right), in a dog's specimen of experimental "bloc bilateral manqué". (Hematoxylin-eosin; × 12 and × 150.)

Mahaim Fibers or AV Bypass Tracts Within the Conduction System

Anderson et al.[33] identified Mahaim fibers or AV bypass tracts mediated within the conduction system (Figs. 22-3 and 22-5) as fasciculoventricular connections and this should apply only for those branching off from the AV node and common bundle, but not for those arising from the proximal and middle course of the bundle branches. Mahaim fibers should better be subdivided into four topographic and anatomofunctional groups: upper or nodoventricular, possibly including the theoretically suggested "overlay" fibers (both superficial and deep[33]) and the proper fasciculoventricular fibers, the subgroups of middle or Hisioventricular included; lower or bifurcating-ventricular, lowermost or bundle branch-ventricular (on both sides).

Altogether, Mahaim fibers represent anomalous "outlet junctions" between the conducting system and the ventricular muscle. Mahaim fibers

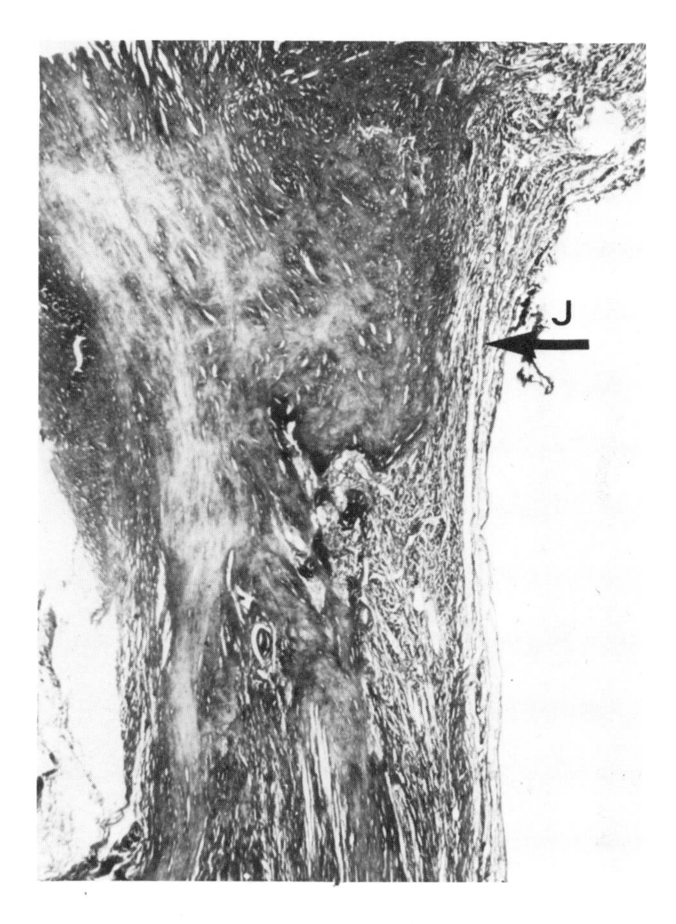

Figure 22–4. Atriofascicular bundle of James (J) impinging the penetrating portion of His bundle (H). (Hematoxylin-eosin; × 25.)

are apparently specific and/or transitional in nature, just as those of the AV junctional or bundle branch myocardium from which they originate. Accordingly, lower Mahaim fibers arising from the right bundle branch can be indistinguishable from the adjacent septal myocardium.

Whether or not Mahaim fibers (particularly upper nodoventricular, or middle or lower fasciculoventricular) are responsible for pre-excitation and reciprocating tachyarrhythmias is still under discussion. They can be present in electrophysiologic studies but their pathologic demonstration is scanty.[24,28] In two of our cases the evidence of Mahaim fibers of different type had a questionable anatomoclinical significance. Indeed, fasciculoventricular (middle and lower) Mahaim fibers were found in a two-month baby and in an adult man not exhibiting pre-excitation nor

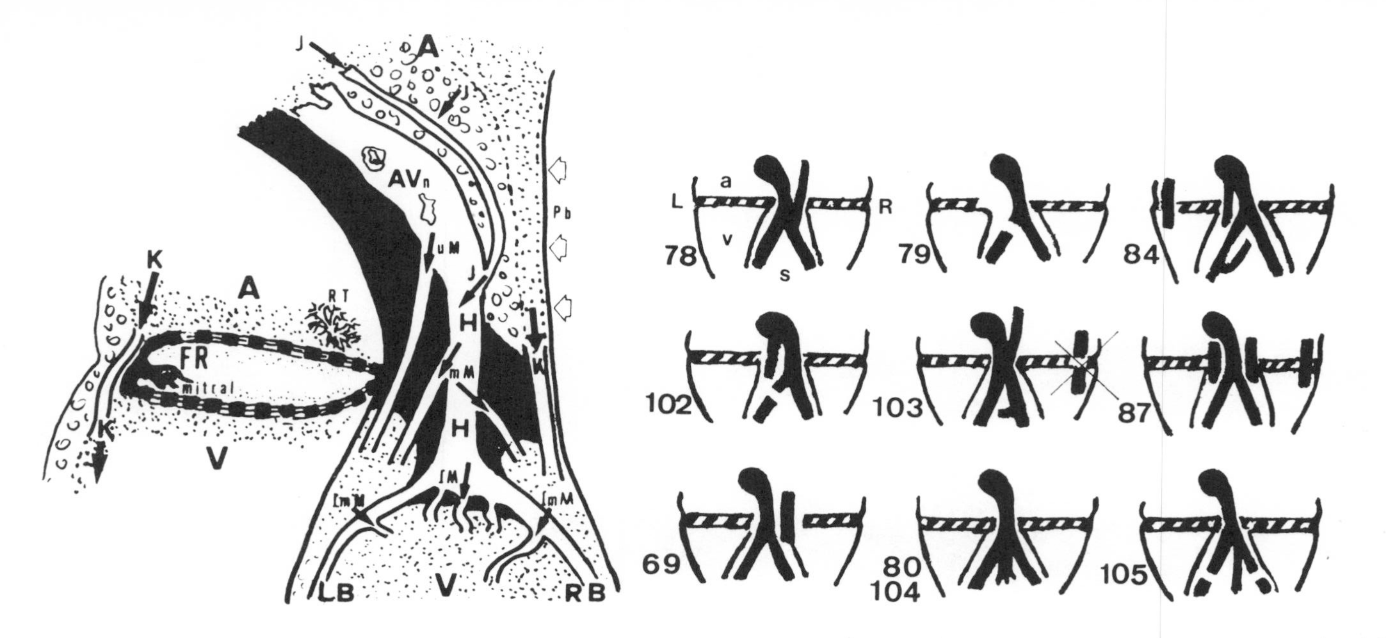

Figure 22–5. *Left*: A semirealistic diagram of conducting system and anomalous A.V. pathways: blank tracts represent the A.V. pathways (arrows); the black bands, central fibrous body and pars membranacea; the dashed line, left annulus fibrosus (the same would apply to the right, not represented): A= atrium, V= ventricle, AVn= atrioventricular node, H= His bundle, L and RB= left and right bundle branch, FR= fibrous ring, RT= ring tissue; K= Kent, J= James, uM= upper Mahaim, mM= middle Mahaim, lM= lower Mahaim, lmM= lowermost Mahaim, and P= Paladino's fibers. *Right*: A synthetic scheme of conducting system and anomalous A.V. communications (black bands), in the present series of cases (see text); the legend (once for all sketches) indicates left (L) and right (R) atrial (a) and ventricular (v) chambers, with the ventricular septum (s), separated by the A.V. ring (dashed line); in case no. 103 the delated right accessory bundle had been surgically divided.

tachyarrhythmias, whereas in a mongrel dog (Fig. 22-3) the experimental cut of both bundle branches, histologically ascertained, had failed to provoke the expected chronic heart block, suggesting the possibility that the Mahaim bypass might be functional.[40]

It has been observed that the AV node may send digitations into the central fibrous body, often very close to the posterior ridge of the muscular ventricular septum (incomplete upper Mahaim tracts?). Likewise, anastomoses of the branching portion of the AV bundle with the adjacent septal muscle is rather common in fetal hearts.[41]

James' Atriofascicular Fibers

James' atriofascicular fibers (Figs. 22-4 and 22-5) belong to the other type of mediate AV bypass by "inlet" of atrial fibers into the AV junctional tissue beyond the impulse delaying core of the Tawara's node. In James' and Sherf's opinion,[42] these mostly represent the terminal fibers of the posterior (Thorel's) internodal tract, circumventing the AV node's convex surface. They enter it distally or join the common bundle directly. Such fibers can show either ordinary atrial or Purkinje-like features, and their presence is far from peculiar to cases of pre-excitation, notwithstanding the current anatomoclinical idea of their relationship with the LGL syndrome. It has been surmised, in this connection, that some conduction impairment in the proximal and middle atrio-AV nodal approaches would be needed to force the impulse exclusively through the distal James fibers and produce pre-excitation without abnormalities of QRS complex.[43] A mechanism of this kind can be relevant to the questions of acquired pre-excitation (cardiomyopathy, myocardial infarction.[12,30,44])

Intranodal (Alternate) Pathways of Specific Myocardium

These are another hypothetical atrio-Hisian bypass, not distinguished from the foregoing "overlay", and not yet demonstrated histologically.

The role of AV ring fenestration or incompleteness, observed in a fairly large number of normal hearts without arrhythmias,[12] with or without pre-excitation should not be thought of as anomalous AV muscular junctions, but they may be relevant to the theory of electrotonic conduction between adjacent atrial and ventricular fascicles.

The same can be said regarding the importance of ring tissue[39] as remanents of specific-looking myocardium (small, interwoven cells) which can be observed within the AV annuli and close to both in normal and pre-excited hearts; its relevance is unclear.

The correlation of electrocardiographic type A and B to pathologic findings is not well established.

Reliable evaluations on the type, site, and function of anomalous pre-exciting AV bypass come from one case studied by surface body potential mapping;[45] in another case with drug-resistant atrial fibrillation triggering bursts of ventricular fibrillation, a right-sided direct AV accessory pathway (Kent's) was identified by epicardial mapping, and surgically divided, with elimination of both pre-excitation and complicating arrhythmias. The histological correlation corroborated the surgical findings.[46]

The frequent pathophysiological demonstration of multiple anomalous AV pathways in individual WPW syndrome hearts has been substantiated by histology. The Kent bundles being the most common.

The findings of abnormal AV connections in our cases with or without pre-excitation syndrome and/or paroxysmal supraventricular tachydysrhythmias are shown in Figure 22-5. It can be observed that in three WPW specimens (No. 84, type A; No. 103, type B; No. 87, types A-B) multiple anomalous and/or accessory AV pathways were found, whereas only one was demonstrated in other two cases (No. 78, type B; No. 012, type A); a wide gap in the AV fibrous ring was seen in the post-infarct pre-excitation case No. 88. In the remaining three cases (No. 69, No. 80, and No. 104), single abnormal AV tracts were found among these, a case of supraventricular tachycardia with a septoseptal (Kent's) accessory pathway and without pre-excitation was seen and it is an histological demonstration of the so-called "concealed WPW syndrome". Case No. 105 is the canine heart with experimental "block bilateral manqué",[47] due to the presence of a lower Mahaim's fasciculoventricular bypass (Fig. 22-3).

Histological as well as pathophysiological abnormalities, peculiar to pre-excitation syndrome, sinoatrial disease[27] and AV or bundle branch block[20,48,49] have been seen to coexist in two of our cases.

REFERENCES

1. Wolff, L., Parkinson, J., and White, P.D.: Bundle branch block with short P-R interval in healthy young people prone to paroxysmal tachycardia. *Am. Heart J.* **5**: 685, 1930.
2. Holzmann, M., and Sherf, D.: Ueber Elektrokardiogramme mit verkürzter Vorhof-Kammer Distanz und positiven P-Zacken. *Z. Klin. Med.* **121**: 404, 1932.
3. Durrer, D., Schuilenburg, R.M., and Wellens, H.J.J.: Pre-excitation revisited. *Am. J. Cardiol.* **25**: 690, 1970.
4. Kent, A.F.S.: The right lateral auriculoventricular junction of the heart. *Proc. Physiol. Soc.* **48**: 22, 1914.

5. Mahaim, I.: Le syndrome de Wolff-Parkinson-White et sa pathogenie. *Helvet. Med. Acta* 8: 483, 1941.
6. James, T.N.: Morphology of the human atrioventricular node, with remarks pertinent to its electrophysiology. *Am. Heart J.* 62: 757, 1961.
7. Rosenbaum, F.F., Hecht, H.H., Wilson, F.N., and Johnston F.D.: Potential variations of the thorax and the esophagus in anomalous atrio-ventricular excitation (Wolff-Parkinson-White syndrome). *Am. Heart J.* 29: 281, 1945.
8. Frank, R.: Apport des investigations endocavitaires et des cartographies epicardiques dans l'etude des syndromes de pre-excitation ventriculaire. Paris, Ed. Medicales Universitaires, 1974.
9. Lown, B., Ganong, W.F., and Levine, S.A.: The syndrome of short P-R interval, normal QRS complex and paroxysmal rapid heart action. *Circulation* 5: 693, 1952.
10. Gallagher, J.J., Kasell, J., Sealy, W.C., et al.: Epicardial mapping in the Wolff-Parkinson-White syndrome. *Circulation* 57: 854, 1978.
11. Mahaim, I., and Bogdanovich, P.: Un cas mortel de syndrome de Wolff-Parkinson-White. Lesions inflammatoires chroniques du faisceau de His-Tawara. *Acta Med. Jugoslav.* 2: 137, 1948.
12. Schumann, G.: Ueber das erworbene WPW syndrome. *Z. Kreislaufforsch.* 59: 1081, 1970.
13. Scherf, D., and Cohen, J.: *The Atrioventricular Node and Selected Cardiac Arrhythmias.* New York, Grune & Stratton, 1964.
14. De la Fuente, D., Sasynjuk, B., and Moe, J.K.: Conduction through a narrow isthmus in isolated canine atrial tissue: a model of the Wolff-Parkinson-White syndrome. *Circulation* 44: 803, 1971.
15. Sherf, L.: The atrial conduction system: clinical implications. *Am. J. Cardiol.* 37: 814, 1976.
16. Moe, J.K., Preston, J.B., and Burlington, H.: Physiologic evidence for a dual A-V transmission system. *Circulation Res.* 4: 357, 1956.
17. Lev, M., Gibson, S., and Miller, R.A.: Ebstein's disease with Wolff-Parkinson-White syndrome. *Am. Heart J.* 49: 724, 1955.
18. Rossi, L.: Histopathology of Cardiac Arrhythmias. Milan, Casa Ed. Ambrosiana, 1978.
19. Oehnell, R.F.: Post-mortem examination and clinical report of a case of the short P-R interval and wide QRS wave syndrome (Wolff, Parkinson and White). *Cardiologia* 4: 249, 1940.
20. Lev, M., Kennamer, R., Prinzmetal, M., and De Mesquita, Q.: A histopathologic study of the atrioventricular communications in two hearts with the Wolff-Parkinson-White syndrome. *Circulation* 24: 41, 1961.
21. Schumann, G., Jansen, H.H., and Anschutz, F.: Zur Pathogenese des WPW Syndroms. *Virch. Arch. path. Anat. Physiol.* 349: 48, 1970.
22. Boineau, J.P., and Moore, E.N.: Evidence for propagation of activation across an accessory atrioventricular connection in types A and B pre-excitation. *Circulation* 41: 375, 1970.
23. Brechenmacher, C., Laham, J., Iris, L., et al.: Etude histologique des voies anormales de conduction dans un syndrome de Wolff-Parkinson-White, et dans un syndrome de Lown-Ganong-Levine. *Arch. Mal. Coeur* 67: 507, 1974.

24. Brechenmacher, C., Coumel, P., Fuchier, J.P., et al.: De subitaneis mortibus XXII. Intractable paroxysmal tachycardias proved fatal in type A Wolff-Parkinson-White syndrome. *Circulation* **55**: 408, 1977.
25. James, T.N., and Puech, P.: De subitaneis mortibus IX. Type A Wolff-Parkinson-White syndrome. *Circulation* **50**: 1264, 1974.
26. Rossi L., Knippel M., and Taccardi B.: Histological findings, His bundle recordings and body-surface potential mapping in a case of Wolff-Parkinson-White syndrome. An anatomoclinical comparison. *Cardiology* **60**: 265, 1975.
27. Dreifus, L.S., Wellens, H.J., Watanabe, Y., et al.: Sinus bradycardia and atrial fibrillation with the Wolff-Parkinson-White syndrome. *Am. J. Cardiol.* **38**: 149, 1976.
28. Lev, M., Fox, S., Bharati, S., et al.: Mahaim and James fibers as a basis for a unique variety of ventricular pre-excitation. *Am J. Cardiol.* **36**: 880, 1975.
29. Brechenmacher, C., Courtadon, M., Jourde, M., et al.: Syndrome de Wolff-Parkinson-White par association de fibres atrio-Hissiennes et de fibres de Mahaim. *Arch. Mal. Coeur* **69**: 1275, 1976.
30. Gavrilescu, S., Gavrilescu, M., and Luca, C.: Accelerated atrioventricular conduction during acute myocardial infarction. *Am. Heart J.* **94**: 21, 1977.
31. Becker, A.E., Anderson, R.H., Durrer, D., and Wellens, H.J.J.: The anatomical substrates of Wolff-Parkinson-White syndrome. A clinicopathologic correlation in seven cases. *Circulation* **57**: 870, 1978.
32. Brechenmacher, C.: Atrio-His bundle tracts. *Br. Heart J.* **37**: 853, 1975.
33. Anderson, R.H., Becker, A.E., Brechenmacher, C., et al.: Ventricular pre-excitation. A proposed nomenclature for its substrates. *Europ. J. Cardiol.* **3**: 27, 1975.
34. Paladino, G.: Contributi alla anatomia, istologia, fisiologia del cuore. *Movimento Medico-Chirurgico (Napoli)* **8**: 428, 1876. Per una questione di priorità sui rapporti intimi tra la muscolatura degli atrii e quella dei ventricoli del cuore. *Rend. Accad. Sc. Fis. Matem.-Sez. Soc. Reale di Napoli* **48**: 268, 1909.
35. Anderson, R.H., and Taylor, I.M.: Development of atrioventricular specialized tissue in human heart. *Br. Heart J.* **34**: 1205, 1972.
36. Barold, S.S., and Coumel, P.: Mechanism of atrioventricular junctional tachycardia. Role of re-entry and concealed accessory bypass tracts. *Am. J. Cardiol.* **39**: 97, 1977.
37. Durrer, D., and Wellens, H.J.J.: The Wolff-Parkinson-White syndrome anno 1973. *Europ. J. Cardiol.* **1**: 347, 1974.
38. Rossi, L.: A histological survey of pre-excitation syndrome and related arrhythmias. *G. Ital. Cardiol.* **5**: 816, 1975.
39. Anderson, R.H., Davies, M.J., and Becker, A.E.: Atrioventricular ring specialized tissue in the normal heart. *Europ. J. Cardiol.* **2**: 219, 1974.
40. Van Dam, T., Rossi, L., and Pozzi, L.: unpublished data.
41. Visioli, O., and Vitali-Mazza, L.: Le connessioni alte del sistema di conduzione atrio-ventricolare. *Riv. Anat. Pat. Oncol.* **13**: 47, 1957.
42. James, T.N., and Sherf, L.: Specialized tissue and preferential conduction in the atria of the heart. *Am. J. Cardiol.* **28**: 414, 1971.
43. Bellet, S.: *Clinical Disorders of the Heart Beat.* Philadelphia, Lea & Febiger, 1971, p. 488.

44. Krikler, D.M., and Goodwin, J.S.: *Cardiac Arrhythmias. The Modern Electro-physiological Approach.* London, W.B. Saunders Co., 1975.
45. De Ambroggi, L., Taccardi, B., and Macchi, E.: Body-surface maps of heart potential: tentative localization of pre-excited areas in forty-two Wolff-Parkinson-White patients. *Circulation* **54**: 251, 1976.
46. Rossi, L., Thiene, G., and Knippel, M.: A case of surgically corrected Wolff-Parkinson-White syndrome. Clinical and histological data. *Br. Heart J.* **40**: 581, 1978.
47. Mahaim, I., and Winston, M.R.: Recherches d'anatomie comparée et de pathologie experimentale sur les connexions hautes du faisceau de His-Tawara. *Cardiologia* **5**: 189, 1941.
48. Lev, M., Leffler, W.B., Langendorf, R., and Pick, A.: Anatomic findings in a case of ventricular pre-excitation (WPW) terminating in complete atrioventricular block. *Circulation* **34**: 718, 1966.
49. Coumel, P., Krikler, D., Slama, R., and Bouvrain, Y.: Anomalous atrioventricular conduction associated with complete block of the nodal-His pathway: an electrocardiographic study. *Br. Heart J.* **36**: 397, 1974.

23

WPW Syndrome: Electrophysiological Studies in Patients With Tachycardias

Jerónimo Farré, M.D., David L. Ross, M.B., B.S., F.R.A.C.P., Isaac Wiener, M.D., Frits W. Bar, M.D., and Hein J.J. Wellens, M.D.

The association of paroxysmal tachycardia and the electrocardiographic features which characterize the Wolff-Parkinson-White (WPW) syndrome was noted in the original description of this condition.[1] The introduction of the technique of programmed electrical stimulation of the heart[2] combined with the recording of multiple intracardiac electrograms, gives us the opportunity to define the mechanisms and electrophysiological determinants of the arrhythmias observed in patients with the WPW syndrome.[3–7]

METHODS

Following informed consent, electrophysiological studies are performed in the postabsorptive state. Cardioactive drugs are discontinued before the investigation according to their expected half-lives unless the stimulation study is performed to test the effects of a drug following chronic oral administration. Electrode catheters are percutaneously introduced via one or both femoral veins and positioned at the following intracardiac locations: high right atrium (HRA), right ventricular apex (RV), tricuspid valve (His region). Coronary sinus (CS) catheterization is accomplished

Dr. Farré has been supported by the Fundación Conchita Rábago de Jiménez Diaz, Madrid, Spain. Dr. Ross is supported by the National Heart Foundation, Australia.

either by the femoral route or by a left antecubital vein approach. The latter permits more extensive mapping of the posterior half of the low left atrium.[4,6]

Electrocardiographic leads I, II, III, V_1 and V_6 are simultaneously recorded with bipolar electrograms from the HRA, CS and His regions on a multi-channel direct ink-jet recorder (Mingograf, Siemens-Elema, Sweden) at a paper speed of 100 mm/sec. All data are stored on magnetic tape (Ampex PR-2200) to enable play back at different paper speeds permitting accurate measurements of conduction time intervals.

Stimulation is performed by means of a programmable electrical stimulator (Janssen Pharmaceutica, Belgium). Impulses which are 2 ms in duration and twice diastolic threshold in amplitude are delivered[6] according to the protocol of stimulation shown in Table 23-1.

Table 23-1. Programmed Electrical Stimulation of the Heart in Patients With WPW

A. BASIC PROTOCOL
1. RV extra-stimulus technique
2. RV pacing at increasing rates
3. HRA extra-stimulus technique
4. CS extra-stimulus technique
5. HRA pacing at increasing rates
6. CS pacing at increasing rates

The extra-stimulus technique is performed, if possible, at three different BCL (500 and 600 ms, and the BCL corresponding to the frequency just above the sinus rate).

Pacing at increasing rates is performed up to
a. induction of tachycardia
b. block in the normal and accessory pathway
c. rates between 200–250/minute are attained
d. signs or symptoms of intolerance develop

B. PROTOCOL DURING TACHYCARDIA
1. RV single and multiple timed premature stimuli
2. HRA single and multiple timed premature stimuli
3. CS single and multiple timed premature stimuli

C. IF THE ANTEGRADE ERP OF THE AP IS SHORT
Atrial pacing at very fast rates or multiple atrial premature stimuli at the shortest possible coupling-interval resulting in atrial capture to induce atrial fibrillation.

Abbreviations: RV= right ventricular apex; HRA= high right atrium; CS= coronary sinus; BCL= basic cycle length; ERP= effective refractory period; AP= accessory pathway.

TACHYARRHYTHMIAS IN WPW

The true incidence of tachyarrhythmias in patients with WPW is unknown, the reported values varying according to the selection of patients in a given series.[8] In our own series of 157 patients with WPW who have undergone electrophysiological investigation, electrocardiographic documentation of tachyarrhythmias (either regular paroxysmal tachycardia or atrial fibrillation) prior to the stimulation study was available in 94 percent of cases.[9]

From a practical point of view, tachyarrhythmias in the WPW syndrome can be divided into two groups: (1) paroxysmal regular tachycardias, and (2) paroxysmal atrial fibrillation. A few patients with the WPW syndrome may present with a chronic atrial fibrillation, generally as a result of associated organic heart disease. The latter group of patients will not be considered in this chapter.

PAROXYSMAL REGULAR TACHYCARDIA IN WPW

Table 23-2 includes the possible mechanisms underlying paroxysmal regular tachycardia in patients with the WPW syndrome. The most frequent form of paroxysmal regular tachycardia in these patients is based on a junctional re-entry mechanism utilizing the accessory pathway (AP). In 69 consecutive patients with WPW admitted to hospital because of a documented paroxysmal regular tachycardia, a subsequent electrophysiological study was able to induce an electrocardiographically similar type of tachycardia which proved to be based on the above mentioned mechanism.[9] In addition, in our series of 157 patients with WPW who underwent an electrophysiological investigation, a circus-movement tachycardia (CMT) incorporating the AP was induced in 103 (65.5%) patients.

A-V JUNCTIONAL CMT IN WPW: ELECTROPHYSIOLOGICAL BASIS

It is well documented that in most patients with WPW, in addition to the normal A-V nodal-His pathway an accessory atrioventricular pathway connects the atria and ventricles.[2–9] In some of these patients the electrophysiological properties of the A-V node-His axis and the accessory pathway are such that an appropriately timed premature beat is blocked in one of the pathways while still being conducted over the other. This phenomenon is observed in those instances in which the refractory period of one of the pathways connecting the atria and ventricles is longer than that of the other. Once this premature impulse is blocked in one of the pathways, a certain degree of "slow conduction" is required to initiate the first echo-beat and maintain the subsequent circusmovement tachycardia.[6]

In the most frequent form of CMT observed in WPW, the AP is utilized as the retrograde (V-A) limb of the re-entry circuit while the normal A-V nodal-His-Purkinje pathway is used for antegrade (A-V) conduction.

Table 23-2. Paroxysmal Regular Tachycardia in the WPW Syndrome

I. A-V Junctional Re-entry Tachycardias (Figure 23-5)
- A. A-V Junctional CMT incorporating the AP
  1. Orthodromic CMT (common type) using the AP in V-A direction and the normal A-V nodal-His axis in A-V direction
  2. Antidromic CMT (reversed or uncommon type) using the AP in A-V direction and the normal pathway in V-A direction
- B. Intra-A-V nodal reciprocating tachycardia
- C. A-V Junctional CMT incorporating two APs

II. Atrial Tachyarrhythmias
- A. Atrial tachycardia
- B. Atrial flutter

III. Ventricular Tachycardia

Abbreviations: CMT= circus movement tachycardia.

This implies that the QRS complexes during tachycardia show normal intraventricular conduction or typical bundle branch block configuration. This form of tachycardia is also known as the "orthodromic" type and its initiation during the stimulation study requires:

1. Dissimilar properties of the A-V node-His axis and the AP in one or both of the following ways: (a) antegrade effective refractory period (ERP) of the AP longer than that of the A-V node, (b) retrograde ERP of the AP shorter than that over the His-A-V nodal axis.
2. Presence of V-A conduction by way of the AP.
3. A revolution time (time required to complete the whole circuit) longer than the longest refractory period of any of the components of the re-entry loop.

In patients with a relatively short antegrade ERP of the AP, initiation of this form of CMT following atrial premature beats (APB) frequently occurs within a zone of premature beat intervals which extends from the ERP of the AP down to the ERP of the atrial myocardium at the site of stimulation (Fig. 23-1). In patients with a long antegrade ERP of the AP, the upper limit of the "zone of tachycardia" is below the value of the longest premature beat interval at which block over the AP is observed.[3,10] The latter feature does not suggest intra-A-V nodal re-entry as formerly postulated by some investigators, but represents the need for "slow conduction" to induce the first atrial echo-beat, since arrival of the impulse at the atrial insertion of the AP must be delayed beyond the atrial refractory period.[10] In a similar way, atrial pacing at increasing rates can induce this type of CMT on reaching a critical rate at which block over the AP occurs while A-V conduction by way of the normal A-V nodal-His pathway is still possible.

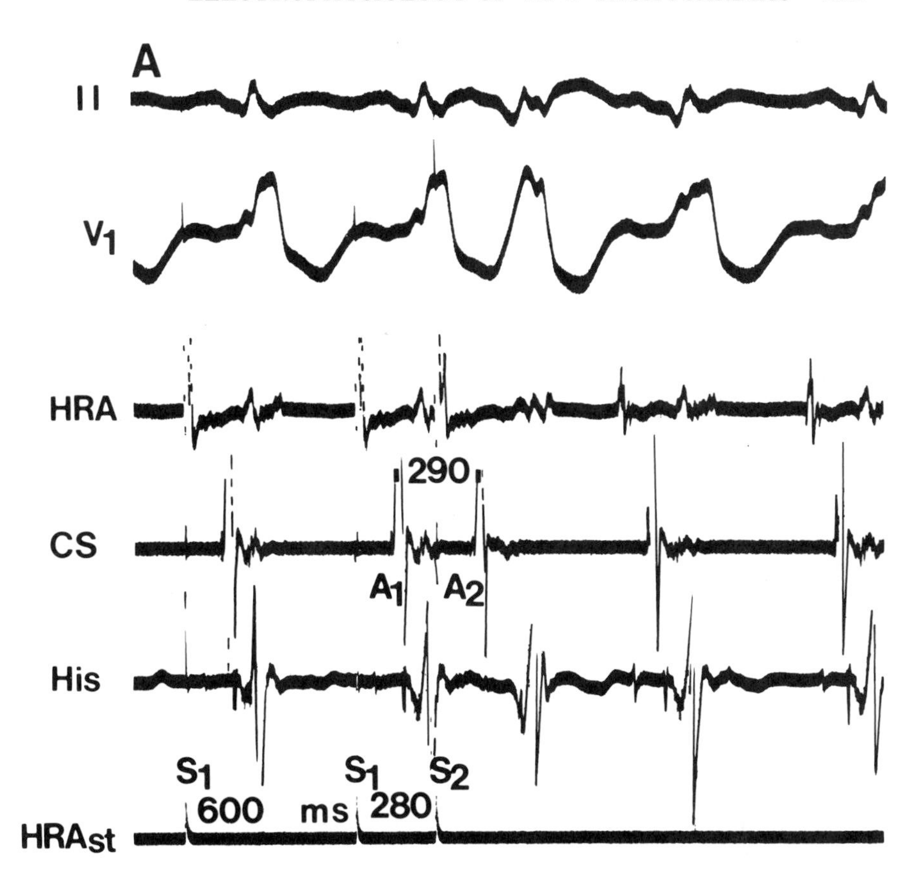

Figure 23-1. Initiation of circusmovement tachycardia utilizing the accessory pathway in V-A direction following an atrial premature beat on reaching the antegrade effective refractory period of the AP. In panel *A* the atrial test-impulse delivered at a premature beat interval of 280 ms is followed by a maximally pre-excited QRS complex.

As recently discussed, stimulation close to the atrial insertion of the AP can be an important determinant of the ease of initiation of CMT incorporating the AP in V-A direction.[6] This statement applies not only to the atrial single test-stimulus technique but also to regular pacing of the atrium at increasing rates. In a few patients, critical discontinuation of the regular atrial pacing after block of the atrial impulses is observed over the AP, may be necessary to initiate tachycardia (Fig. 23-2).

Initiation of the orthodromic type of CMT by single ventricular premature beats (VPB) is observed when the ventricular test-stimulus is blocked within the normal pathway while V-A conduction by way of the

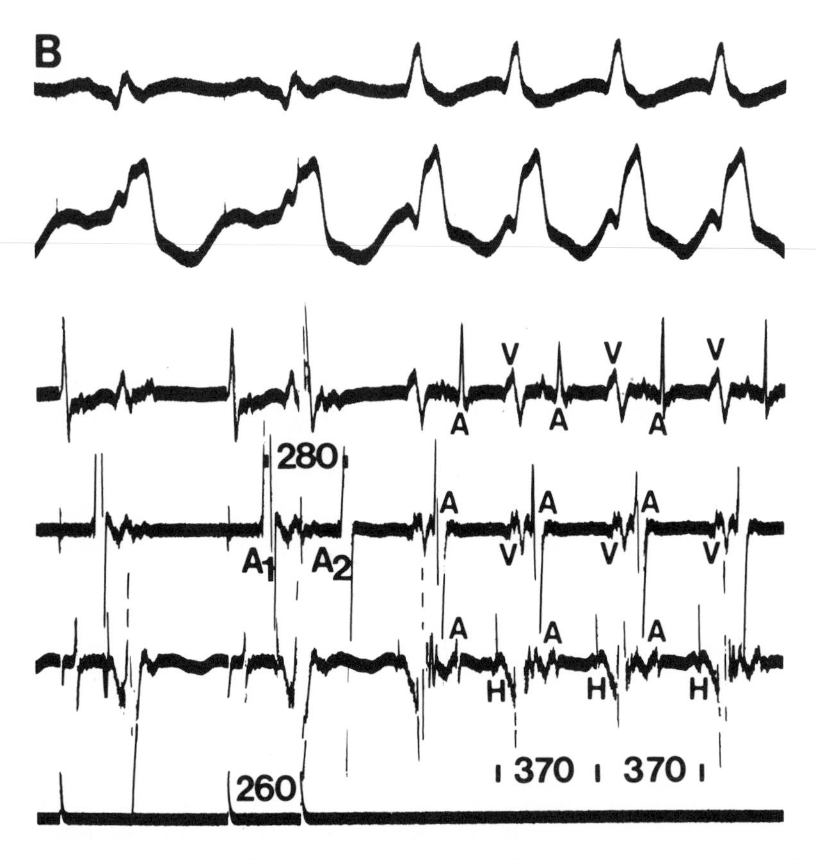

Figure 23-1 *(Continued).* In panel *B* the atrial test-impulse is antegradely blocked in the AP and atrioventricular conduction occurs by way of the normal A-V nodal-His pathway. Due to the presence of right bundle branch block, QRS complexes during tachycardia show the typical configuration of this intraventricular conduction disorder. Due to intra-atrial conduction delay with increasing prematurity of the atrial test-stimulus, A_1-A_2 close to the atrial insertion of the AP is 280 ms for an S_1-S_2 delivered at the HRA level of 260 ms. During CMT the sequence of retrograde atrial activation is eccentric (starting in the CS lead which was positioned laterally in the left A-V groove).

AP is still possible. In some patients in whom CMT using the AP in V-A direction cannot be induced following APBs because the antegrade ERP of the AP is shorter than that of the A-V node, VPBs will frequently elicit reciprocating tachycardia by creating block in the normal pathway while conduction to the atrium over the AP is still possible. Similar electrophysiological considerations apply to the initiation of this tachycardia during ventricular pacing at increasing rates.[6] The modes of ini-

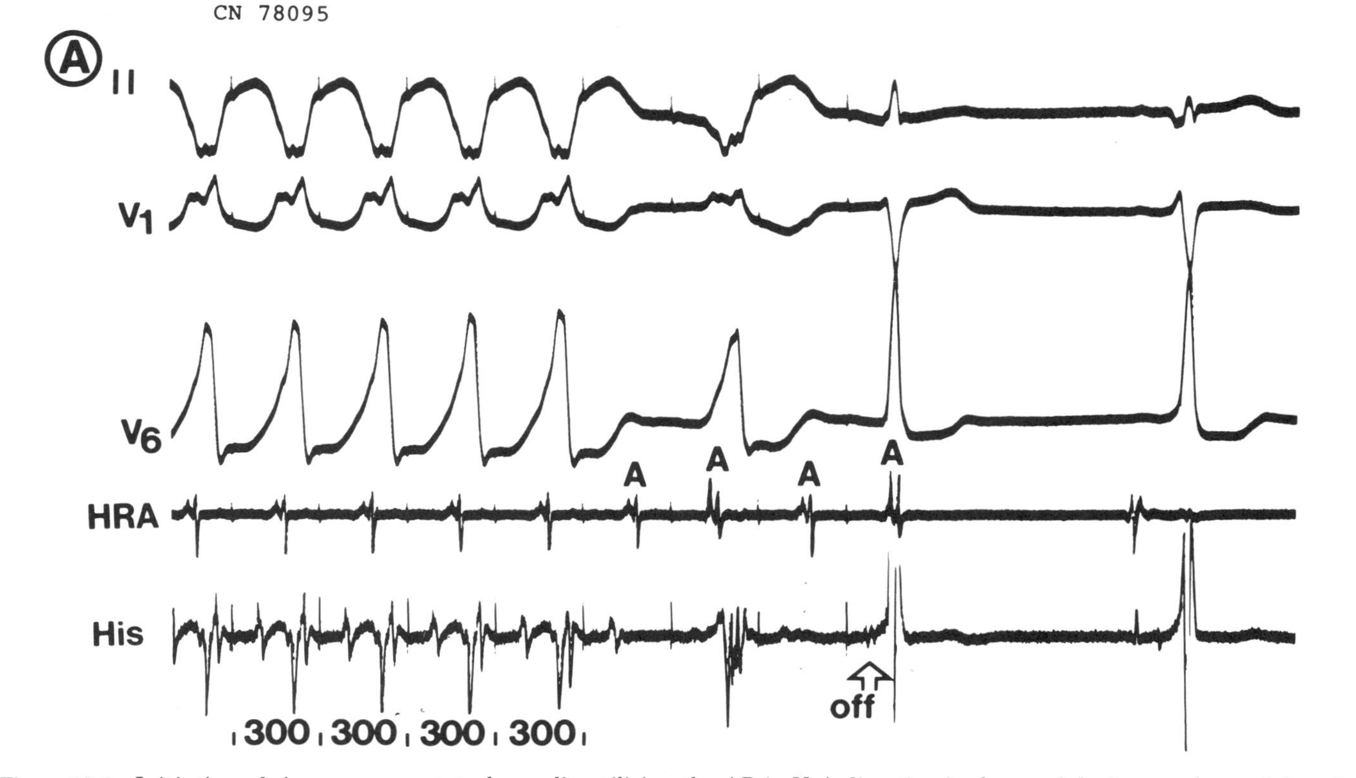

Figure 23–2. Initiation of circusmovement tachycardia utilizing the AP in V-A direction is observed during regular atrial pacing on reaching a rate at which block over the AP occurs. As illustrated, not only a critical pacing rate plays a role, but also the timing of discontinuation of pacing. In panel *A* initiation of tachycardia is prevented because the last atrial paced beat is blocked both in the normal (A-V node-His) and accessory pathway.

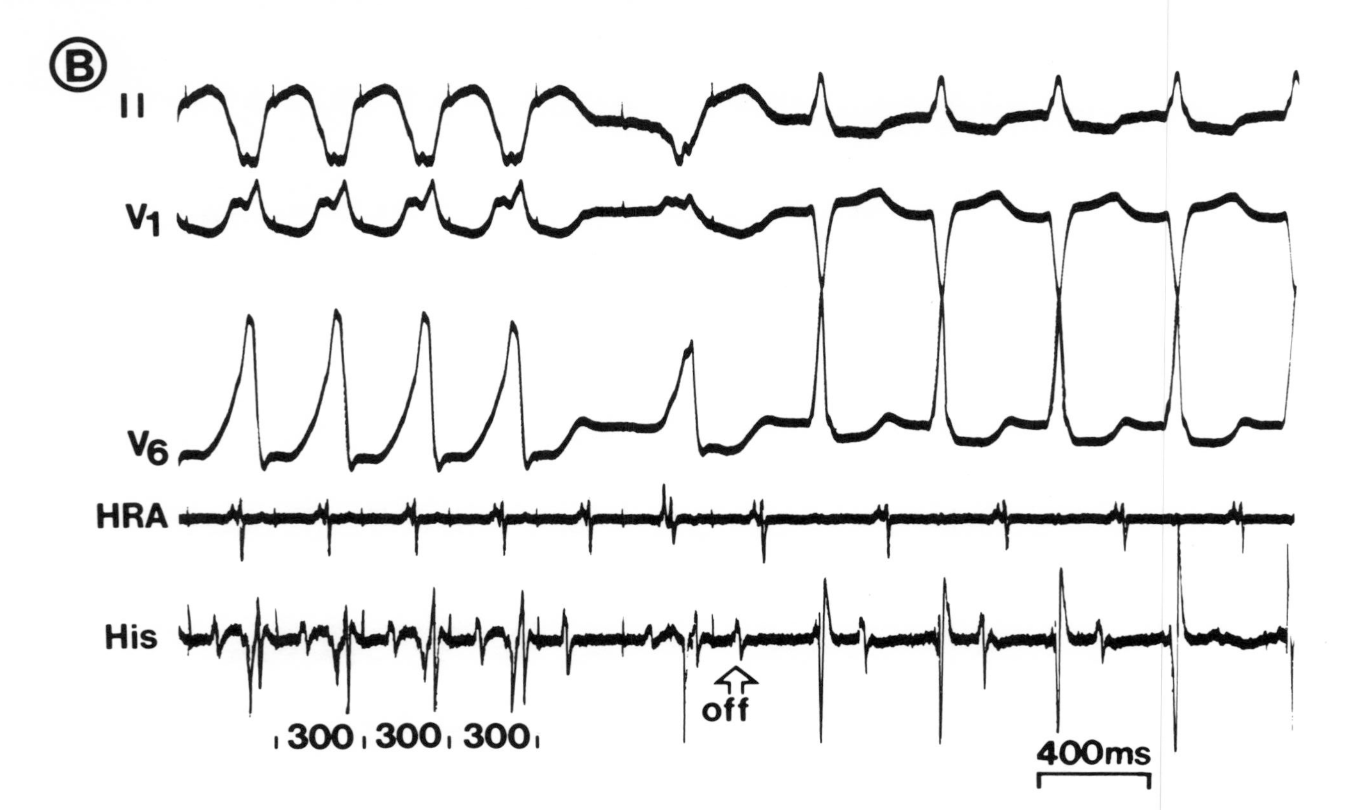

Figure 23–2 *(Continued).* In panel *B* the last atrial paced beat is exclusively conducted by way of the normal A-V pathway and is followed by initiation of tachycardia. Coronary sinus pacing at a rate of 200/min is being performed in both panels.

tiation of CMT incorporating the AP in V-A direction in patients with WPW have been recently reviewed.[11]

In a few patients the reversed (antidromic) form of CMT can be induced during the stimulation study. A-V conduction in this reciprocating tachycardia is by way of the AP and V-A conduction is over the normal His-A-V nodal axis. Therefore, QRS complexes during tachycardia show maximal pre-excitation. Initiation of the antidromic junctional CMT utilizing the AP in WPW requires:

1. Dissimilar properties of the normal and AP in one or both of the following ways (a) antegrade ERP of the AP shorter than that of the A-V node, and (b) retrograde ERP of the AP longer than that of the normal pathway.
2. Presence of V-A conduction by way of the normal pathway.
3. A revolution time longer than the longest refractory period of any of the components of the re-entry circuit.

During the stimulation study, this reversed CMT has been more frequently initiated following APBs than by VPBs.[11] The differential diagnosis of this reciprocating tachycardia is complex and we have recently discussed it in length elsewhere.[6]

OTHER FORMS OF PAROXYSMAL REGULAR TACHYCARDIAS IN WPW

Atrial tachycardia, A-V nodal re-entrant tachycardia, CMT utilizing two accessory pathways, and ventricular tachycardia have been induced during stimulation studies in patients with WPW.[3,4,6,8] Atrial flutter with 1:1 or 2:1 A-V conduction by way of the AP can also give rise to a regular tachycardia (Fig. 23-3).

The most important of all these less frequent forms of tachycardia is that based on an intra-A-V nodal reciprocating mechanism. In the eight instances of intra-A-V nodal re-entrant tachycardia encountered in our series, the QRS complexes showed normal intraventricular conduction or typical bundle branch block configuration. Therefore, the differential diagnosis in these patients had to be made with a CMT utilizing the AP in V-A direction. As discussed elsewhere, intranodal reciprocating tachycardias in WPW could also produce pre-excited ventricular complexes[6] as postulated in the left panel of Figure 23-4. However, either atrial fusion or cancellation within the AP itself usually occurs so that the QRS complex shows absence of pre-excitation during tachycardia (right panel, Fig. 23-4). Criteria diagnostic and suggestive for V-A conduction by way of an AP during junctional CMT are listed in Table 23-3 and should be used to differentiate the orthodromic CMT using the AP and the intranodal reciprocating tachycardia in WPW.

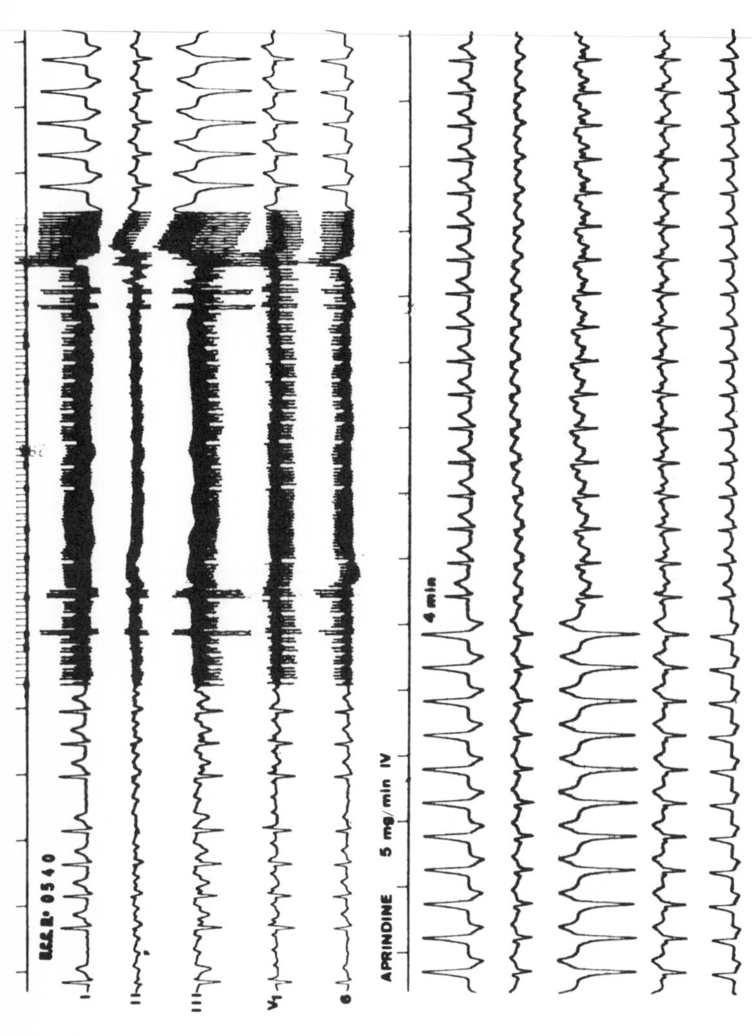

Figure 23-3. Atrial flutter in a patient with type B WPW-syndrome. In the upper panel the typical flutter waves are observed (F) while A-V conduction is by way of the normal A-V nodal-His pathway as a result of the administration of ajmaline intravenously (not illustrated). When the effect of ajmaline declines, 2:1 A-V conduction by way of the AP is observed giving rise to a regular tachycardia with wide (completely pre-excited) QRS complexes. Following the intravenous administration of aprindine, antegrade block over the AP is observed and atrial flutter with 2:1 A-V conduction by way of the normal A-V node-His axis is demonstrated. The upper and lower panels are not continuous.

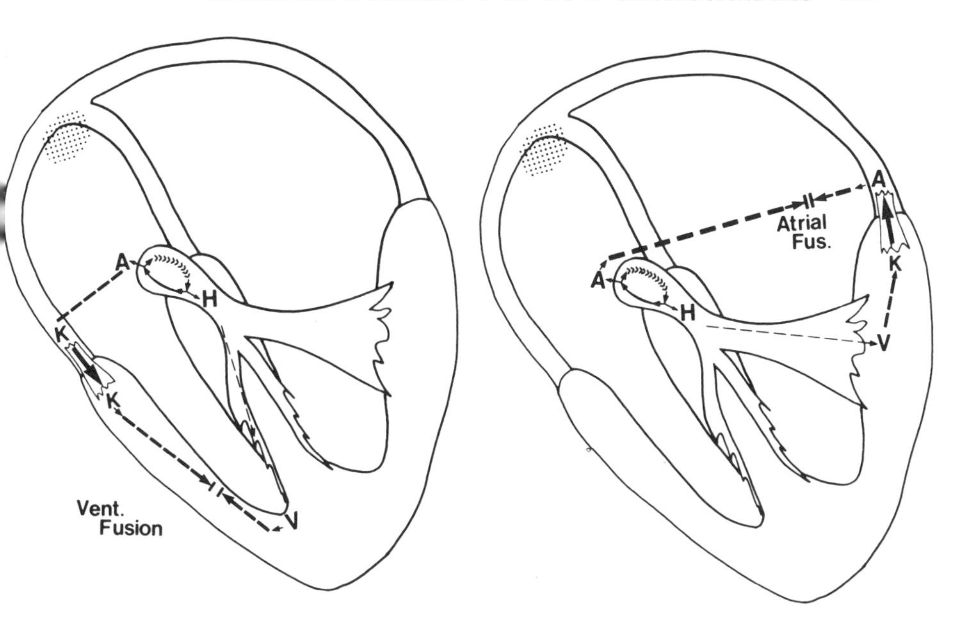

Figure 23-4. Intra-AV nodal reciprocating tachycardias in patients with the WPW syndrome. QRS complexes during tachycardia can be pre-excited (left panel) or show normal configuration due to exclusive ventricular activation by way of the normal intraventricular conducting system (right panel). Among the factors influencing QRS configuration during this form of tachycardia in WPW are: (1) mode of initiation of tachycardia and relationship between the ERP of the fast intranodal pathway and the AP in antegrade direction, (2) intra-atrial conduction times, (3) location of the AP, (4) conduction times over the AP, and (5) presence of bundle branch block ipsilateral to the AP.

ATRIAL FIBRILLATION IN WPW

Paroxysmal atrial fibrillation is not rare in patients with the WPW syndrome. It has been suggested that atrial fibrillation is more frequent in WPW than in the general population.[3] Whether this is real or a result of selection in the series of patients with WPW is a matter or debate.[8] During paroxysmal atrial fibrillation, very rapid, life-threatening, ventricular rates can develop in patients with WPW if the antegrade ERP of the AP is short.[5] A good correlation has been found between the shortest R-R interval during atrial fibrillation and the antegrade ERP of the AP.[5] The development of ventricular fibrillation has been documented in some patients with WPW and atrial fibrillation with very rapid ventricular rates due to exclusive A-V conduction by way of an AP which has a short antegrade ERP.[5,8]

Table 23-3. Criteria for the Diagnosis of V–A Conduction By Way of an Accessory Pathway During Tachycardia or Ventricular Pacing

A. DIAGNOSTIC

1. Eccentric retrograde atrial activation during V-A conduction.
2. VPB during tachycardia able to advance the atrial activity at a time when the His bundle is refractory, the sequence of the advanced atrial activity being identical to that observed during tachycardia.
3. V-A time prolongation after the development of functional BBB ipsilateral to the AP during tachycardia.
4. V-A time following a VPB during tachycardia equal to or less than the basal V-A time during tachycardia.
5. Prolongation of H-A time whenever H-V time prolongation occurs during tachycardia.
6. Termination of tachycardia following block in or distal to the bundle of His.

B. VERY SUGGESTIVE

7. Retrograde atrial activation in all intracavitary leads during tachycardia starting after termination of the QRS complex*

Abbreviations: VPB= ventricular premature beat; BBB= bundle branch block.

*Except during BBB contralateral to the AP in which case the earliest atrial activity can be within the terminal forces of the QRS complex

The development of ventricular fibrillation in patients with the WPW syndrome is unrelated to the age of the patient, previous history of paroxysmal tachycardia and presence of associated cardiac disease.[8] Ventricular fibrillation may be the presenting symptom in some patients with WPW.[8] The group from Duke University has reported on 18 patients with WPW who had a documented attack of ventricular fibrillation. On comparing the latter group of patients with those in whom atrial fibrillation never degenerated into ventricular fibrillation, the only significant different was the occurrence in the ventricular fibrillation group of consecutive pre-excited R-R intervals equal to or less than 205 ms during atrial fibrillation.[8]

In view of these arguments, our present approach to patients with the WPW syndrome and a short antegrade ERP of the AP (equal to or less than 270 ms) includes the induction of atrial fibrillation during the stimulation study (Table 23-1). Observations of both the ventricular rate and the shortest R-R interval of consecutively pre-excited beats during atrial fibrillation, may have prognostic and therapeutic implications.[9]

IMPLICATIONS OF THE STIMULATION STUDIES IN THE SELECTION OF THERAPY IN PATIENTS WITH WPW

The therapeutic implications of the stimulation studies can be considered under three different headings: (1) investigation of the action of drugs on the properties of the AP and the rest of the cardiac structures

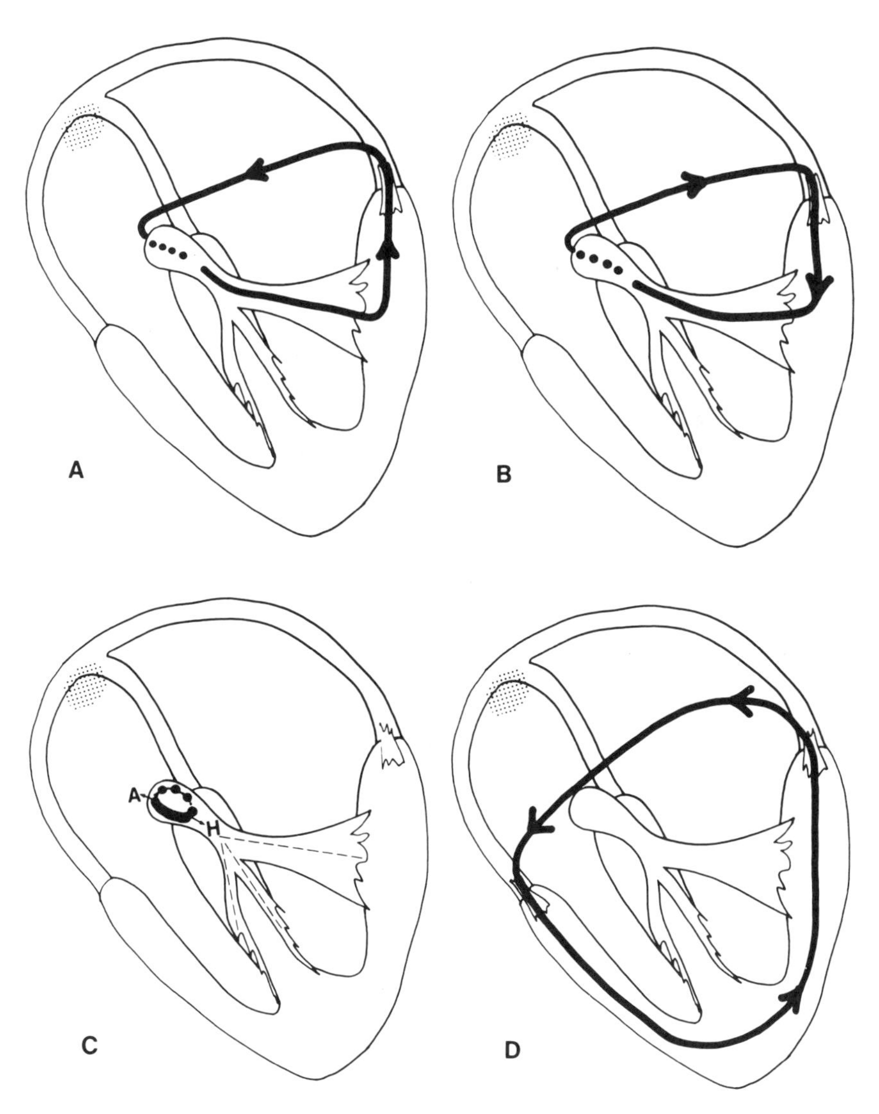

Figure 23-5. Different forms of A-V junctional reciprocating tachycardias described in patients with the WPW syndrome (Table 23-2 and text). Panel *A*: CMT incorporating the AP in V-A direction (orthodromic CMT). Panel *B*: CMT utilizing the AP in A-V direction (antidromic CMT). Panel *C*: Intra-AV nodal reciprocating tachycardia. Panel *D*: CMT incorporating two accessory pathways in the re-entry circuit.

which play a role in the tachycardias of these patients; (2) investigation of the mechanism, modes of initiation and termination of tachycardia in a given patient in order to select the most appropriate form of therapy; (3) investigation of the patient considered refractory to medical treatment to determine whether other forms of therapy (pacemakers or surgery) could be of help in controlling the arrhythmias.

Investigation of the Electrophysiological Effects of Drugs

The effects of several antiarrhythmic drugs have been tested during the stimulation study in patients with WPW.[3,6,8] A few general principles have been learned from these investigations:

1. *Drugs which shorten the ERP of the AP:* Digitalis may shorten the antegrade ERP of the AP. In approximately one third of patients with atrial fibrillation and WPW, the administration of digitalis resulted in an increase in the ventricular rate due to facilitation of A-V conduction by way of the AP.[12] Administration of digitalis to patients with WPW should be avoided during paroxysmal atrial fibrillation as well as in patients with a known short antegrade ERP of the AP.

2. *Drugs which prolong the ERP of the AP:* Several drugs have been shown to prolong the refractory period of the AP (ajmaline, amiodarone, aprindine, disopyramide, lidocaine, lorcainide, procainamide, quinidine).[3,6,8] There are several principles to be remembered in relation to these drugs: (a) the shorter the ERP of the AP prior to drug administration, the smaller the increment in refractoriness induced following most of these agents; (b) drugs which significantly prolong the antegrade ERP of the AP frequently induce less significant increments in the refractory period of the AP in V-A direction; (c) some of these drugs slow conduction velocity in several structures participating in the re-entry mechanism leading to tachycardia in these patients. The implications of these facts are as follows: (a) patients with the greatest need for prolongation of the antegrade ERP of the AP because of their very short basal value, will frequently obtain little benefit from currently available drugs. Of all drugs which prolong the antegrade ERP of the AP, amiodarone seems to be the most efficient to protect patients with WPW against the development of life-threatening ventricular rates during atrial fibrillation;[13] (b) prolongation of the antegrade ERP of the AP without adequate lengthening of refractoriness in V-A direction may facilitate initiation of CMT;[6,9] (c) initiation and perpetuation of CMT may be facilitated following the administration of drugs which slow conduction velocity in the re-entry circuit so that the revolution time is made longer than the longest refractory period of any of its components.[3,6,9]

3. *Effects of drugs on the tachycardia-zone:* During the stimulation study the effects of drugs on the zone of premature beat intervals resulting in tachycardia (tachycardia-zone) can be evaluated. Inability to induce tachycardia following the administration of a drug is considered as a positive and potentially relevant response from the therapeutic point of view. Drugs which induce complete antegrade block over the AP or significantly prolong the antegrade ERP of the AP can, however, enlarge the zone of tachycardia following atrial premature beats. This occurs when the drug does not induce V-A block over the AP or a very significant prolongation of its retrograde ERP. As stated before, the tachycardia-zone can be particularly enlarged if the drug also slows conduction velocity in the re-entry circuit. This phenomenon, reported after amiodarone administration[14] but observed with many other drugs, does not necessarily mean that the drug will exacerbate the episodes of tachycardia in the clinical situation. Frequently, spontaneous termination of the induced tachycardias after a few beats or a single echo are observed, which were not present prior to drug administration. When these spontaneous terminations occur after a certain drug has been administered, independently of the effects on the zone of tachycardia, the drug may improve the clinical situation of the patient by preventing the perpetuation of the episodes of tachycardia.

Therapeutic Implications of the Investigation of Mechanism, Modes of Initiation and Termination of Tachycardia

There are patients with WPW in whom the definition of the mechanism of tachycardia may play an important role in the selection of therapy. This occurs in patients in whom tachycardia is based on an intra-A-V nodal re-entry mechanism since these tachycardias can frequently be prevented by propranolol whereas this drug, given alone, is less effective to prevent episodes of CMT utilizing the AP. If the antegrade ERP of the AP is long (above 300 ms) digitalis could also be used in the prophylaxis of A-V nodal reciprocating tachycardias in these patients.[12]

In patients with a history of paroxysmal tachycardia and electrocardiographically documented episodes of atrial fibrillation, the stimulation study will be useful in determining the presence of other arrhythmias, particularly CMT using the AP. If during the stimulation study CMT is also initiated, it is very likely that the arrhythmia will clinically exist.[7,9] If in patients with atrial fibrillation no form of V-A conduction is observed during ventricular pacing, a junctional reciprocating mechanism can be excluded. If V-A conduction by way of the AP is not demonstrated, the common (orthodromic) form of CMT utilizing the AP can be ruled out to develop in this patient. When CMT cannot be induced during the stimulation study because of equal refractoriness in the A-V node-His axis and AP in spite of V-A conduction over both pathways, it is wise not to exclude the possibility of development of CMT under different electrophysiological circumstances, such as following the administration of a drug which is prescribed to prevent the development of life-threatening ventricular rates during atrial fibrillation. Thus, in these patients, a repeat stimulation study should be done after the administration of the drug considered to be given to the patient to prevent rapid ventricular rates during atrial fibrillation.

In some patients the identification of the weakest link of the re-entry circuit can be accomplished by studying the modes of termination, spontaneous and/or pacing-induced, of tachycardia. Drugs known to act on that segment of the circuit identified as the weakest link, should then be tested.

Electrophysiological Investigations in Patients Refractory to Medical Treatment

In the U.S.A. propranolol and quinidine, quinidine alone, digitalis and more recently disopyramide, are the most widely used drugs in patients with WPW and paroxysmal tachycardias. In Europe, although these drugs are frequently employed, most cardiologists prefer amiodarone as the most successful and convenient antiarrhythmic drug for control of arrhythmias in patients with this syndrome.[6,9,13,14]

In patients with "refractory" paroxysmal tachycardias, an electrophysiological investigation should be performed and based on the findings obtained during the stimulation study the effects of drugs should be tested. Chronic drug studies may be particularly useful in patients considered refractory to conventional drug treatment to establish the effectiveness of different drugs or combination of drugs to prevent initiation and/or perpetuation of tachycardia.[15]

Patients suffering from intractable junctional CMT can occasionally be controlled by a combination of antiarrhythmic drugs and a specially designed pacemaker. In these patients a stimulation study must be performed to define the modalities of pacing which most easily terminate the tachycardia. If single premature beats are capable of terminating the reciprocating tachycardia, a conventional demand unit may be implanted which can be converted into fixed rate pacing when the patient holds a magnet over the generator after recognizing the onset of tachycardia. "Burst" pacemakers can also be used when multiple premature stimuli (either atrial or ventricular) are required to stop tachycardia.[16]

Surgical Treatment

In patients in whom neither drugs nor combination of drugs and pacing techniques can obtain satisfactory control of the arrhythmias, surgical techniques should be considered. A pre-operative electrophysiological investigation is required to define the number and location of the accessory pathways. The more comprehensive the pre-operative evaluation the better the selection of patients for surgery and the better the planning of the surgical procedure. Furthermore, in some patients pre-excitation cannot be elicited during the operation for a number of reasons and in these patients the results of the preoperative catheter mapping become of paramount inportance.[17] Surgery for the WPW syndrome should be performed only in centers acquainted with the technical aspects of endocardial and epicardial intraoperative mapping, by surgeons experienced with this type of investigation.[8,18] The surgical approach to patients with WPW should probably still be considered investigational and reserved for carefully selected patients. The role of a wider application of surgical techniques in the WPW syndrome remains to be defined.

REFERENCES

1. Wolff, J., Parkinson, J., and White, P.D.: Bundle branch block with short P-R interval in healthy young people prone to paroxysmal tachycardia. *Am. Heart. J.* 5: 685, 1930.
2. Durrer, D., Schoo, L., Schuilenburg, R.M., and Wellens, H.J.J.: The role of premature beats in the initiation and termination of supraventricular tachycardia in the Wolff-Parkinson-White syndrome. *Circulation* 41: 399, 1967.
3. Wellens, H.J.J.: The electrophysiological properties of the accessory pathway in the Wolff-Parkinson-White Syndrome. In Wellens, H.J.J., Janse, M.J., and Lie, K.I. (eds.): *The Conduction System of the Heart.* Philadelphia, Lea and Febiger, 1976, p. 567.
4. Gallagher, J.J., Sealy, W.C., Wallace, A.G., and Kasell, J.: Correlation between catheter electrophysiological studies and findings on mapping of ventricular excitation in the WPW syndrome. In Wellens, H.J.J., Janse, M.J., and Lie, K.I. (eds.): *The Conduction System of the Heart.* Leiden, Stenfert-Kroese, 1976.
5. Wellens, H.J.J., and Durrer, D.: Relation between refractory period of the accessory pathway and ventricular frequency during atrial fibrillation in patients with the Wolff-Parkinson-White syndrome. *Am. J. Cardiol.* 33: 178, 1974.
6. Wellens, H.J.J., Farré, J., and Bar, F.W.: Value and limitations of programmed electrical stimulation in patients with the Wolff-Parkinson-White Syndrome. In Narula, O. (ed.): *Cardiac Arrhythmias: Electrophysiology, Diagnosis and Management.* Baltimore, Williams & Wilkins, 1979.

7. Denes, P., Wu, D., Amat-y-Leon, F., et al.: Determination of atrioventricular reentrant paroxysmal tachycardia in patients with Wolff-Parkinson-White Syndrome. *Circulation* **50**: 415, 1978.
8. Gallagher, J.J., Pritchett, E.L.C., Sealy, W.C., et al.: The preexcitation syndromes. *Prog. Cardiovasc. Dis.* **20**: 285, 1978.
9. Wellens, H.J.J., Farré, J., and Bar, F.W.: The Wolff-Parkinson-White Syndrome. In Mandel, W.J. (ed.): *Cardiac Arrhythmias.* Philadelphia, J.B. Lippincott Co., in press.
10. Pritchett, E.L.C., Gallagher, J.J., Scheinman, M., and Smith, W.M.: Determinants of Antegrade Echo Zone in the Wolff-Parkinson-White Syndrome. *Circulation* **57**: 671, 1978.
11. Wellens, H.J.J.: Modes of initiation of circusmovement tachycardia in 139 patients with the Wolff-Parkinson-White syndrome studied by programmed electrical stimulation. In Kulbertus, H.E. (ed.): *Re-entrant Arrhythmias.* Lancaster, MTP Press, 1977.
12. Sellers, T.D., Bashore, T.M., and Gallagher, J.J.: Digitalis in the pre-excitation syndrome: Analysis during atrial fibrillation. *Circulation* **56**: 260, 1977.
13. Wellens, H.J.J., Bar, F.W., and Gorgels, A.N.: Effect of drugs in the WPW syndrome. Importance of initial length of effective refractory period of accessory pathway. *Am. J. Cardiol.* **41**: 372, 1978.
14. Wellens, H.J.J., Lie, K.I., Bar, F.W., et al.: Effect of amiodarone in the Wolff-Parkinson-White Syndrome. *Am. J. Cardiol.* **38**: 189, 1976.
15. Wu, D., Amat-y-Leon, F., Simpson, R.J., et al.: Electrophysiological studies with multiple drugs in patients with atrioventricular re-entrant tachycardias utilizing an extranodal pathway. *Circulation* **56**: 727, 1977.
16. Wellens, H.J.J., Bar, F.W., Gorgels, A.P., and Farré, J.: Electrical management of arrhythmias with emphasis on the tachycardias. *Am. J. Cardiol.* **41**: 1025, 1978.
17. Gallagher, J.J., Kasell, J., Sealy, W.C., et al.: Epicardial mapping in the Wolff-Parkinson-White Syndrome. *Circulation* **57**: 854, 1978.
18. Gallagher, J.J., Sealy, W.C., Anderson, R.W., et al.: The surgical treatment of arrhythmias. In Kulbertus, H.E. (ed.): Re-entrant Arrhythmias. Lancaster, MTP Press, 1977.

24

Natural History of the Pre-excitation Syndrome

Libi Sherf, M.D.

During the last decade, a large number of papers dealing with pre-excitation have appeared in the literature. They covered special areas of this syndrome, such as the electrophysiological profile of patients with tachycardia, surgical reports and pathological studies.

In this study, the natural history of the syndrome derived from the follow-up study of 215 consecutive cases seen at the Heart Institute, Chaim Sheba Medical Center in Tel-Aviv and a review of the literature is presented.

Four aspects of the pre-excitation syndrome will be reviewed: general considerations, morbidity, mortality, and treatment.

GENERAL CONSIDERATIONS

Prevalence

The prevalence of pre-excitation is difficult to determine because the ECG patterns may be absent in cases of intermittent pre-excitation at the time of recording. The diagnosis is usually made (1) by the incidental finding of the typical pattern on a routine ECG, in the absence of arrhythmias, (2) in 5 to 10 percent of cases suffering from paroxysmal tachycardias, or (3) in cases admitted to hospital because of misinterpretation of a routine ECG revealing this anomaly.

In a report among 429,300 subjects, 666 cases had pre-excitation (0.155%). The average prevalence of pre-excitation among hospital in-patients was similar to that among healthy individuals undergoing routine examination. The below-16 age group did not differ from the over-16 group. The only outstanding finding is that children below the age of 16 under care for different cardiac conditions had a prevelence of pre-excitation approximately three times higher than any of the other groups. This higher incidence in the child heart clinics may be due to the association of congenital heart disease with the pre-excitation syndrome, and is not carried over into the general population since many of these children die during childhood.

Sex

In Wolff-Parkinson-White's classic paper,[1] eight of their 11 patients were males and three were females. Every series of cases published since then has shown a similar male preponderance (60–70%). Of a total of 1,011 patients with pre-excitation collected from the literature, where the sex was mentioned, 657 were males (65%) and 364 females (35%). Among the 215 cases from our hospital, 157 were males and 58 females.[2]

Age

Although Wolff-Parkinson-White[1] assumed that the pre-excitation syndrome is a disorder of young adults only, it has by now been reported in all ages, from early childhood[3–5] including neonates to old age.

Our youngest patient was three days old and the oldest was 80 years. There were relatively few cases at the two extremes of the age spectrum in our patients: 24 in children under the age of 16 and 18 in adults over 60. Patients from 11 to 20 years of age were twice as numerous (66 cases) as the mean (26.8). This may be due to the fact that this group includes many children and young adults sent for cardiac investigation because of a functional murmur or nonspecific chest pain discovered by the school or army physician.

Familial Occurrence

Pre-excitation in two or more members of the same family does occur, although rarely. We detected such cases in 21 families from the literature and one from our own series. The number of affected members in any family may vary, from two (the majority) to six. Harnischfeger[6] reported a particularly interesting family with five cases, two of which were monozygotic twins. Ohnell[7] reported families where some members had classic pre-excitation ECG's while others had partial forms of the syndrome. Pre-excitation in our series occurred in a mother and a son.

THE PRE-EXCITATION SYNDROME ASSOCIATED WITH CONGENITAL HEART DISEASE

From 122 cases from the literature, the following conclusions can be made: (1) Pre-excitation occurs in many types of congenital heart disease. (2) The number of cases with VSD (as an isolated malformation, 20 of 122 cases) and of transposition of the great vessels (not always specified if corrected or complete, 7 of 122 cases) exceeds the expected percentage. (3) The association of pre-excitation and Ebstein's anomaly of the tricuspid valve is far greater than expected. If we add to this last group cases with tricuspid atresia (4 of 122), it may be suggested that the pre-excitation syndrome has some relationship to lesions of the tricuspid valve.

In our series six cases of pre-excitation with associated congenital heart disease, one had Ebstein's anomaly of the tricuspid valve, one had PDA (associated with pulmonary hypertension), one had discrete and muscular subaortic stenosis, the fifth had fibroelastosis and the sixth had an anomalous origin of both great vessels from the right ventricle. Donzelot et al.[8] reported three cases among 1,100 patients (0.27%), while Hecht[9] reported three among 350 consecutive patients (0.86%) and the association of pre-excitation and cardiac congenital disease. However, when pre-excitation is taken as the point of reference, the following is seen: 15 cases of congenital heart disease among 28 patients with pre-excitation (53%),[4] 19 cases of congenital heart disease among 48 children with pre-excitation (40%),[5] and 20 cases of congenital heart disease among 62 cases with pre-excitation.[3] If these figures are considered definitive, we can expect congenital cardiac malformation in one-third to one-half of all children with pre-excitation. The high mortality rate from congenital heart disease in these children (8 out of 20 died during Giardin's follow-up study[3]) reduced the number of adults with concurrence of the two disorders.

PRE-EXCITATION SYNDROME ASSOCIATED WITH CARDIAC DISEASES OTHER THAN CONGENITAL

In an analysis of 11 series[2] covering 593 cases of pre-excitation collected from the literature and from our files, in which the incidence and associated heart disease were available in a general population (Table 24-1), no cardiac involvement was detected in the vast majority (68.3%) and these cases are considered "isolated pre-excitation". In the remaining cases (31.7%), the percentage of heart disease ranged from 19 to 62.9 percent. Rheumatic disease was found in 32 of the 593 patients. Atherosclerotic heart disease included anginal syndrome, coronary insufficiency, myocardial ischemia and myocardial infarction. Fifty-four patients suffered from these diseases including 14 from our own series. Hypertensive cardiovascular disease was another relatively large group with 45 cases, many of them also had atherosclerotic heart disease but were classified under the heading of "hypertension" only. Twelve were from our series, including one case of juvenile hypertension. Myocarditis and/or "acute rheumatic fever" were found in 17 patients in this group, of which two were ours. In 20 patients there was no definite diagnosis of heart disease, although the authors felt that there was some type of cardiac involvement.

Morbidity

Without Tachyarrhythmias: A distinction is made between cases of pre-excitation alone and those with signs of associated heart diseases. Differences between adults and children are also noted.

Isolated Pre-excitation: Individuals with pre-excitation and no history of tachycardia or other heart disease who are asymptomatic.

Patients With Associated Heart Disease: About 30 percent of people with pre-excitation have associated heart disease. In cases with tachyarrhythmias, the health status is related to the underlying heart disease. Many patients with pre-excitation have undergone surgery without ill effects.

With Tachyarrhythmias: It occurs in about half the cases. The effect of the tachyarrhythmias on prognosis is not well known. In nine series from the literature and our own group in which there was long-term follow-up, three dealt with children only[3–5] (including newborns and infants), one mainly with elderly people, and the rest contained material from general populations. Among the 717 cases collected, 327 (45.60%) had attacks of tachycardia (in our own series 109 of 215) (Table 24-2).

Age of Onset of Paroxysmal Tachycardias: Palpitations can make their first appearance at any time. Pre-excitation behaves differently in newborns than in older children, in whom the syndrome behaves like in adults. There is a high incidence of tachycardias in babies under the age of 10 months, ranging between 77 and 84 percent depending on the study, while in older children and adults it is between 40 and 60 percent. In babies, pre-excitation is discovered because of attacks of tachycardias and its occurrence is much higher than in all the other age groups. Fifty percent of all the infants seen with paroxysmal tachyarrhythmias also had pre-excitation (as compared to 5–10% of older children and adults).

The age of first attack of tachycardia in the older population is such that we found in eight cases the onset occurred over the age of 50. This late onset of rhythm disturbances raises the question of whether they are

Table 24-1. Pre-excitation and Cardiovascular Diseases

	No. of cases with pre-excitation	Associated heart disease	Rheumatic valve disease	ASHD	Hypertension	Myocarditis (+ rheumatic fever)	Uncertain cardiac involvement	Congenital heart disease
TOTAL	593	188 (31.7%)	32	54	45	17	20	20

Table 24-2. Studies from the Literature with Long-term Follow-up

No. Series	No. of Cases	Lost to Follow-up	Years of Follow-up	Associated Heart Disease	Tachycardia	Death	
						Sudden	Tachycardia
10	717 100%	38 5.29%	0 – 28	161 22.45%	327 45.60%	3 0.4%	9 1.25%

related to the pre-excitation or to a basic degenerative heart disease. This question cannot be answered definitively at present, but one can assume a direct connection to pre-excitation if the documented tachycardia is of the pseudo-ventricular type where the QRS complexes are broad and deformed. The same can be said apparently for repeated PAT in the absence of other kinds of tachycardias. But, when the attacks are simply paroxysmal atrial fibrillations, they are more likely related to the basic heart disease than to pre-excitation.

The Duration of the Tachycardias: Eighty-five percent of infants with tachycardias have no recurrences of paroxysms after 6 to 12 months of age.[3] Recurrence of PAT beyond 18 months of age is very rare. Thus, the prognosis seems excellent, and the period of rhythm disturbances short. For children and adults it is usual for paroxysms of palpitations to continue for years and even decades.

A salient feature of the pre-excitation syndrome is the unpredictability of the frequency of tachycardias and the variation in their duration.

The 98 patients in the Tel-Hashomer group with paroxysmal tachycardias available for follow-up were questioned as to the frequency and duration of their attacks. The largest group reported suffering between one and five attacks in a year (32 patients); only 12 had the same number in one week. The paroxysms of tachycardia continued for only several seconds or minutes in almost half, or 42, of these 98 patients. In 24, the pattern was mixed—sometimes seconds, sometimes hours, and sometimes the patient could not recall the duration. In a minority of cases (10 patients) the palpitations continued for hours and even days, and they usually required admission to the hospital. On follow-up, forty-nine reported no noticeable change; 23 reported feeling better because the paroxysms became shorter or less frequent; nine stated that the palpitations had stopped completely, and six were convinced that they felt worse.

Types of Tachyarrhythmias: No ECG was recorded during attacks of palpitations in 58 of the 98 Tel-Hashomer cases, mostly because of their short duration. ECG documentation was obtained in 40 patients, 16 had atrial tachycardia (PAT) with narrow[13] or broad[3] QRS complexes. Atrial fibrillation was seen in 15 patients, with narrow ventricular complexes in four and broad in 11. Atrial flutter was documented in two patients and sinus tachycardia in six.

Mortality

The introduction of surgery in the treatment of patients with pre-excitation turned this syndrome from an academic matter into a clinical problem requiring critical decisions. Surgery is directed to control intractable arrhythmias and/or to prevent sudden and unexpected death. Since these unexpected deaths have become a *raison d'etre* for surgery, they must be carefully analyzed to clarify whether the mortality rate in the disease itself is smaller or greater than that in surgery. The results may dictate a second look at what the optimal treatment should be in a given case, conservative or surgical.

Definite statistics on the mortality rate in pre-excitation cannot be derived from the literature due to lack of data and insufficient follow-up. Nevertheless, an impression can be gained from a few follow-up studies published. Orinius[10] followed 50 patients with pre-excitation and paroxysmal tachycardia for 21 years and did not find a higher mortality rate when calculating their life expectancy rate. The Aetna Life and Casualty Company followed 49 patients with pre-excitation covering 314 patient years. A precise statistical evaluation is pending, but at the moment the mortality rate appears to be within the predicted normal range.

Deaths Associated With Tachycardia: Prolonged periods of tachycardias were the only or the main contributing factor to death in some patients. The question is only how often this occurs. A search for the literature for cases of death directly resulting from tachycardias yielded the following: 23 cases reported by Okel,[11] ten cases by Dreifus et al.,[12] eight others found by us in the literature and two patients from our series of 215, bringing the total to 43. Fourteen died in shock or congestive heart failure due to the long periods of tachyarrhythmia and 29 died a sudden death.

While this tabulation gives a figure for the number of cases who died as a direct result of pre-excitation, it is of little help in illuminating the incidence of such deaths in the whole population of pre-excitation cases. Firstly, the exact number of cases is unknown (it is estimated somewhere between 1,500 and 2,000), and secondly, many of the reported cases suffered from additional heart diseases which by themselves may be complicated by tachycardias.

Seven hundred seventeen cases were followed from one to 25 years (Table 24-2), most for more than ten years, 327 suffered from palpitations and tachycardias (45.60%) and 91 cases are known to have died. Twelve were suspected to have died as a direct result of the pre-excitation syndrome, nine during attacks of tachycardia and three of sudden death. Death during tachycardia was certain in only two of the nine suspected cases; an infant with Fallot who died during repeated attacks of PAT and one case of Swidersky.[5] In the other seven cases it was more an assumption than a proven fact.

Sudden Death: Sudden death is directly connected with pre-excitation. In some cases ventricular fibrillation was documented, and probably accounted for the sudden death. The ventricular fibrillation usually appears in the ECG tracing as a continuation of a paroxysm of atrial fibrillation with broad QRS complexes pseudo-ventricular tachycardia) at a very fast rate. Among the 43 cases of death in patients with pre-excitation collected from the literature, described above, 29 died a sudden death. In 17 cases accompanying factors were present which by themselves can cause sudden death, mainly additional heart diseases and some medications. At least eight of them suffered from a cardiomyopathy, and one of each: Ebstein's anomaly of the tricuspid valve, myocarditis, mitral stenosis and lipoma of the interatrial septum. One patient received intravenous digitalis during an attack of pseudo-ventricular tachycardia and died.[11] For calculating the mortality incidence we can only use cases collected from the literature and included in long-term follow-up studies. If we consider all 12 of the 717 cases previously mentioned, as representing death secondary to features of the pre-excitation syndrome, we find a mortality incidence of 1.67 percent in these series. But, since it is obvious that not all the cases died solely as a result of their electrical disturbance, the incidence of mortality in pre-excitation seems to be closer to that calculated Lepeshkin[13] namely, one percent.

Treatment: The great majority of episodes of paroxysmal tachycardia requires no special treatment, being very brief and terminating spontaneously. Occasionally, however, the paroxysms are longer and may produce considerable hemodynamic deterioration and symptoms. In such cases treatment is indicated. Until recently, many physicians preferred to administer digitalis intravenously in cases of pseudo-ventricular tachyarrhythmias, considering the paroxysm a simple rapid atrial fibrillation for which digoxin is known to be the most effective drug. Recent evidence, however, suggests that this treatment may acutely shorten the refractory period of the accessory pathway by 10 to 50 m/sec, thereby increasing the already fast cardiac rate of the tachycardia. This very fast atrial fibrillation has been known to induce ventricular fibrillation, with fatal outcome in some patients and successful resuscitation in others. It is generally agreed at the present time that digitalis preparations are strictly contraindicated in such conditions. This statement applied, however, only to adult patients and older children, and not newborns and infants. In newborns the danger of irreversible heart failure and death is great.[5] The tachycardia in babies is always the reentrant type (PAT) (to the best of our knowledge no pseudo-ventricular tachycardia has been reported in an infant). Thus, the drug of choice is digitalis.

Beta-blockers are contraindicated in pre-excitation with signs of sinus node dysfunction (bradycardia-tachycardia syndrome). These patients may present spontaneous dizziness or syncope, not as a result of their tachycardias, but rather due to overdrive malfunction of the sinus node (or AV node) and with poor escape mechanisms. The administration of beta-blockers in such patients may induce periods of iatrogenic asystole and syncope.[14] Therefore, their use is contraindicated.

Surgery: Two major approaches characterize this surgical intervention in pre-excitation: (a) the interruption of anomalous conduction by section of an accessory muscle bundle connecting an atrium with a ventricle, and (b) the interruption of normal conduction by section of the His bundle and production of complete atrioventricular block, always combined with the insertion of an artificial pacemaker.

Results of Surgery: The clinical and electrocardiographic results of operations undertaken for the treatment of tachycardias in the pre-excitation syndrome must, however, be approached with caution. The findings reported comprise 83 patients and 94 operations (Table 24-3). The delta wave disappeared in 43 patients (53.75%) after surgery and remained unchanged or slightly changed in 36 (43.27%) (one patient died before a clear finding could be recorded and 3 others had no delta wave from the beginning). Tachycardia did not recur after the first operation in 47 patients (56.62%), and recurred in 29 (34.43%). Eight patients (9.63%) died during or soon after the surgical procedures, bringing to 37 (44.56%) the total number of patients who did not enjoy positive results (both first and second operations are included in this figure. Results have been more favorable in those cases with pathways in the left or right free wall portion (right or left ventricle) or the AV groove than in those with septal connections. In cases operated at Duke University,[15] the free wall accessory bundle was successfully divided in 20 of 22 patients as judged by disappearance of the delta wave and abolition of tachycardias, while it was successful in only five of 14 septal connections. Additional bypass pathways were discovered in at least 13 operated cases, usually after section of the main accessory bundle: seven were most probably multiple muscular AV connections, three Mahaim bundles, and three conducting James' bypass fibers.

There seems to be general consensus that surgical intervention should be considered only in a small group pf patients with intractable episodes of supraventricular tachycardias who are unresponsive to medical and/or electrical therapy, or cases with life-threatening arrhythmias, especially atrial fibrillation with an extremely rapid ventricular response. Surgery should be attempted in those medical centers equipped with the electrophysiological techniques necessary to locate the site of the AV bypass. In approaching a patient for surgery, the following considerations should be made: The surgical mortality rate is 10 percent as compared to one to two percent mortality in pre-excitation in general. The tachycardias ceased after surgery in only a little more than half of the patients. The success of surgery is less when the accessory bundle is located near the

Table 24-3. Results of Surgery

Series N	No. of patients operated	"Kent bundle" dissection	His bundle dissection	Elective	Secondary
16	34	71	23	12	11

Delta Wave remained unchanged	Delta wave disappeared	Tachycardia remained (after 1 operation)	Tachycardia disappeared	Death operative
36	43	29	47	8
43.27%	53.75	34.93%	56.62%	9.63%

septum than when it is on the free wall of the ventricles. Multiple connections including Mahaim or James' fibers can be present but are silent and identifiable only after the main bypass bundle has been sectioned, in many cases. When the His bundle is interrupted, reentry for supraventricular tachycardias is eliminated, but not AV conduction over the accessory pathway which can be utilized in atrial fibrillation. The documentation of paroxysmal atrial tachycardia does not exclude the possibility of a fast pseudo-ventricular tachycardia developing in the same patient at another time.

REFERENCES

1. Wolff, L., Parkinson, J., and White, P.D.: Bundle branch block with short P-R internal in healthy young people prone to paroxysmal tachycardia. *Am. Heart. J.* 5: 685, 1930.
2. Sherf, L., and Neufeld, H.N.: *The Pre-excitation Syndrome: Facts and Theories.* New York, Yorke Medical Books, 1978.
3. Giardina, A.C.V., Ehlers, K.H., and Engle, M.A.: Wolff-Parkinson-White syndrome in infants and children. A long-term follow-up study. *Br. Heart. J.* 34: 839, 1972.
4. Shiebler, G.L., Adams, P.J., and Anderson, R.C.: The Wolff-Parkinson-White syndrome in infants and children. A review and a report of 28 cases. *Pediatrics* 24: 585, 1959.
5. Swiderski, J., Lees, M.H., and Nadas, A.S.: The Wolff-Parkinson-White syndrome in infancy and childhood. *Br. Heart J.* 24: 561, 1962.
6. Harnischfeger, W.W.: Heredity occurrence of the pre-excitation (Wolff-Parkinson-White) with re-entry mechanism and concealed conduction. *Circulation* 19: 28, 1959.

7. Ohnell, R.E.: Pre-excitation, a cardiac abnormality. *Acta Med. Scand.* **Suppl. 152**, 1944.
8. Donzelot, E.: Traite des cardiopathies congenitales. Paris, Masson, 1954, r. 1025.
9. Hecht, H.H.: Anomalous atrioventricular excitation. Panel discussion. *Ann. N.Y. Acad. Sci.* **65**: 826, 1959.
10. Orinius, E.: Pre-excitation. Studies on criteria, prognosis and heredity. *Acta Med. Scand.* **Suppl. 465**, 1966.
11. Okel, B.B.: The Wolff-Parkinson-White syndrome, report of a case with fatal arrhythmia and autopsy findings of myocarditis, inter-atrial lipomatous hypertrophy, and prominent right moderator band. *Am. Heart J.* **75**: 673, 1968.
12. Dreifus, L.S., Hait, R., Watanabe, Y., et al.: Ventricular fibrillation. A possible mechanism of sudden death in patients and Wolff-Parkinson-White syndrome. *Circulation* **43**: 520, 1971.
13. Lepeschkin, E.: The Wolff-Parkinson-White syndrome and other forms of pre-excitation in cardiology, edited by A.L. Luisade, New York, McGraw-Hill, 1962.
14. Berry, E.M., and Hasin, Y.: Propranolol-induced dysfunction of the sinus node in Wolff-Parkinson-White syndrome. *Chest* **73**: 873–875, 1978.
15. Tonkin, A.M., Gallagher, Y.Y., and Wallace, A.G.: Tachyarrhythmias in Wolff-Parkinson-White syndrome treatment and prevention. *J.A.M.A.* **235**: 947, 1976.

25

Relationship Between Alternating Wenckebach Periods and Paroxysmal Block in the A–V Node

Agustin Castellanos, M.D., Victor M. Alatriste, M.D., and Ruey J. Sung, M.D.

Although several articles have dealt with A-V nodal alternating Wenckebach periods, few have dealt with its relationship with paroxysmal A-V nodal block, as will be discussed in this chapter.

MATERIAL AND METHODS

Methods

Electrophysiological studies were performed as previously outlined,[1,2] in 19 patients who, among other problems, had recurrent supraventricular tachyarrhythmias. The procedure was explained to the patients and their relatives, and witnessed informed consent was obtained. As in other laboratories,[3,4] part of our work-up on patients with recurrent supraventricular tachyarrhythmias includes attempts to reinduce these arrhythmias in the cardiovascular laboratory under controlled conditions, as well as the evaluation of the response to intravenously administered drugs[1,2].

Definitions and Intervals of Conduction

Unless otherwise specifically stated, the terminology used in reference to the various deflections, intervals of conduction, and disturbances in conduction, as well as in the ladder diagrams that incorporate His bundle electrograms, has been discussed previously.[2] Normal values for the P-R, atrio-His (A-H), and His-ventricle (H-V) intervals in our laboratory range from 120 to 210 msec, from 55 to 120 msec, and from 35 to 55 msec, respectively. Normal values of atrioventricular nodal refractory periods during pacing with extrastimulus technique were those given by Denes et al.[5] For the purposes of this presentation atrioventricular nodal alternating Wenckebach periods were episodes of 2:1 A-H blocks, during which there was a progressive prolongation of the A-H interval of the conducted beats, terminating in 3:1, 4:1, 5:1 or 6:1 A-H block.

Patients

The patients (none of whom had coronary arterial disease) were divided into four groups, Group 1 consisted of eight nonmedicated patients without atrioventricular nodal disease (normal P-R intervals, A-H intervals, and atrioventricular nodal refractory periods) in whom rapid atrial pacing was performed at gradually increasing rates until the occurrence of intra-atrial Wenckebach periods. Data concerning this pattern of conduction in these cases has been presented elsewhere.[1] Group 2 included four patients with pacing-induced sustained episodes of atrial flutter with 2:1 atrioventricular conduction in whom intracardiac electrograms were recorded 30 minutes after the intravenous administration of ouabin (0.01 mg/kg of body weight). Group 3 consisted of four patients in whom rapid atrial pacing was performed either 30 minutes after the administration of ouabain as outlined previously (three patients) or ten minutes after having received 10 mg of verapamil intravenously (one patient).[6] These drugs had been given (successfully) to abolish previously present reciprocating atrioventricular nodal tachycardias. Group 4 included three patients with narrows QRS complexes who had the sick sinus syndrome, recurrent atrial tachyarrhythmias, and atrioventricular nodal disease manifested by prolonged P-R and A-H intervals and atrioventricular nodal refractory periods. In these cases, atrial pacing at increasing rates was performed only at cycle lengths between 600 and 350 msec.

RESULTS

Atrioventricular nodal (A-H) alternating Wenckebach periods ending in 5:1 atrioventricular block occurred in one of the eight patients in group 1, in all four patients in group 2, in all four patients in group 3, and in two of the three patients in group 4 (Table 25-1). This pattern of conduction had not been observed in the four patients in group 2 and the four

Table 25-1. Disturbances in Atrioventricular Nodal Conduction Coexisting With Alternating Wenckebach Periods Ending in 5:1 Atrioventricular Block*

DATA	GROUP 1	2	3	4
No. of patients in group	8	4	4	3
Atrioventricular block ending alternating Wenckebach periods				
5:1 block	1	4	4	2
3:1 or 4:1 block	6	4	4	3
Paroxysmal block	0	0	3	2

*Table values are numbers of patients.

patients in group 3 prior to the administration of ouabain or verapamil. In addition, six of the eight patients in group 1, and all of the patients in groups 2, 3 and 4, also had atrioventricular nodal alternating Wenckebach periods ending in 3:1 and 4:1 block.

Figures 25-1 and 25-2 were recorded for the only patient in group 1 who had atrioventricular nodal alternating Wenckebach periods ending in 5:1 atrioventricular block during atrial stimulation. This was preceded by alternating Wenckebach periods terminating in 4:1 atrioventricular block. The latter, as diagrammed in Figure 25-1, has been attributed (with penetration of all atrial impulses into, at least, the uppermost parts of the atrioventricular node) to the coexistence of 2:1 block in a "proximal" atrioventricular nodal level and Wenckebach periods in a "distal" level.[1,2,7-11] Partial penetration excludes true atrioventricular nodal entrance block and implies the existence of a third atrioventricular nodal level, located "more proximally" to the previously mentioned "proximal" level (represented diagrammatically immediately below the horizontal level separating A from A-H) with a shorter effective refractory period.

Thus, the first half of Figure 25-1 shows (A-H) block of every other atrial impulse (A5, A3, and A5) with progressively increasing (A-H) delays of the conducted impulses (A2, A4, and A6) due to 4:3 Wenckebach in the distal level. Completion of the latter during inscription of A8 (with persistence of 2:1 block at the proximal level) converts the 2:4 block into 4:1 atrioventricular block.

An alternating Wenckebach period ending in 5:1 atrioventricular block (obtained from the same patient) is shown in Figure 25-2. The diagram depicts the basic sequence postulated to explain alternating Wenckebach periods ending in 4:1 atrioventricular block as influenced by erratic variations in the A-H interval. As a consequence of these fluctuations, one atrial impulse (A7 in Fig. 25-2) appeared so soon (205 msec) after another (A6) that it arrived at the atrioventricular node early enough to have been unable to penetrate the "more proximal level" (true atrioven-

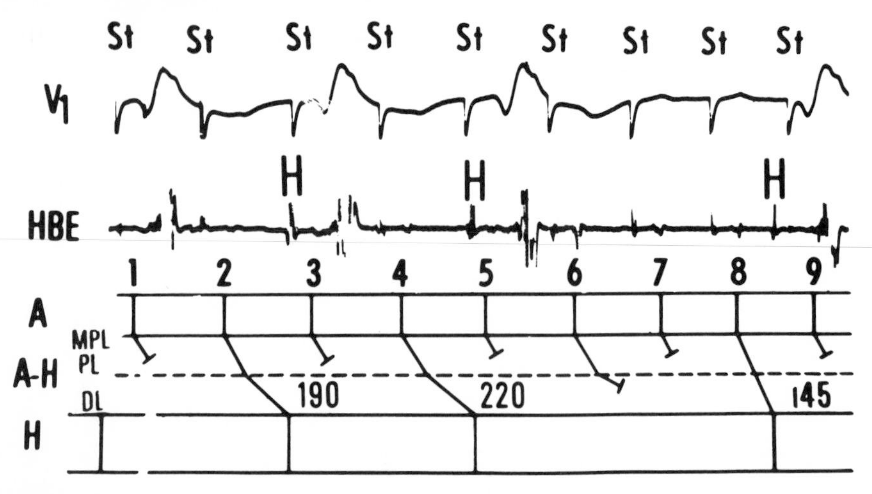

Figure 25–1. Atrioventricular nodal alternating Wenckebach period ending in 4:1 atrioventricular block during rapid atrial stimulation in a nonmedicated patient without atrioventricular nodal disease. According to conventional electrographic theory this results from the existence of a Wenckebach period in the distal level (DL) with a 2:1 block in the proximal level (PL), with penetration of all impulses through the more proximal level (MPL). St = stimulus artefact. HBE = His bundle electrographic lead. A = atrial deflection recorded by the HBE lead. H = His bundle electrogram. Numbers on top of the A level indicate consecutive atrial impulses. Numbers below indicate the duration (in msec) of the corresponding (conducted) A-H intervals.

tricular nodal entrance block) or to have decremented within it. In any case, this occurred during inscription of an atrial impulse (A7) which would (had the alternating Wenckebach sequence persisted) otherwise have been able to reach the His bundle. Therefore, the alternating Wenckebach period ended in 5:1 atrioventricular block. It is postulated that the events in this case, as well as those occurring in nine patients from group 2 whose tracings are shown in Figure 25-3, were due to the coexistance of 7.6 block in the "more proximal level" with 2:1 block in the "proximal" level and a 3:2 Wenckebach period in the "distal" level.

Figures 4 and 5 were obtained from a patient in group 3. In Figure 4 there is an alternating Wenckebach period ending in 3:1 atrioventricular block which occurred (after propagation through the "more proximal" level) because of the coexistance of Wenckebach periods in the "proximal" level with 2:1 block in the "distal" level. During the first half of the record A2 and A6 were blocked, but A1, A3 and A5 were conduction with progressively increasing atrioventricular nodal (A-H) delays. Two consecutively blocked atrial impulses occurred after A5 because the cycle of the Wenckebach period was completed (as the "proximal" level) during

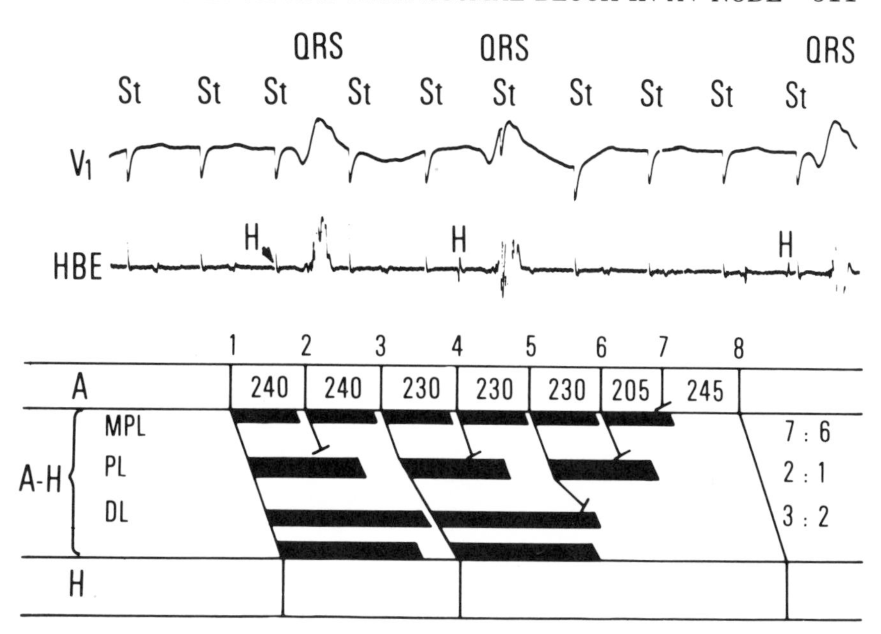

Figure 25-2. Same patient as in Figure 25-1, showing atrioventricular nodal alternating Wenckebach period ending in 5:1 atrioventricular nodal block. Diagram depicts 7:6 block in the MPL level, 2:1 block in the PL and 3:2 Wenckebach in the DL.

the inscription of an impulse (A7) which would have been conducted if the 2:1 sequence had persisted. In this cycle of the alternating Wenckebach periods, the maximum increment in A-H conduction did not occur at the beginning, but at the end of the period. Thus, the R-R intervals progressively increased, instead of decreasing, as in cycles of "classic" Wenckebach periods; however, this is not a constant feature of alternating Wenckebach periods, since other cycles show the characteristic R-R sequence.

Figure 25-5 (obtained from the same patient) shows an alternate Wenckebach period ending in 5:1 block due to the coexistence of a 7:6 Wenckebach period in the most proximal level; 6:4 block in the proximal level and 3:2 Wenckebach in the distal level.

All four patients in group 3 and two of the three patients in group 4 had episodes of pacing-induced paroxysmal atrioventricular block[12] occurring at the atrioventricular node.[13–15] The block was tachycardia-dependent and emerged either directly from sinus rhythm with 1:1 atrioventricular conduction (Figure 25-6) or from brief episodes of 2:1 atrioventricular nodal block showing alternating Wenckebach sequences (Figure 25-7).

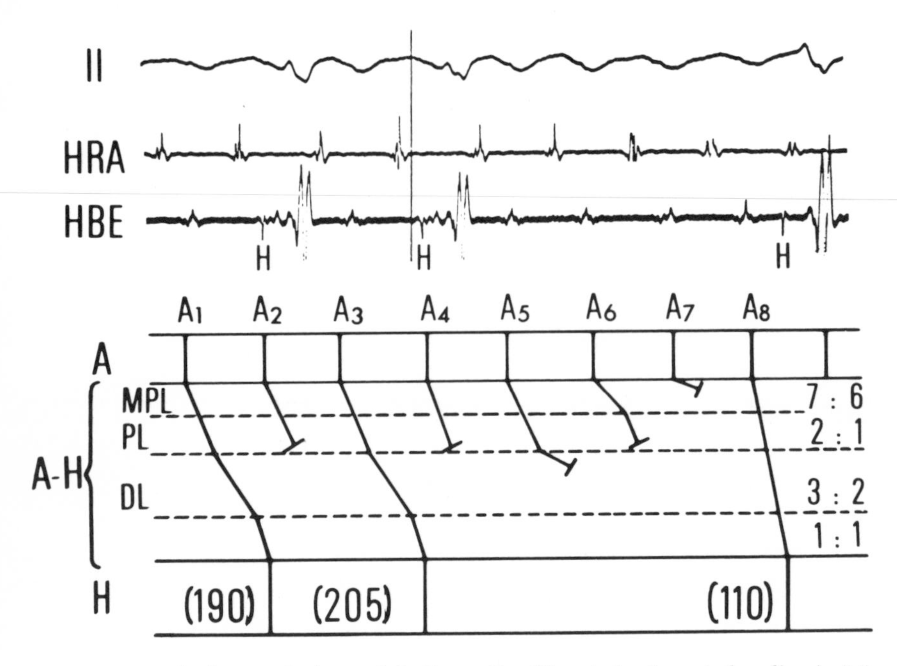

Figure 25–3. Atrioventricular nodal alternating Wenckebach period ending in 5:1 atrioventricular nodal block in a patient with atrial flutter.

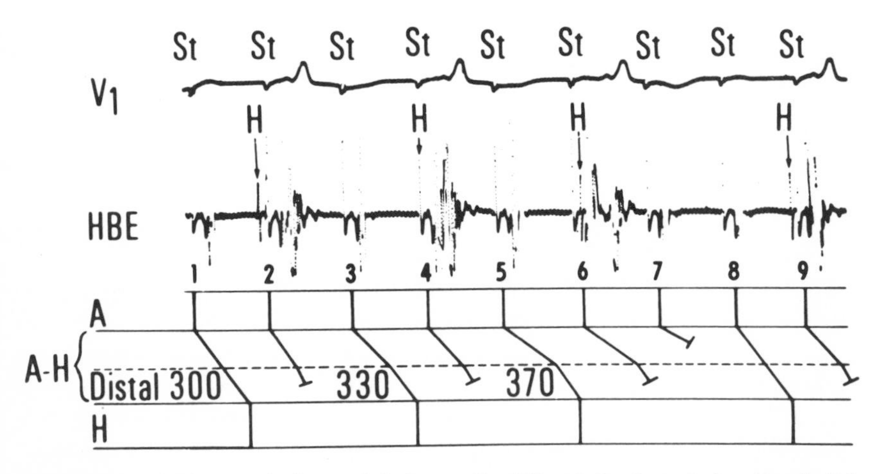

Figure 25–4. Atrioventricular nodal alternating Wenckebach period ending in 3:1 atrioventricular nodal block during rapid atrial stimulation. This has been attributed to the coexistence of a 2:1 block in the distal level and a Wenckebach period in the proximal level.

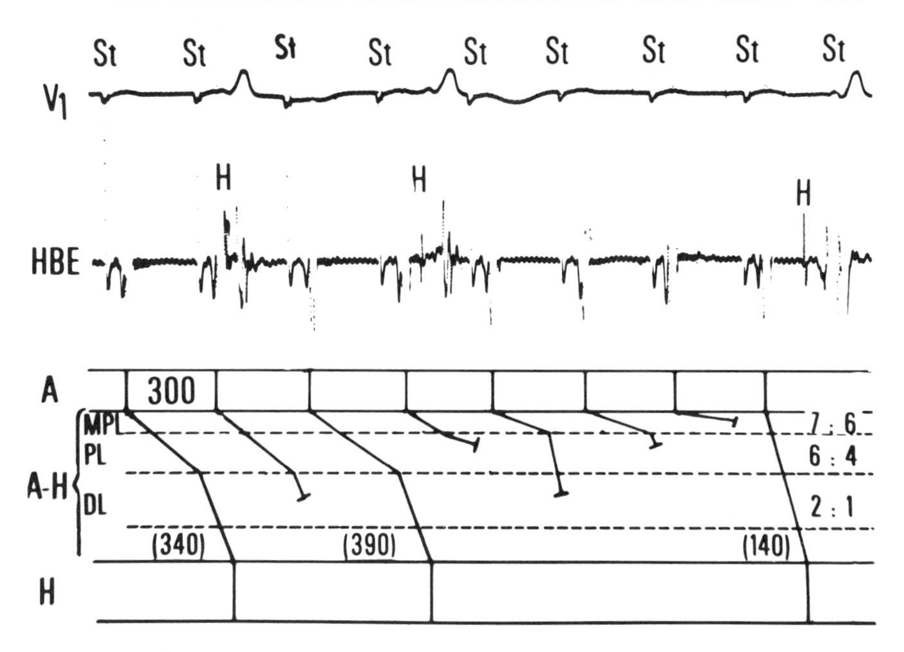

Figure 25–5. (Same patient as in Figure 25-4). Atrioventricular nodal alternating Wenckebach period ending in 5:1 atrioventricular nodal block during artificial atrial stimulation. Because the alternating Wenckebach period had been immediately preceded by one terminating in 3:1 (not 4:1, as in Figures 25-1 and 25-2), it is postulated that the events in this Figure resulted from the coexistence of a 7:6 Wenckebach or the MPL; a 6:4 block in the 11 and a 2:1 block in the DL.

DISCUSSION

Values of His Bundle Recordings

As in previous reports discussing alternating Wenckebach periods ending in 3:1 and 4:1 atrioventricular block, His bundle recordings were important in the evaluation of 5:1 atrioventricular block only because they permitted the localization of the disturbances in conduction to the atrioventricular node (A-H region).[1,2,9–11] The exact location of the atrioventricular nodal levels and the type of disturbances in conduction occurring in each level were impossible to determine, since only the input into the atrioventricular node (given by the atrial deflection) and its output (given by the His deflection) could be recorded with the conventional technique using a catheter-electrode.[1,2,9–11]

The 5:1 atrioventricular block need not have occurred as depicted diagrammatically in Figures 25-2, 25-3 and 25-5; however, several authors have postulated that block of more than three consecutive atrial

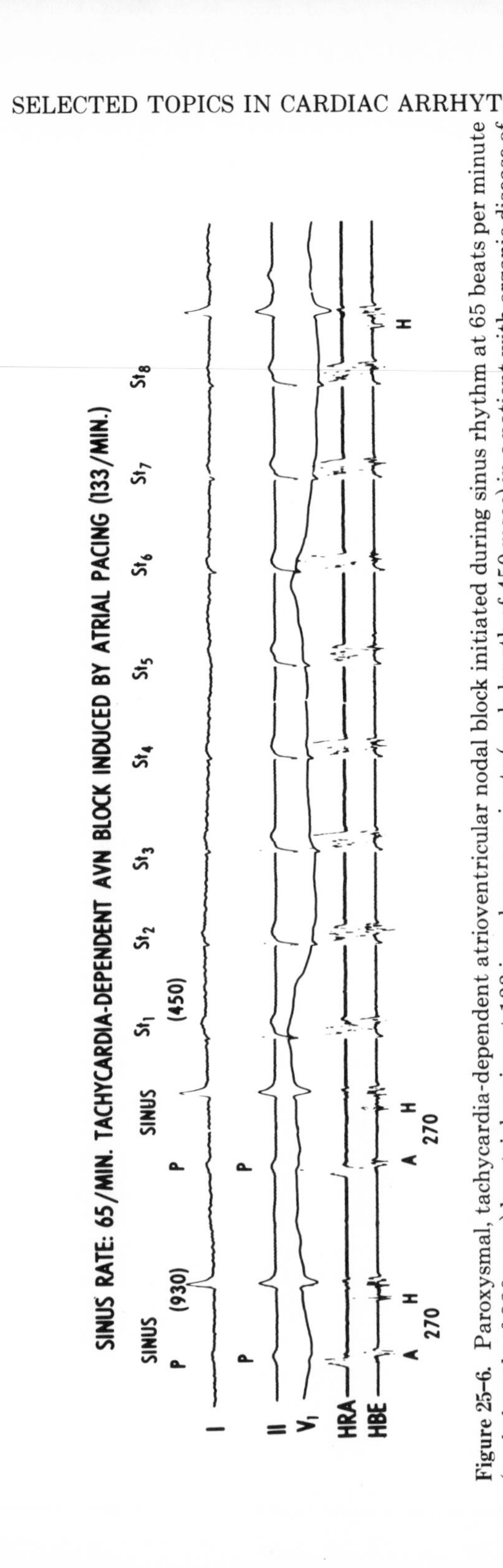

Figure 25–6. Paroxysmal, tachycardia-dependent atrioventricular nodal block initiated during sinus rhythm at 65 beats per minute (cycle length of 930 msec) by atrial pacing at 133 impulses per minute (cycle length of 450 msec) in a patient with organic disease of atrioventricular node. Values are expressed in milliseconds. St = artifact from pacemaker stimulus. HRA = bipolar electrogram from high right atrium.

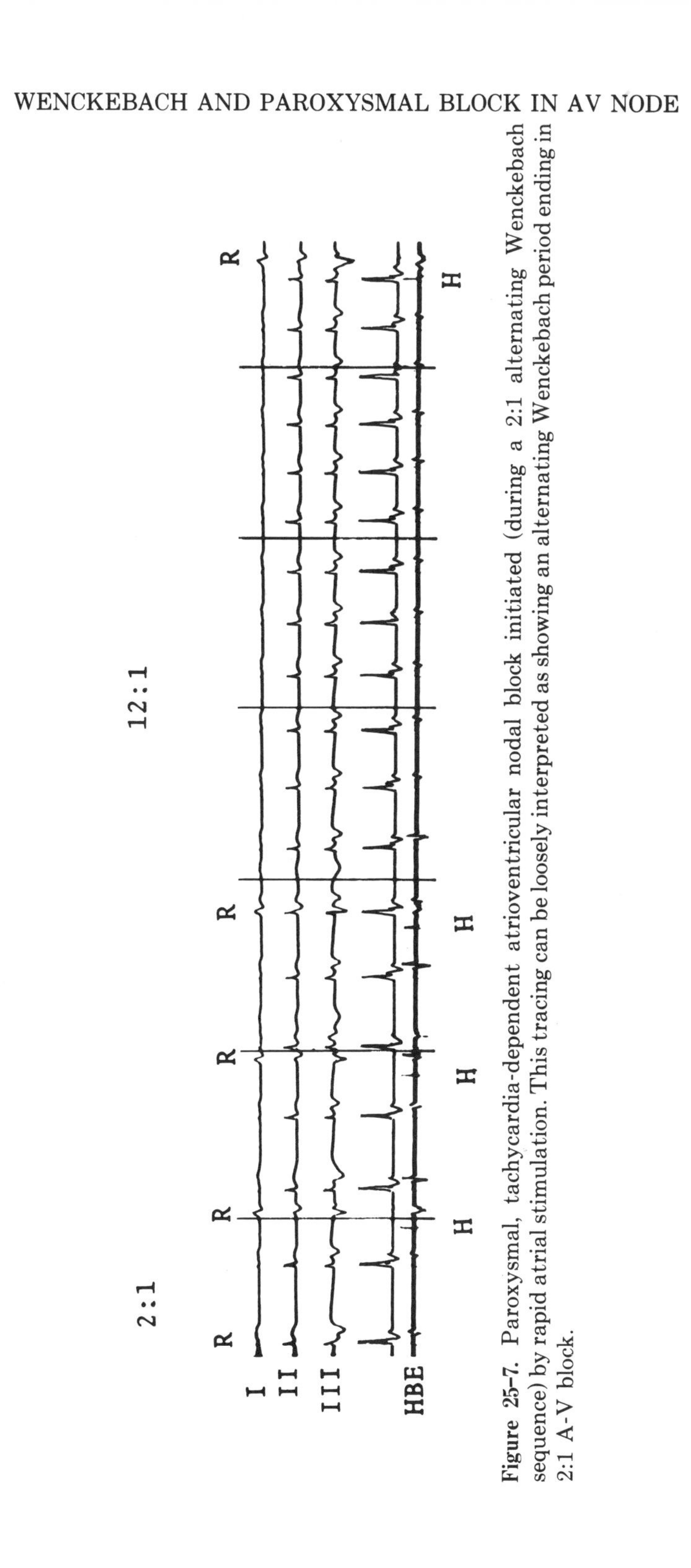

Figure 25-7. Paroxysmal, tachycardia-dependent atrioventricular nodal block initiated (during a 2:1 alternating Wenckebach sequence) by rapid atrial stimulation. This tracing can be loosely interpreted as showing an alternating Wenckebach period ending in 2:1 A-V block.

impulses can indeed result from three levels of block in the atrioventricular node.[1,9,16–20] These assumptions have been validated by a study in which a three-level disturbance in conduction occurred in three different anatomic structures.[1] Specifically, it was observed that high right atrial pacing at very fast rates could produce a type of 5:1 stimulus-His (St-H) block resulting from the association of Wenckebach periods in the atria with second-degree block in both the atrioventricular node and in the His-Purkinje system.[1] These findings can be extrapolated to the atrioventricular node by considering the atria equivalent to the "more proximal level", the A-V node to the "proximal" level and the His-Purkinje system to the "distal" level.[1]

Alternating Wenckebach Periods Ending in 4:1 and 5:1 Atrioventricular Block

In Figure 25-2, the 5:1 atrioventricular block appeared because the impulse that was blocked at the "more proximal" level was one which had reached the His bundle during the previously present alternating Wenckebach sequence. On the contrary, had this block at the "more proximal level" occurred during inscription of an impulse otherwise blocked in a lower atrioventricular nodal level (such as the atrial impulse labelled A6 in Figure 25-1), then the alternating Wenckebach period would have terminated in 4:1 (not 5:1) atrioventricular block as a consequence of a three-level disturbance in conduction, rather than as a result of the classic two-level block usually postulated to explain alternating Wenckebach periods ending in 4:1 atrioventricular block (as shown in Figure 25-1).

That some types of 4:1 atrioventricular block can be due to more than two levels of block has been postulated before,[9,16–18] and is supported by the previously mentioned study in which some episodes of 4:1 St-V block resulted from the association of intra-atrial Wenckebach periods with atrioventricular nodal and His-Purkinje block.[1]

Paroxysmal Atrioventricular Nodal Block

Although both clinical reports[13] and electrophysiologic studies utilizing the microelectrodes[21–23] have demonstrated repetitive concealed conduction in the atrioventricular node, paroxysmal atrioventricular nodal block is a less well known entity, in spite of occasional reports of its occurrence in man.[13] Watanabe and Dreifus[23] showed an example (their Figure 5-3) of paroxysmal block in the rabbit's atrioventricular node, which they attributed to "incomplete repolarization of the N region". Recently, El-Sherif and associates[24] documented the existence of tachycardia-dependent block in the ischemic atrioventricular node of the dog.

The genesis of paroxysmal atrioventricular nodal block in man is unclear. That there are mechanisms other than those operating in Figure 25-1 is suggested by the fact that the enhancement of vagal tone produced by massage of the carotid sinuses can produce this disturbance in conduction in some patients (Fig. 25-8).[8,25,26] As in the His-Purkinje system, some of the episodes of paroxysmal atrioventricular nodal block emerged from alternating Wenckebach periods occurring during 2:1 atrioventricular conduction.[15,27–31] This suggests (but does not prove) a related electrogenetic mechanism, which could very well be repetitive concealed conduction. According to Elizari et al.,[31] the fact that the action potentials within the injured His-Purkinje system resembled those of the atrioventricular node and that refractoriness outlasted repolarization, with excitability and conduction not being completely reversed after the end of the preceding action potentials, suggested repetitive concealed conduction in the affected portions of the His-Purkinje system (or the atrioventricular node); however, less and less penetration of each succeeding beat is unlikely, since this requires the levels of block to equal the number of consecutively blocked impulses.

On the other hand, the 8:1 paroxysmal atrioventricular nodal block in Figure 25-7 can be explained by assuming only block at three levels, the same number of levels postulated to explain the alternating Wenckebach periods ending in 5:1 atrioventricular block in Figures 25-1 and 25-2. Yet, for this to occur, the block at each level should be of the 2:1 type. Whenever the ratio of atrioventricular conduction doubles, with 2:1 block in each additional level, the number of consecutive beats is simply one less than the ratio. With 2:1 block in only one level, the ratio of atrioventricular conduction is obviously 2:1, and the number of consecutively blocked beats is one. With 2:1 block in two levels, the ratio is 4:1, and the number of consecutively blocked beats is three. With 2:1 block in three levels, the ratio of atrioventricular conduction is 8:1, and the number of consecutively blocked beats is seven.

Clinical Implications

In this study, atrioventricular nodal alternating Wenckebach periods ending in 5:1 atrioventricular block and paroxysmal atrioventricular nodal block were only rarely due to rapid atrial rates per se. On the contrary, most episodes occurred in patients who had received ouabain or verapamil or who had organic atrioventricular nodal disease. Therefore, pharmacologic effects or organic disease can be suspected from clinical tracings alone (without concomitant recording of the activity of the His bundle) wherever these patterns of conduction appear during atrial tachyarrhythmias or rapid atrial stimulation in patients with narrow

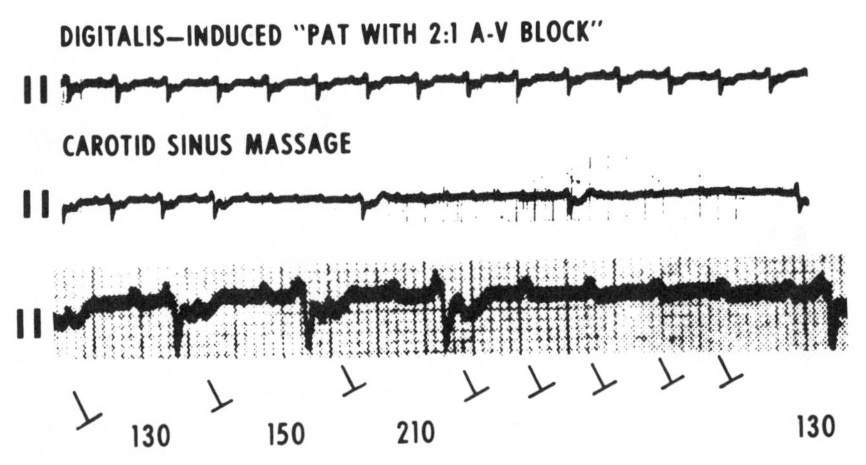

Figure 25-8. Paroxysmal atrioventricular block produced (presumably at atrioventricular node) by massage of carotid sinus in patients with digitalis-induced "paroxysmal" atrial tachycardia (PAT) with 2:1 atrioventricular block. Bottom strip (enlargement of the first part of the middle strip) shows that paroxysmal atrioventricular block emerged from alternating Wenckebach sequence. Hence, this strip can also be interpreted as an alternating Wenckebach period ending in 6:1 A-V block.

QRS complexes. Although the mechanisms of paroxysmal atrioventricular nodal block following administration of ouabain most probably resulted from the direct effects of this drug on the atrioventricular node, the role of vagal stimulation requires further studies (Fig. 25-8); for example, both paroxysmal atrioventricular nodal block and alternating Wenckebach periods can be produced by massage of the carotid sinuses in some patients with sinus rhythm (Figure 5-29 of Watanabe and Dreifus[23]), atrial flutter with 2:1 atrioventricular conduction (Figure 228 of Katz and Pick[8] and Figure 56-4 of Bellet[25]), and digitalis-induced "paroxysmal" atrial tachycardia with atrioventricular block.[26]

SUMMARY

Atrioventricular nodal alternating periods ending in 5:1 atrioventricular block during rapid atrial rhythms were explained by postulating the presence of block in three levels of the atrioventricular node. This pattern of conduction occurred in 10 of 11 patients who either had received ouabain or verapamil (9 patients) or who had organic atrioventricular nodal disease (2 patients). In contrast, this pattern of conduction occurred in only one of eight nonmedicated patients without organic atrioventricular nodal disease. The frequent association of this pattern with paroxysmal, tachycardia-dependent atrioventricular nodal block suggested a similar, but no necessarily identical, mechanism. In conclusion, atrioventricular nodal alternating Wenckebach periods ending in 5:1 atrioventricular block, as well as paroxysmal atrioventricular nodal block, were only rarely the result of rapid atrial rates per se, their occurrence indicating organic or pharmacologic effects on the atrioventricular node. Since both can be produced by carotid sinus pressure, further studies appear to be necessary to determine the role that vagal effects can have in their genesis.

REFERENCES

1. Castellanos, A., Sung, R.J., Mallon, S.M., et al.: Effects of proximal intra-atrial Wenckebach on distal atrioventricular nodal, and His-Purkinje, block. With special reference to the theory of alternating Wenckebach periods. *Am. Heart J.* **97**: 228–234, 1978.
2. Castellanos, A., Sung, R.J., Aldrich, J.L., et al.: Electrocardiographic manifestations and clinical significance of atrioventricular nodal alternating Wenckebach periods. *Chest* **73**: 69–74, 1978.
3. Sellers, T.D., Jr., Campbell, R.W.P., Bashore, T.M., et al.: Effects of procaineamide and quinidine sulfate in the Wolff-Parkinson-White syndrome. *Circulation* **55**: 15–22, 1977.

4. Wellens, H.J.J.: The electrophysiological properties of accessory pathway in Wolff-Parkinson-White syndrome. In Wellens, H.J.J., Lie, K.I., and Janse, M.J. (eds.): *The Conduction System of the Heart: Structure, Function, and Clinical Implications.* Leiden, the Netherlands, HE Stenfert Kroese NV, 1976, pp. 567–587.
5. Denes, P., Wu, D., Dhingra, R., et al.: The effects of cycle length on cardiac refractory periods in man. *Circulation* **49**: 32–41, 1974.
6. Rizzon, P., DiBiase, M., Calabrese, P., et al.: Electrophysiological evaluation of intravenous verapamil in man. *Eur. J. Cardiol.* **6**: 179–194, 1977.
7. Besoain-Santander, M., Pick, A., and Langendorf, R.: A-V conduction in auricular flutter. *Circulation* **2**: 604–616, 1950.
8. Katz, L.N., and Pick, A.: *Clinical Electrocardiography: The Arrhythmias* (Part I). Philadelphia, Lea and Febiger, 1956, pp. 413–418, 421.
9. Kosowsky, B.D., Latif, P., Radoff, A.M.: Multilevel atrioventricular block. *Circulation* **54**: 914–921, 1976.
10. Amat-y-Leon, F., Chuquimia, A., Wu, D., et al.: Alternating Wenckebach periods: A common electrophysiological response. *Am. J. Cardiol.* **36**: 757–764, 1957.
11. Hartzler, G.O., and Maloney, H.D.: Supra-His alternate beat Wenckebach dysrhythmia. *Mayo Clin. Proc.* **50**: 475–481, 1975.
12. Sachs, A., and Traynor, R.L.: Paroxysmal complete auriculo-ventricular block. *Am. Heart J.* **9**: 267–271, 1933.
13. Rosen, K.M., Loeb, H.S., and Rahimtoola, S.H.: Mobitz type II block with narrow QRS complex and Stokes-Adams attacks. *Arch. Intern. Med.* **132**: 595–596, 1973.
14. El-Sherif, N., Scherlag, B.J., and Lazzara, R.: An appraisal of second degree and paroxysmal atrio-ventricular block. *Eur. J. Cardiol.* **4**: 117–130, 1976.
15. El-Sherif, N., Scherlag, B.J., and Lazzara, R.: The pathophysiology of tachycardia dependent paroxysmal atrioventricular block after myocardial ischemia: Experimental and clinical observations. *Circulation* **50**: 515–528, 1974.
16. Langendorf, R., and Pick, A.: Concealed conduction. Further evaluation of a fundamental aspect of propagation of the cardiac impulse. *Circulation* **13**: 381–399, 1956.
17. Langendorf, R.: New aspects of concealed conduction of the cardiac impulse. In Wellens, H.J.J., Lie, K.I., and Janse, M.J. (eds.): *The Conduction System of the Heart: Structure, Function, and Clinical Implications.* Leiden, the Netherlands, HE Stenfert Kroese NV, 1976, pp. 410–423.
18. Schindler, S., and Albers, W.: A-V block (letter to editor). *Circulation* **56**: 689, 1977.
19. Langendorf, R., Pick, A., Edelist, A., et al.: Experimental demonstration of concealed A-V conduction in the human heart. *Circulation* **32**: 386–393, 1965.
20. Pick, A.: Mechanisms of cardiac arrhythmias: From hypothesis to physiologic fact. *Am. Heart J.* **86**: 249–269, 1973.
21. Moe, G.K., Abildskov, J.A., and Mendez, C.: An experimental study of concealed conduction. *Am. Heart J.* **67**: 338–356, 1964.

22. Moore, E.N.: Microelectrode studies on concealment of multiple premature atrial responses. *Circ. Res.* **18**: 660–672, 1966.
23. Watanabe, Y., and Dreifus, L.S.: *Cardiac Arrhythmias: Electrophysiologic Basis for Clinical Interpretation.* New York, Grune and Stratton, 1971, pp. 187–188.
24. El-Sherif, N., Scherlag, B.J., and Lazzara, R.: Experimental production of "Mobitz II" and paroxysmal block in the A-V node (Abst.). *Clin. Res.* **23**: 181A, 1975.
25. Bellet, S.: *Clinical Disorders of the Heart Beat,* 3rd ed. Philadelphia, Lea and Febiger, 1971, p. 1160.
26. Calvino, J.M., Azan Cano, L., Castellanos, A., Jr.: Valor de las derivaciones esofagicas en las arritmias complejas. *Rev. Cubana Cardiol.* **16**: 293–316, 1955.
27. Rosenbaum, M.B., Elizari, M.V., Levi, R.J., et al.: Paroxysmal atrioventricular block related to hypopolarization and spontaneous diastolic depolarization. *Chest* **63**: 678–688, 1973.
28. Halpern, M.S., Nau, G.J., and Levi, R.J.: Wenckebach periods of alternate beats: Clinical and experimental observations. *Circulation* **48**: 41–49, 1973.
29. Cohen, H.C., D'Cruz, I., and Pick, A.: Concealed intraventricular conduction in the His bundle electrogram. *Circulation* **53**: 776–783, 1976.
30. Castellanos, A., Sung, R.J., Aldrich, J.L., et al.: Alternating Wenckebach periods occurring in the atria, His-Purkinje system, ventricles and Kent bundle. *Am. J. Cardiol.* **40**: 853–859, 1977.
31. Elizari, M.V., Novakosky, A., Quintero, R.A., et al.: The experimental evidence for the role of phase 3 and phase 4 block in the genesis of A-V conduction disturbances. In Wellens, H.J.J., Lie, K.I., and Janse, M.J. (eds.): *The Conduction System of the Heart: Structure, Function, and Clinical Implications.* Leiden, the Netherlands, HE Stenfert Kroese NV, 1976, pp. 360–377.

26

Arrhythmias in the Mitral Valve Prolapse Syndrome

Joseph H. Yahini, M.D., Zvi Vered, M.D., Pierre Atlas, M.D., and Henry N. Neufeld, M.D.

The frequency, severity and significance of arrhythmias in the mitral valve prolapse syndrome (MVP) have been studied in a number of publications[2,4,5] but some controversies have remained. We report here our experience with 114 patients with this syndrome, 48 of whom also suffered from arrhythmias.

MATERIALS AND METHODS

One hundred and fourteen consecutive, nonselected patients seen between 1973 and 1977 at the Heart Institute (Tel Aviv) form the basis of this report. The presence of MVP was suspected on clinical grounds and confirmed by echocardiography in all.

Left heart catheterization was deemed to be justified and carried out in two patients only. Twenty-two hour Holter monitoring was performed on 105 and stress tests on 102 patients.

RESULTS

The frequency of the syndrome was practically equal among Sephardi and Ashkenasi Jews. In contrast to most reports, males predominate in our series—68 to 46 (59.6% vs. 40.4%). "Palpitations" constituted the chief complaint in only 26 patients (22.8%), the others suffering mainly from atypical chest pain (29.8%) and dyspnea (9.6%). Five patients complained of syncopal attacks. One third of patients were diagnosed as

MVP on routine examination (Table 26-1). A midsystolic click (MSC), with or without a late systolic murmer (LSM) was heard in 78 (68.5%). A pansystolic murmur was heard in 13 (10.5%). LSM only was detected in 20 (18.4%). Three patients had no auscultatomy findings, and were discovered by echocardiography performed on account of atypical chest pains. ECG changes (inverted T wave in the inferior, right and/or left chest leads, or tall and peaked T waves in V leads) were frequent and encountered in 53 patients (46.6%). A prolonged Q-T interval was seen in seven patients; none related the presence of syncopal attacks.

Arrhythmias (Table 26-2) were apparent on routine ECG in 50 percent, and on Holter monitoring and/or stress testing in the rest, the former being twice as sensitive as the latter. Forty-eight (42.1%) (31 males and 17 females) suffered from arrhythmias, the ventricular being twice as frequent as the atrial arrhythmias.

Ventricular arrhythmias (VA) were equally distributed among males and females, and showed a clearcut increase of frequency with age (Table 26-3) until 60 years of age.

Supraventricular arrhythmias (SVA) were less frequent (14.9%). They showed a distinct male predominance (26.6% vs. 6.1%). Seven out of nine patients with atrial premature beats (APBs) and/or paroxysmal atrial tachycardia (PAT) and all six patients with atrial fibrillation (AF) were males. All except two were over 40 years of age (Tables 26-4 and 26-5). No statistically significant correlation was found between the patients' complaints, e.g., palpitations, atypical chest pain or ECG changes, and the presence of arrhythmia.

DISCUSSION

Barlow[1] found an increased incidence of the MVP among the black population of South Africa. No significant difference was found in this series among Jews of Western (Ashkenasi) or Eastern (Sephardi) origin as far as frequency of the syndrome is concerned.

Curiously, and in contrast to previous reports, males predominate in our series, the possible reasons being:

1. We examine routinely twice as many men than women at the Heart Institute.
2. Only 68.5 percent of our patients had a midsystolic click with or without LSM. The remaining, although showing a prolapsed mitral valve on echocardiography, may not represent genuine cases of the Barlow's syndrome.[1]

It is relevant to stress that the predominance of women was not readily apparent in a recent report on arrhythmias in the MVP as well.[2] It may be that analysis of a large series may case doubt on the assumptions that

Table 26-1. Mitral Valve Prolapse with Presenting Symptoms

Sex	No. of Patients	Atypical Chest Pain	Palpitations	Dyspnea	Syncope	Routine Examination
Male	68	20 (29.4%)	16 (23.5%)	7 (10.3%)	1 (1.5%)	24 (35.3%)
Female	46	14 (30.4%)	10 (21.8%)	4 (8.7%)	4 (8.7%)	14 (30.4%)
TOTAL	114	34 (29.8%)	26 (22.8%)	11 (9.6%)	5 (4.4%)	38 (33.4%)

Table 26-2. Mitral Valve Prolapse Classification of Arrhythmias

		ATRIAL				VENTRICULAR			
Sex	No. of Patients	A.P.B.s	A.F.	P.A.T.	Total No. of Sup. Vent. Arrhythmias	V.P.B.s	V.T.	Total No. of Vent. Arrhythmias	Total No. of Patients with Arrhythmias
Male	68	7 (10.3%)	6 (8.8%)	1 (1.5%)	14 (20.6%)	20 (29.4%)	2 (2.9%)	22 (32.3%)	31 (45.6%)
Female	46	2 (3.1%)	0	1 (2.2%)	3 (6.1%)	15 (32.6%)	1 (2.2%)	16 (34.8%)	17 (36.9%)
TOTAL	114	9 (7.9%)	6 (5.3%)	2 (1.8%)	17 (14.9%)	35 (30.7%)	3 (2.6%)	38 (33.3%)	48* (42.1%)

*Note: Seven patients (5 males and 2 females) suffered from both VA and SVA.

Table 26-3. Mitral Valve Prolapse with Percentage of Ventricular Arrhythmias Correlated With Age

Age	11–20 (43)*	21–30 (25)*	31–40 (11)*	41–50 (16)*	51–60 (10)*	>61 (7)*
No. of Patients with V.A.	7 (16.3%)	7 (28.0%)	5 (45.4%)	10 (62.5%)	7 (70.0%)	2 (28.6%)

*Number of patients with M.V.P. in age group.

Table 26-4. Mitral Valve Prolapse in Patients With APBs

No.	Sex	Age	Associated Disease	Present Symptoms	Auscul-tation	ECG	Associated Arrhythmias
1	M	24	—	PP	MSC	Normal	—
2	F	42	—	Palpitations	LSM	Normal	VPBs, SVT
3	F	52	—	Routine Exam.	LSM	Inverted TII; III; AVF	VPBs
4	M	45	—	Palpitations Dyspnea	MSC+ LSM	Normal	—
5	M	45	—	PP	LSM	IRBBB	VPBs
6	M	60	—	PP	LSM	Inverted T V2-V4	SVT
7	M	40	—	PP	LSM	Normal	VPBs
8	M	41	—	PP	LSM	Normal	VPBs
9	M	60	—	Dyspnea	LSM	Inverted T V1-V4	—

Abbreviations: PP = precordial pain; MSC = midsystolic click; LSM = late systolic murmur; IRBBB = incomplete right bundle branch block; SVT = supraventricular tachycardia.

the syndrome clearly predominates in women. It may be stressed here that our series of 48 patients with MVP and arrhythmias is one of the largest reported.

As described by others,[3] many of our patients with MVP (33%) were asymptomatic and discovered on routine examination only (Table 26-1). An important point to emphasize is that only 22.8 percent of our patients complained of "palpitations", militating against any bias in favour of arrhythmias, which perhaps explains our low percentage of arrhythmias when compared to similar reports.

In accordance with others no statistically significant correlation was found between the patients' complaints (e.g., palpitations, atypical chest pain) or ECG changes, and the frequency or type of arrhythmias. Also in accordance with others, no correlation between arrhythmias and syncopal attacks could be found in five cases of syncope (Table 26-1) except for one patient, who fainted during paroxysmal atrial fibrillation.

As stated, we found twice as many ventricular than supraventricular arrhythmias, the reason for which not being readily apparent. No significance could be attached to coupled or multifocal VPBs in this report; however, VPBs originating from the left ventricle were seven times more frequent in women than in men, for which we have no explanation. Only three patients had ventricular tachycardia (VT) but none reported syncopal attacks.

An interesting point is the increased frequency of VA with age. Table 26-3 shows no significant difference of VA in absolute numbers among the various age subgroups, but reveals a definite increase in the percent-

Table 26-5. Mitral Valve Prolapse in Patients With Atrial Fibrillation

	No.	Sex	Age	Presenting Symptom	T Wave Changes	Associated Arrhythmia	Holter	ECG Stress	Angio-graphy	Auscultation
CHRONIC	1	M	56	PP	+	V. BGMN.	VPBs BGMN.	Not Done	—	Pans. M.
	2	M	65	PP	—	—	—	Not done	Normal Cor.	Pans. M.
	3	M	68	PP	+ (IRBBB)	—	—	Not done	—	L.S.M.
	4	M	61	CHF	—	VT;VPBs	VT VPBs	Not done	Lt. Ventr.	Pans. M.
PAROXYSMAL	1	M	24	PP	+	—	A. Fibril-lation	Normal	—	L.S.M.
	2	M	79	CHF	—(LVH)	VPBs	VPBs	Not Done	—	L.S.M.

Note: no ejection click detected in any patient.
Abbreviations: V. BGMN. = ventricular begimini; VT = ventricular tachycardia; VPBs = ventricular premature beats; LSM = late systolic murmur; Pans. M. = pansystolic murmur; LVH = left ventricular hypertrophy.

age of patients presenting VA when related to the total number of patients with MVP in that age subgroup.

The following also deserve special emphasis: as already stated, most of our patients with SVA were males, mainly above 40 years of age, and only two had a MSC in auscultation. These features strongly suggest that atrial arrhythmias in the MVP result from an associated process (atherosclerotic ? degenerative ?) rather than from the MVP. MVP per se may however be held responsible in some instances of SVA, as evident in the case of the 24-year-old patient with spontaneous attacks of paroxysmal AF and syncope.

It is tempting to extend these considerations to the VA, which as stressed, show a tendency to increase with age and it may well be that an associated process rather than the MVP is the responsible etiologic factor for the arrhythmias in these patients as well.

CONCLUSIONS

Arrhythmias were encountered in 48 of 114 (42.1%) patients with MVP seen between 1973 and 1977 at the Heart Institute. Their frequency was similar in men and women (45 vs. 37%). They were discovered on routine ECG in only half, and by Holter monitoring or stress testing in the other half; Holter monitoring being twice as sensitive as stress testing.

No correlation was established between patients' complaints and/or ECG changes and frequency of arrhythmias.

Ventricular arrhythmias were more frequent than atrial arrhythmias in males (32.6 vs. 20.6%) and especially in females (34.8 vs. 6.1%).

Ventricular arrhythmias were encountered in only 33.3% of patients. They were equally distributed between males and females and showed a clearcut increase of frequency with age.

The great majority of patients with APBs and PAT were male, over 40 years and had a pansystolic or late-systolic murmur without midsystolic click, suggesting associated ASHD, on a degenerative process.

All patients with atrial fibrillation were males, five of whom were over 50 years of age. None had a click. In a middle-aged man with chest pains, T-wave changes and AF, mitral insufficiency may be due to either mitral valve prolapse or papillary muscle dysfunction.

REFERENCES

1. Barlow, J.B., and Pocock, W.A.: The problem of non-ejection clicks and associated mitral systolic murmurs: emphasis on the billowing mitral leaflet syndrome. *Am. Heart J.* 5: 636–655, 1975.

2. De Maria, A.N., Amsterdam, E.A., et al.: Arrhythmias in the mitral valve syndrome. *Ann. Intern. Med.* **84**: 656–660, 1976.
3. Procacci, P.M., Sarvan, M.S.V., et al.: Prevalence of clinical mitral valve prolapse in 1169 young women. *N. Eng. J. Med.* **294**: 1086–1088, 1976.
4. Winkle, R.A., Lopes, M.G., et al.: Life threatening arrhythmias in the mitral valve prolapse syndrome. *Am. J. Cardiol.* **60**: 961–967, 1976.
5. Campbell, R.W.F., Godman, M.G., et al.: Ventricular arrhythmias in syndrome of balloon deformity of mitral valve. *Br. Heart J.* **38**: 1053–1057, 1976.

27

Paroxysmal Ventricular Tachycardia Without Organic Heart Disease

Yehezkiel Kishon, M.D., Marion Hefer, M.D., and Henry N. Neufeld, M.D.

Paroxysmal ventricular tachycardia (PVT) is always considered an expression of grave underlying organic heart disease. It is found associated with cardiomyopathies, ventricular aneurysm, digitalis intoxication and electrolyte imbalance, among other conditions. Its presence with prolapse of the mitral leaflet or prolonged QT interval is well established. In these cases, PVT is frequently a serious complication with grave, often fatal outcome.

About eight percent of the patients with PVT have no evidence of cardiac lesions and the prognosis seems to be more favorable.[1] Lewis[2] reported the first tachycardia of this type in 1909. This arrhythmia occurred in a seaman who experienced single premature contractions and runs of as many as 11 abnormal beats in a row. In 1922, Gallavardin made a distinction between the "terminal pre-fibrillatory ventricular tachycardia" and the milder form of "ventricular extra systoles with paroxysmal tachycardia." While the number of reported cases of this type of tachycardia increased with time,[3–5] and new classifications were introduced,[1,6] very little attention was paid to the various clinical aspects of this arrhythmia, as its relation to physical stress and the response to active and preventive medical treatment. These aspects, as well as other clinical data have been studied in seven patients with PVT without evidence of organic heart disease. Patients younger than five years or older than 45 years were excluded from this study because of possible undetected congenital or ischemic heart diseases.

All patients had normal physical findings, laboratory data, electrocardiograms at rest and during exercise (except for the arrhythmia under discussion), chest x-ray and fluoroscopy. In four patients, with equivocal findings, cardiac catheterization was performed, including left ventriculograms and coronary angiograms. All findings were within normal limits.

RESULTS

The main clinical and electrocardiographic data are summarized in Tables 27-1 and 27-2. There were five males and two females, four patients were younger than 20 years. In two patients, the arrhythmia was precipitated by emotional stress, in one patient it was triggered by rise in body temperature, while in another patient it was precipitated by drinking coffee and smoking. Precipitating factors could not be detected in four patients.

The main symptoms were dizziness, palpitations, shortness of breath, sweating and chest pain, in this order of frequency. Only one patient had syncopal attack while another complained of anorexia and vomiting. One patient remained entirely asymptomatic. The patients were followed for a period of one to ten years and no deaths occurred during this period.

Ventricular premature beats, when present, were graded according to the classification of Lown and Wolff[7] (Table 27-2). Three of the patients

Table 27.1
P.V.T. WITHOUT ORGANIC HEART DISEASE
CLINICAL DATA

CASE No.	SEX	AGE OF ONSET OF ARRHYTHMIA	PRECIPITATING EVENT	SYMPTOMS	FOLLOW-UP PERIOD (YS)
1	M	43	EXCITEMENT, STRESS	PALPITATIONS, CHEST PAIN, DYSPNEA, DIZZINESS, SWEATING.	2
2	M	13	- - -	DIZZINESS, SYNCOPE.	10
3	F	6	EFFORT, FEVER, STRESS	PALPITATIONS, DYSPNEA, ANOREXIA, DIZZINESS, NAUSEA.	7
4	M	39	- - -	PALPITATIONS, DIZZINESS, DYSPNEA, SWEATING.	1
5	M	44	COFFEE, SMOKING	DIZZINESS, BLURRED VISION	5
6	M	18	- - -	NONE	5
7	F	19	- - -	PALPITATIONS	1

Table 27.2

P. V. T. WITHOUT ORGANIC HEART DISEASE
ELECTROCARDIOGRAPHIC FINDINGS

CASE No.	GRADE OF VPBs	VENTRICULAR TACHYCARDIA				INCIDENCE	DURATION
		CONFIG.	QRS AXIS	RATE/min.	TYPE	(OF PAROXYSMS)	
1	5	LBBB	+ 90	210	CONTIN.	1 / mo	15 min.-6 hr.
2	5	LBBB	+ 80	280	CONTIN.	2 / yr	15 min.
3	0	RBBB	- 110	180	CONTIN.	4 / mo	1hr.-4 d.
4	2	LBBB	+ 60	180	INTERMIT.	3 / yr	1hr.
5	5	LBBB	+ 80	280	INTERMIT.	1 / yr	5 min.
6	4a	LBBB	+ 110	130	INTERMIT.	?	5 min.
7	4a	?	?	65 - 150	INTERMIT.	1 / yr	15 min.

had the R on T phenomenon. All ectopic beats were monoformic.

The QRS complex of the tachycardia was of the LBBB pattern in five patients (with the electrical mean axis in the frontal plane between +80° and +110°). The QRS was of the RBBB pattern in one patient (No. 3) with electrical axis of −110°, and could not be determined in one patient. The tachycardia was monoformic in all cases, with the ventricular rate between 130 to 280 beats per minute except in one patient with relative slow tachycardia.

Two different types of tachycardia could be distinguished (Fig. 27-1). The *continuous* type of ventricular tachycardia was characterized by prolonged paroxysms of tachycardia, separated by long periods of sinus rhythm sometimes lasting for weeks. Only very few premature beats, if any, could be detected between the attacks.

The *intermittent* type was characterized by frequent and short paroxysms, interrupted by few sinus beats and constant presence of ventricular premature beats.

The response to physical stress is presented in Table 27-3. Only one patient was treated with antiarrhythmic agent, while performing the ergometric test, and was excluded from this table. The rest of the patients could be subdivided into three small groups on the basis of their response to effort. In patients Nos. 1 to 3, all with the continuous type of tachycardia, maximal effort of 125 watts had no effect on the arrhythmia, although the basic sinus rhythm increased by 75 to 100 percent. On the other hand, patients Nos. 5 to 7 (with the intermittent type of tachycardia) were affected by effort: In patient No. 5, mild effort of 50 watts only, triggered the appearance of ventricular premature beats

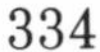

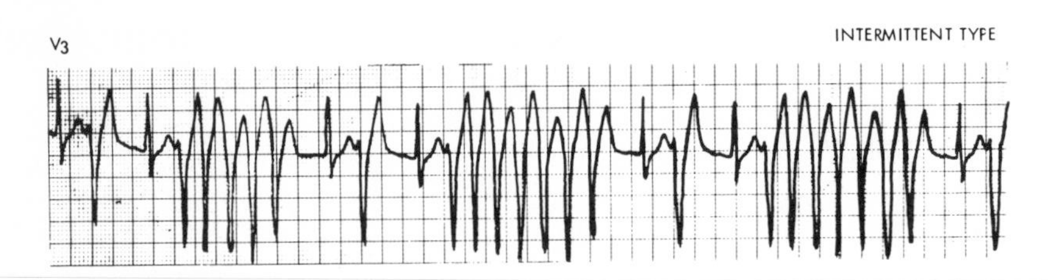

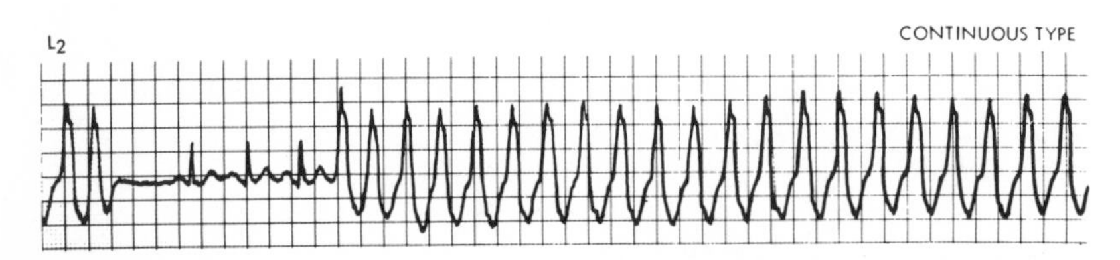

Figure 27-1. Two types of ventricular tachycardia encountered in cases without organic heart disease: *A,* The "intermittent type" (upper tracing) with frequent short runs of tachycardia, few sinus beats and multiple premature beats. *B,* The "continuous type" (lower tracing) with prolonged attacks of tachycardia, separated by long periods of sinus rhythm.

Table 27.3

P. V. T. WITHOUT ORGANIC HEART DISEASE
ERGOMETRIC FINDINGS

CASE No.	AT REST		AT MAXIMAL EFFORT		DURING RECOVERY
	H.R./min.	RHYTHM	MAX. EFFORT (WTS.)	RHYTHM H.R.	RHYTHM
1	57	SINUS	125	SINUS 100	SINUS
2	80	3/min. VPBs	125	3/min. VPBs 140	3/min. VPBs
3	75	SINUS	125	SINUS 150	SINUS
5	100	SINUS	50	25/min. VPBs 150	20/min. VPBs (1st. min., 110/min.)
6	120	SALVES OF VT	75	SINUS 200	PVT RE-APPEARED AT H.R. < 200
7	70	SALVES OF VT	125	SINUS 170	SALVES OF VT RE-APPEARED AT H.R. < 80

and even short runs of tachycardia, while in the last two patients, runs of VT, present at rest, disappeared during exercise, only to reappear later, as the basic heart rate slowed down. Numbers, however, are too small to draw any conclusions regarding the correlation between the response to effort and the type of the tachycardia.

The arrhythmia was successfully treated by intravenous bolus of 100 mg of lidocaine in four patients. In two patients, the arrhythmia stopped spontaneously. In one patient, the only patient with the RBBB type complex of the tachycardia, the arrhythmia was totally refractory to various antiarrhythmic agents as lidocaine, verapamil and ajmaline and electrical countershocks were necessary.

Quinidine sulphate, taken orally in daily doses of 1.2 gm, was the most effective agent in the prevention of the paroxysms but not the premature beats. On the whole, patients with PVT without organic heart disease seem to be relatively nonresponsive to prophylactic treatment. Again, patient No. 3, was completely refractory to the various prophylactic agents, as was also patient No. 1 (Table 27-4). Facing the potential hazards involved with increased doses of the antiarrhythmic drugs, one should weigh those hazards against the frequency of the paroxysms, their duration, and the hemodynamic effects involved. It should be kept in mind that in most cases, but probably not in all, the arrhythmia under discussion has a benign course. If the tachycardia is rapid and prolonged, lowered cardiac output may lead to disabling symptoms (i.e., syncope, pulmonary edema) and death. Such was the case in a 19-year-old, otherwise normal healthy woman, who died following 32 days of unrelieved ventricular tachycardia.[8]

Table 27.4

P.V.T. WITHOUT ORGANIC HEART DISEASE: PROPHILACTIC TREATMENT (ORAL)

DRUG \ CASE No.	1	2	3	4	5	6	7
QUINIDINE SULPH. (0.2 X 6/d.)	N.E.	P.E.	N.E.	P.E.	P.E.	P.E.	P.E.
PRAJMALIUM BITAR. (00.2 X 6/d.)	N.E.	-	-	P.E.	-	-	-
PROCAINAMIDE HCl (0.5 X 6/d.)	N.E.	-	N.E.	-	N.E	-	-
VERAPAMIL HCl (0.04 t. i. d.)	N.E.	-	N.E.	-	-	N.E.	N.E.
DILANTIN (0.1 X 6/d.)	N.E.	-	N.E.	-	-	-	-
DIGOXIN (0.25 mg./d.)	-	-	N.E.	-	-	-	-
PROPRANOLOL (0.01 q.i.d.)	-	N.E.	N.E.	-	P.E.	N.E.	N.E.

N.E. = NO EFFECT. P.E. = PARTIAL EFFECT

SUMMARY

The relatively rare entity of PVT without evidence of organic heart disease is probably not a homogenous one. Two different types of tachycardia can be recognized:

1. The "continuous" type, not affected by exercise, and relatively refractory to antiarrhythmic agents. This type of PVT probably corresponds to type IV tachycardia of Gallavardin, known also in the French literature as "Bouveret Ventriculaire".
2. The "intermittent" type, with frequent bursts of ventricular premature beats, seems to be affected by effort and by medical treatment and resembles type II tachycardia of Gallavardin. More studies of this type are needed in order to establish the relationship of both effort and response to medical treatment to the arrhythmia under discussion, a facet which remains untouched so far.

REFERENCES

1. Sebastien, P., Waynberger, M., Beaufils, P., et al.: Les tachycardies ventriculaires isolées sans cardiopathie patente. *Arch. Mal. Coeur* **69**: 919, 1976.
2. Ambrust, C.A., and Levine, S.A.: Paroxysmal ventricular tachycardia. A study of 107 cases. *Circulation* **1**: 28, 1950.
3. Hair, T.E., Jr., Eagen, J.T., and Orgain, E.S.: Paroxysmal ventricular tachycardia in the absence of demonstrable heart disease. *Am. J. Cardiol.* **9**: 209, 1962.
4. Cass, R.M.: Repetitive tachycardia. A review of 40 cases with no demonstrable heart disease. *Am. J. Cardiol.* **19**: 597, 1967.
5. Lesch, M., Lewis, E., Humphries, J.O.N., and Ross, R.S.: Paroxysmal ventricular tachycardia in the absence of organic heart disease. *Ann. Intern. Med.* **66**: 950, 1967.
6. Froment, R., Gallavardin, L., and Cahen, P.: Paroxysmal ventricular tachycardia. A clinical classification. *Br. Heart J.* **15**: 172, 1953.
7. Lown, B., and Wolf, M.: Approaches to sudden death from coronary heart disease. *Circulation* **44**: 130, 1971.

28

Intra-atrial Reentrant Tachycardias

Philippe Coumel, M.D., Daniel Flammang, M.D., and Michael Rosengarten, M.D.

Reentry is a very common mechanism of tachycardias. A number of studies have shown that it may occur anywhere in the heart though most frequently in the atrioventricular (A-V) junction. Experimental studies have demonstrated that reciprocation can occur in the sinoatrial node[1,11] and that a *sustained* reciprocating tachycardia can be obtained in fact anywhere in the atrium.[2] In humans, Narula[13] first demonstrated the possibility of such a phenomenon, but a relatively few cases only of *established* tachycardia have been published so far by different authors.[3,4,6,7,10,13–17,19–21] They form a total of about 40 cases, to which we have the opportunity to add 20 cases in the present study. These cases have in common several identifying clinical and electrophysiological characteristics. (Fig. 28-1).

CASE MATERIAL

Clinical Data

Eight males and 12 females were studied. Ages were between 12 and 80 years. Twelve had no detectable heart disease, five had valvular diseases (4 mitral, 1 aortic), three had other conditions (1 hypertension, 1 myocardial infarction, 1 myocardiopathy). In 12 cases palpitations were either isolated or associated with dyspnea (7 cases), dizziness (3 cases) syncope (2 cases) and were the cause of the first examination. But in eight cases, the tachycardia was found in the course of a systematic examination, the arrhythmia being well tolerated, particularly if not

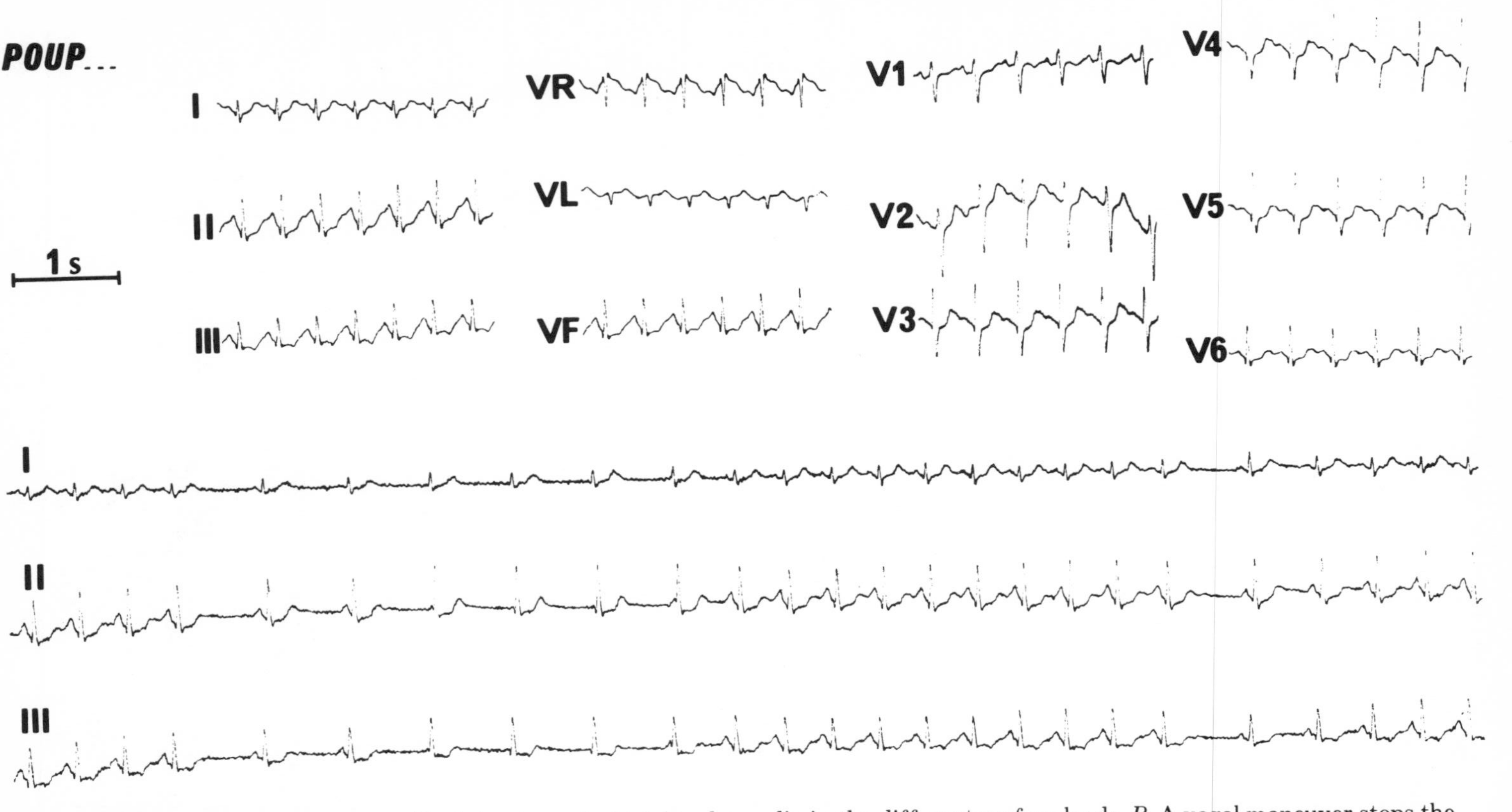

Figure 28–1. Intra-atrial reentry. Basic tracings. *A*, Atrial tachycardia in the different surface leads. *B*, A vagal maneuver stops the tachycardia, which restarts after a few beats.

rapid or of long duration. Atrial arrhythmias (flutter or fibrillation) were observed either spontaneously or during the electrophysiologic study in five patients. Finally, two patients had not only a reentrant atrial tachycardia, but also an A-V junctional one.

Electrophysiological Data Other Than Those Related to the Tachycardia

The pattern of the sinus P waves was normal, or nearly normal in 13 cases (65%), whereas an intra-atrial conduction disturbance was present in seven cases. Sinus P wave duration was equal to or less than 90 msec in ten cases, between 100 and 120 msec in seven cases, and more than 160 in three. The sequence of right atrial activation, and particularly the high left atrium to low right atrium interval was definitely prolonged in only three cases (80 msec in two, 180 in one) but the mean value of the P-A interval, calculated from the 17 remaining patients was slightly prolonged with respect to normal of 35. Evidence of a second-degree sinoatrial block was found in two patients. The A-V nodal conduction time was normal (A-H interval ≤ 140 msec in most patients) as well as the H-V interval (≤ 50 msec) so that in only 4 patients was the A-V conduction altered either at the proximal or distal level (2 cases respectively).

In order to rule out accurately the diagnosis of A-V junctional tachycardia, particular attention was paid to the A-V conduction, both anterograde and retrograde. The stimulation frequency at which second-degree block was produced was carefully evaluated, and compared to the rate of the tachycardia. In 11 cases the second-degree type I A-V block was obtained at an atrial pacing rate slower than that of the tachycardia, thus suggesting that the A-V node did not participate in the reentry circuit. But in nine cases this criterion could not be met, and the atrial location of the tachycardia could not be established by this fact. The retrograde VA conduction was also studied (Fig. 28-2). A third degree (10 cases) or a second degree block (7 cases) was present at a ventricular pacing rate identical to that of the tachycardia: this argument allowed ruling out the possibility of an A-V junctional reentrant tachycardia, so that in only three patients was this mechanism still possible at that time of study.

In the ten patients having a retrograde V-A conduction, and particularly in the three who did not have second degree A-V block at a ventricular pacing rate identical to that of the tachycardia, the morphology of the retrograde P′ waves was carefully compared to that of the atrial tachycardia, both in surface and endocavitary leads. In nine cases (including the 3 patients with no V-A block at fast pacing rates), these morphologies were clearly different, thus eliminating a junctional reentry as the mechanism of the atrial tachycardia. In only one case the retro-

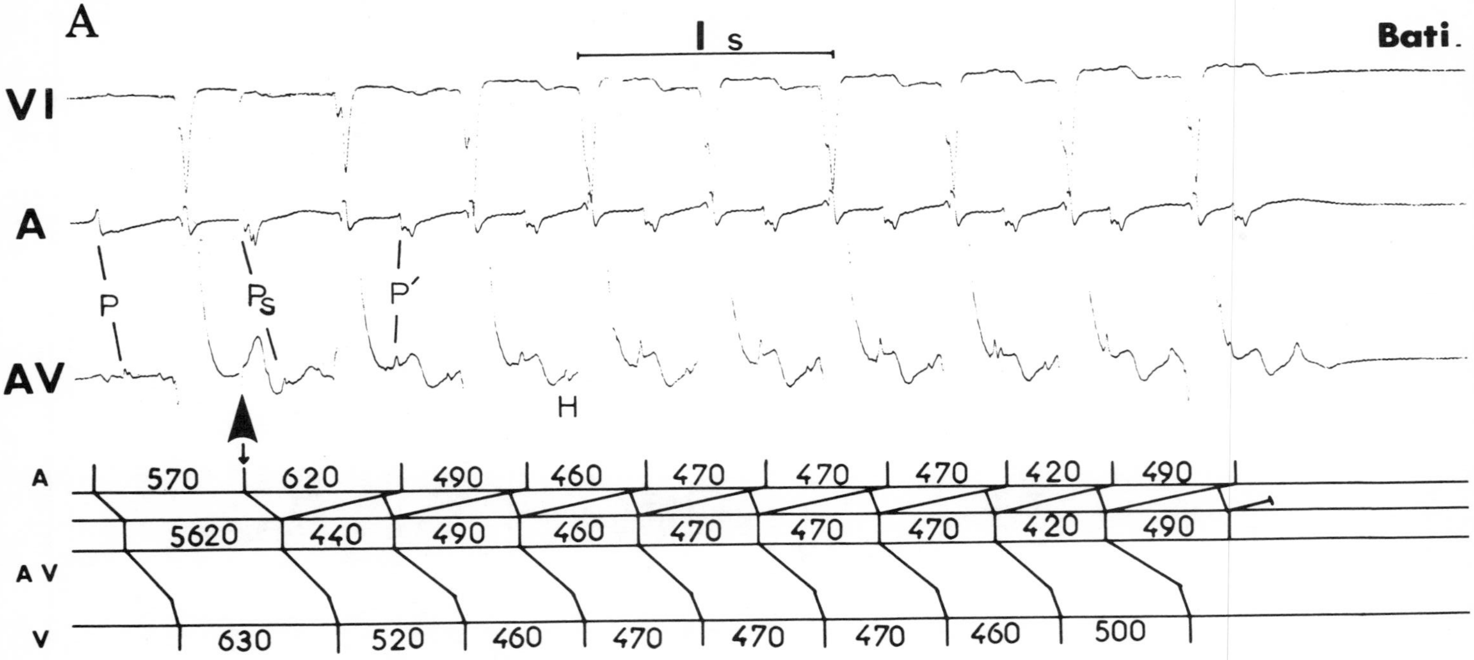

Figure 28–2. Anterograde and retrograde A-V conduction. A, An atrial stimulation (labelled Ps) initiates a run of supraventricular tachycardia, the atrial or junctional origin of which cannot be determined.

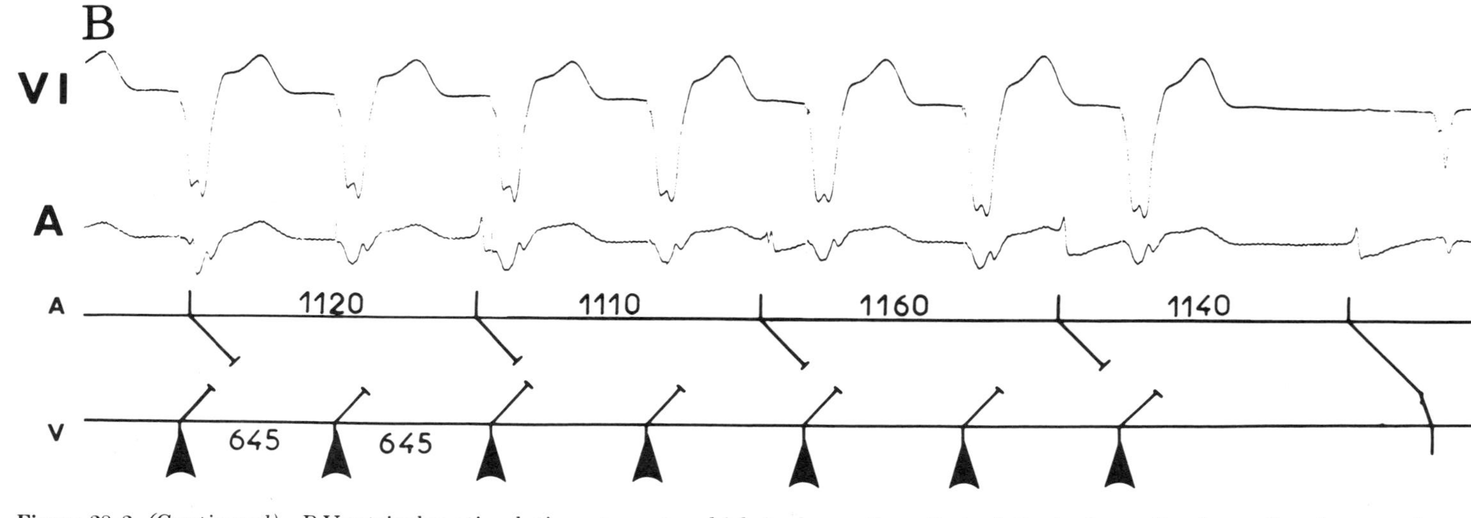

Figure 28–2. *(Continued).* *B,* Ventricular stimulation at a rate which is slower than that of the tachycardia shows the absence of retrograde V-A conduction in the basic conditions, thus proving that the tachycardia is indeed atrial. *Abbreviations:* A = intra-atrial lead; A-V = atrioventricular junctional bipolar lead recording the His bundle electrogram; P = sinus P waves; Ps = stimulated P wave; P′ = P waves of the tachycardia. Arrows point to the stimulation artefacts.

grade P wave morphology was the same as that of the "atrial" tachycardia, so that its junctional origin could not be accurately ruled out, even in the presence of a transient second-degree A-V block during the tachycardia. Finally, in two cases (Fig. 28-3) a true A-V junctional reciprocating tachycardia was demonstrated in addition to the atrial one, and it was possible to alternate from one to the another.

Modes of Initiation of the Atrial Tachycardia

The most common way to induce atrial tachycardia was the extrastimulus technique, or more simply to apply an appropriately-timed premature atrial stimulus during sinus rhythm (Fig. 28-4). This procedure was successful in 19 out of our 20 patients. A single premature atrial stimulation was sufficient in 17 cases, and 2 were necessary in two cases only. According to other authors, a definite echo zone can be determined in the cardiac cycle, situated approximatively between 30 and 60 percent of the cardiac period. We did not attempt to define precisely the inner and outer limits of the echo-zone in every patient, because we do not find it relevant. The existence of the phenomenon itself is very significant as far as the reentry mechanism is concerned, but the limits of the tachycardia zone vary according to the pacing rate or the sinus frequency, the level of the sympathetic tone or the drugs given, and the site of stimulation with respect to the site of origin of the tachycardia.[4] There was only one exception to this mode of initiation; regardless of the site or the coupling of the stimulation the arrhythmia could not be started. This occurred in our only case of true sinus node reentry.

Two other modes of initiation are rather specific of atrial reentry. In nine cases, the progressive acceleration of the atrial pacing rate initiated the tachycardia every time a definite frequency was reached, whatever the site of stimulation (Fig. 28-5). The interval between the last driven P wave and the first P wave of the tachycardia can be either shorter or longer than, or equal to the cycle length of the tachycardia which follows. This mode of initiation was unsuccessful in 11 patients. On the other hand, in one case, pacing the atrium was the best means to prevent the tachycardia.

Escape rhythms were a good way to obtain the tachycardia: a mode of initiation as common as the preceding one (10 patients). An important fact is that the escape P wave initiating the tachycardia is identical to the P waves of the following tachycardia; thus the atrial escape beat seems to come from the reentry circuit, explaining why it can start the tachycardia without any prematurity.

Characteristics of the Tachycardia

The tachycardia rate was less than 150/min in most cases, with a mean value of 128.6/min (extremes 180 and 95/min): in some cases the cardiac frequency was slow enough to interfere with the sinus rhythm. In four cases, two, four, and up to five rates of tachycardia were present, ranging from 100 to 320/min. But the "dominant" tachycardia, i.e., the most frequent or the spontaneous one was the slower one, the others being artificially induced during the electrophysiological study.

The P-R interval was related to the rate of the atrial tachycardia and the conditions of the A-V conduction. In other words, it can vary with the rate, particularly at the beginning of the episodes without influencing the cardiac rate: a very striking difference with what is observed in A-V junctional tachycardias. A second degree A-V block was present in 11 cases: in all cases it was proximal to the His bundle, with Wenckebach periods. It was observed either spontaneously or thanks to ventricular extrastimuli: without capturing the atrium, they were able to modify for a few beats the P-to-R relationships.

In all cases it was possible to obtain, either spontaneously or with the use of drugs (Atropine, Isuprel) a sustained tachycardia, even though the episodes were initially limited to a few beats. Generally speaking, the faster the tachycardia, the longer the spontaneous episodes.

Careful attention was paid to the pattern of the tachycardia P waves, as compared to the sinus P waves. In some cases, where P waves were superimposed to the T waves of the preceding beat thanks to the prolongation of the P-R interval, one or two ventricular stimulations were delivered: this method allowed verifying the absence of atrial capture (thus contributing to eliminate an A-V junctional tachycardia), but overall making the next P wave free of artefact (Fig. 28-6). With this maneuver, sinoatrial P waves and tachycardia P waves appeared to differ in morphology in all cases except in one case. This fact was confirmed by the endocavitary mapping: a unipolar lead allowed to establish exactly the timing of onset of atrial activation, and several (nonfiltered) bipolar electrograms were then recorded to localize as precisely as possible the earliest point of activation in either the right or left (explored through the coronary sinus or the pulmonary artery) atrium, or in the interatrial septum. This first depolarized atrial area was found only once in the HRA (sinus node area). Most often (9 cases) it was found in the mid-right atrium, and in two cases in the low right atrium at the junction with the inferior vena cava. In four cases the left atrium was depolarized before the right atrium and the interatrial septum. The latter was first activated in two cases. Finally, in two cases, the low right atrium recorded by the His bundle electrode was first activated during

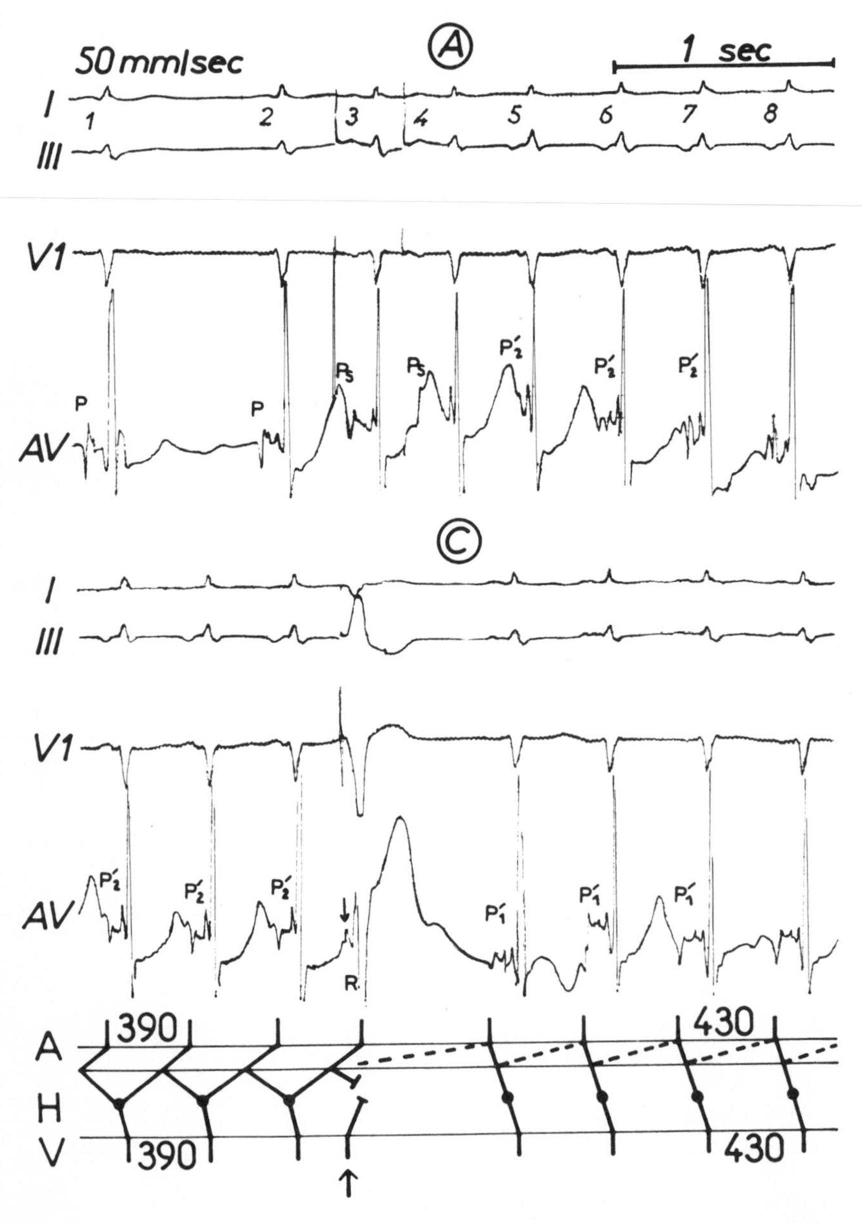

Figure 28-3. Intra-atrial and junctional reentries (on facing pages). Panel A: a paired atrial stimulation initiates a proxysmal junctional tachycardia with negatives P waves (labelled P'_2) in standard lead III. Panel B: a paired ventricular stimulation is able to initiate the same tachycardia, thus proving its junctional origin.

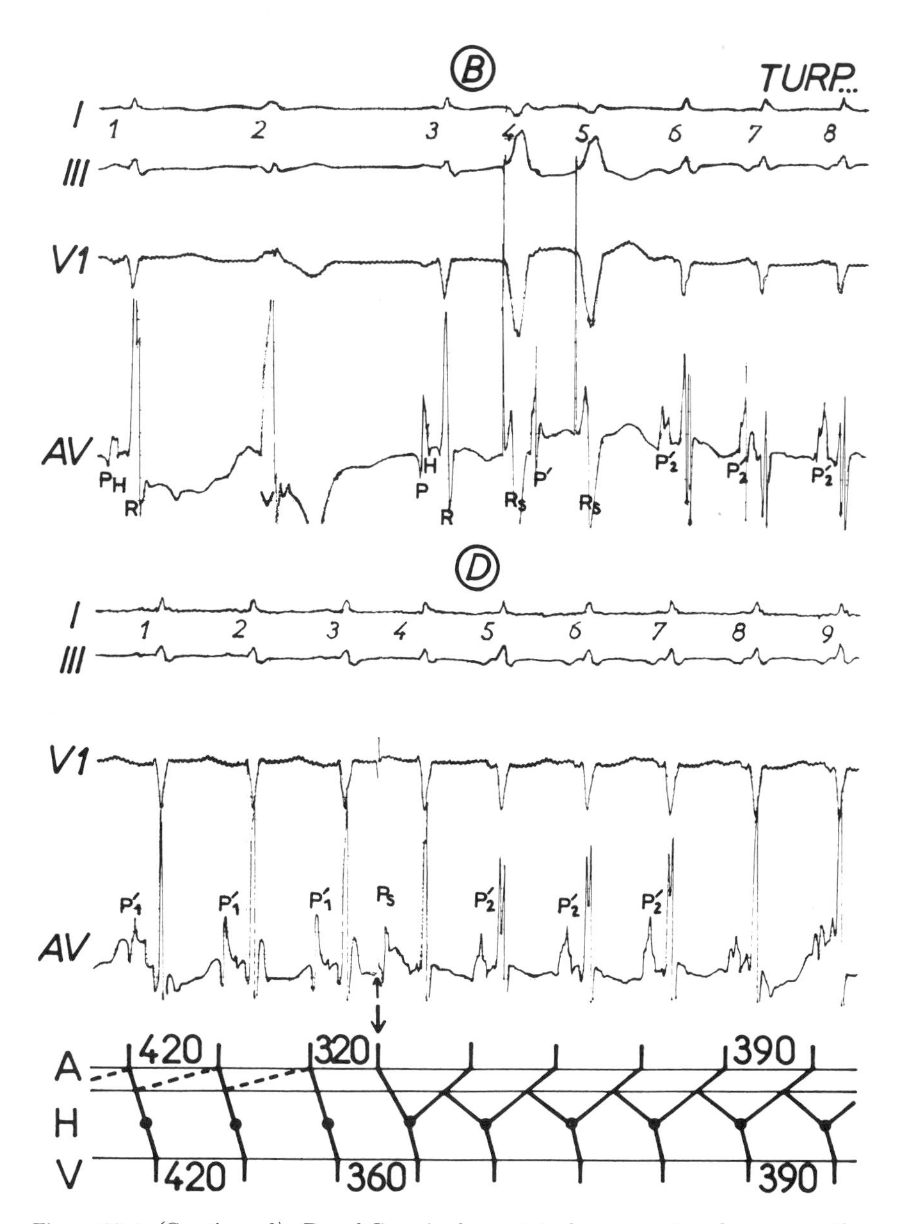

Figure 28–3. *(Continued).* Panel C: a single ventricular premature beat stops the tachycardia without capturing the atrium (see the diagram), proving again the junctional location of the reentry. Then an atrial tachycardia starts directly from the first atrial escape beat: P'_1 waves are clearly different in rate as well as in morphology from both sinus P waves and junctional P'_2 waves. Panel D: a single atrial stimulation during the atrial reentry triggers the junctional one.

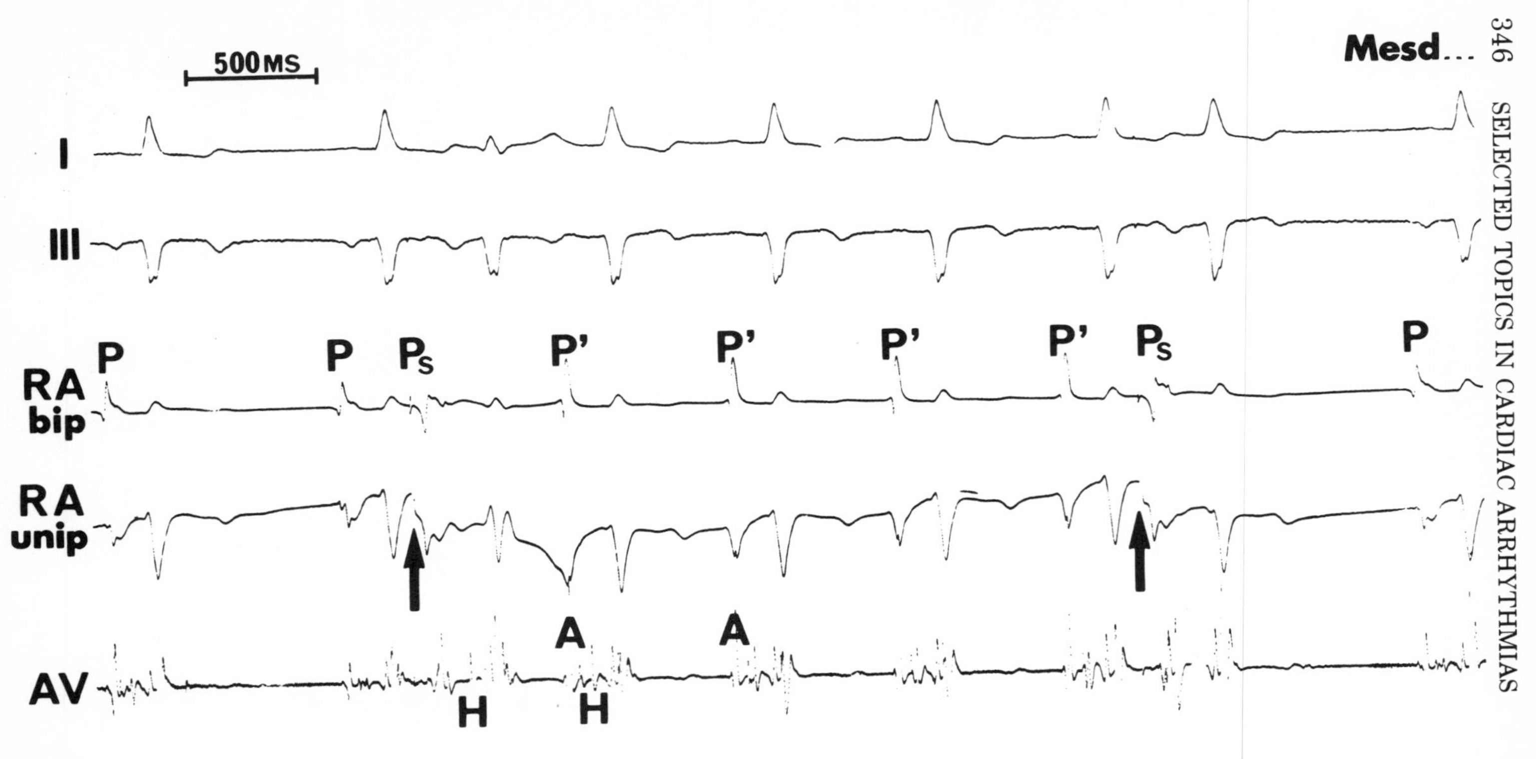

Figure 28–4. Initiation and termination of the tachycardia. A short run of a rather slow "tachycardia" is started and stopped by a single atrial stimulus. Note that the pattern of P′ waves in surface and endocavitary leads are only slightly but indeed different, particularly in the unipolar right atrial lead. (RA bip = bipolar right atrial recording, RA unip = unipolar right atrial recording).

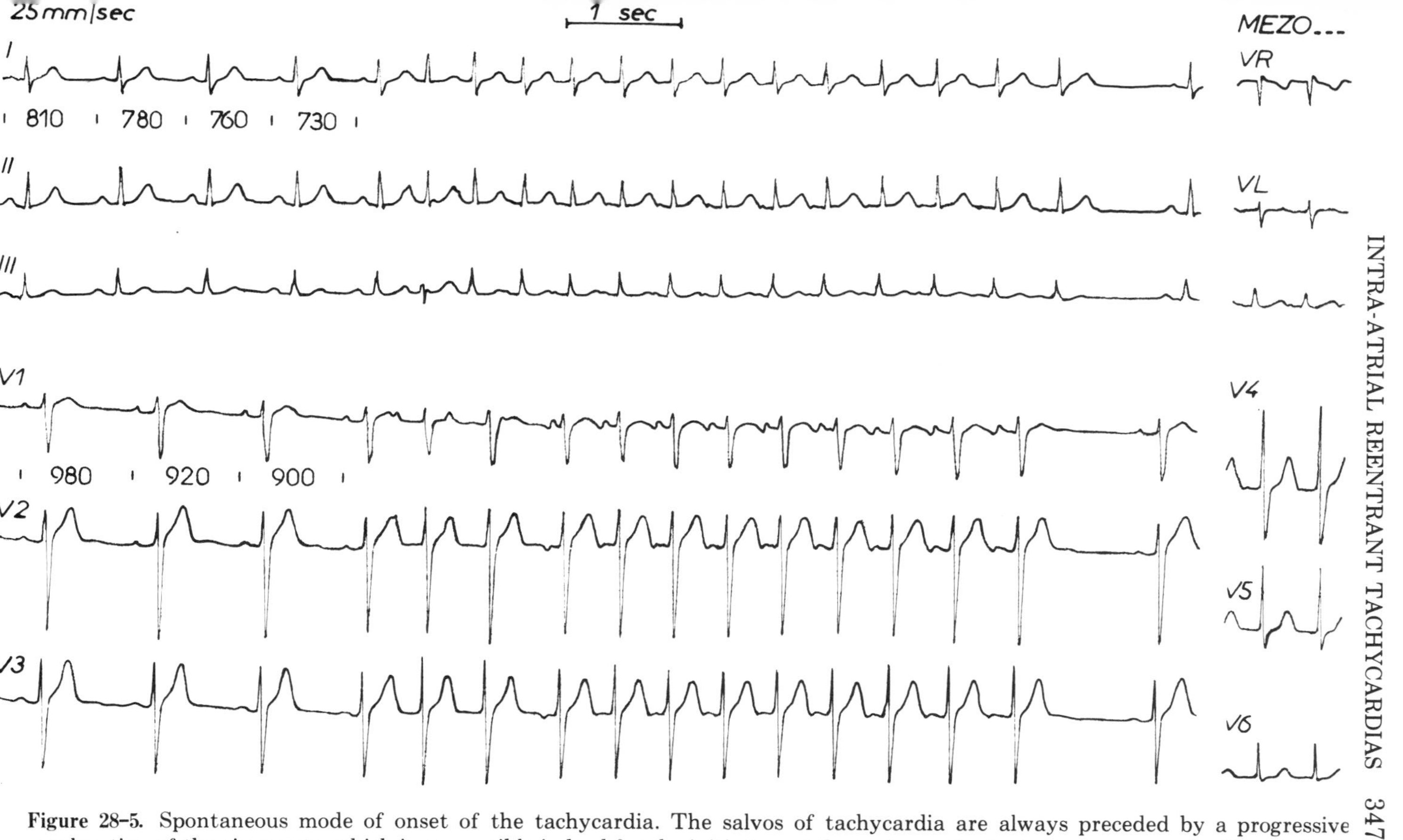

Figure 28–5. Spontaneous mode of onset of the tachycardia. The salvos of tachycardia are always preceded by a progressive acceleration of the sinus rate, which is responsible indeed for the initiation of the tachycardia. Note the presence of a Wenckebach period at the beginning of the tachycardia (lead V1), suggesting the proximal location of the reentry circuit.

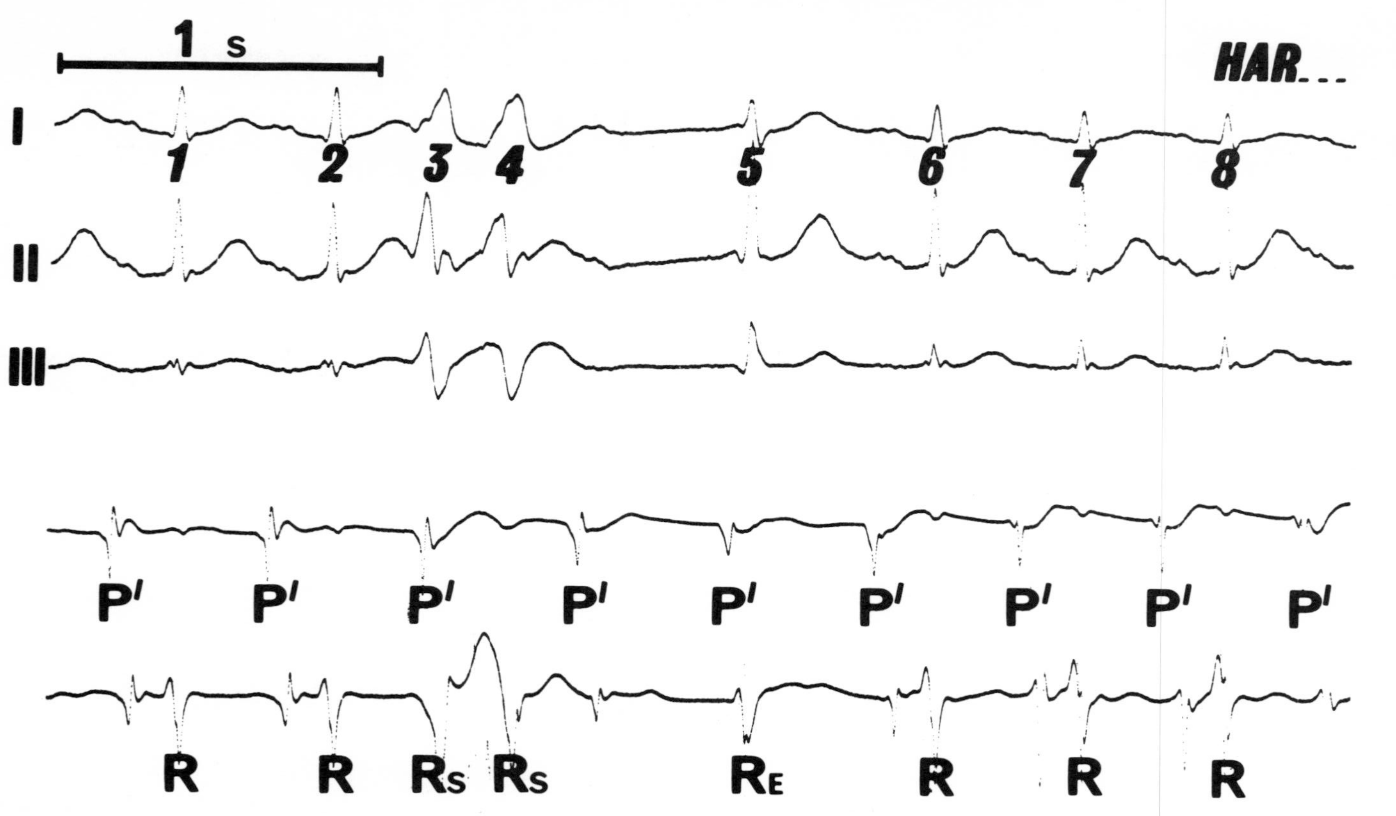

Figure 28–6. Ventricular stimulation during the tachycardia. A paired ventricular stimulation during the course of the tachycardia.[1] The absence of atrial capture, the presence of a blocked P' without any modification of the tachycardia, and a craniocaudal and right-to-left atrial sequence of activation.

the tachycardia (Fig. 28-7), suggesting the participation of the A-V node in the circuit, even though a proximal second-degree AV block excluded the participation of the entire A-V node. The sequence of activation between the earliest point of depolarization, the HRA (sinus node) and the LRA His bundle electrogram was carefully compared for sinus P waves, tachycardia P waves, and retrograde P′ waves when a V-A conduction could be obtained. If only the direction of activation is taken into account, the sequence HRA-to-LRA was unchanged 12 times during the tachycardia, and inverted eight times. If the time relationships between HRA and LRA are also taken into account, in one case only they were strictly identical during sinus rhythm and during the tachycardia, thus proving the existence of a true sinus node tachycardia, and in 11 cases the HRA to LRA interval was shorter during the tachycardia than during sinus rhythm. In cases where retrograde P′ waves could be obtained (10 cases), the LRA to HRA sequence of activation differed from that of the tachycardia in all cases except one, again suggesting the participation of the AV node in this case.

Termination of the Tachycardia

In all patients, the termination of the tachycardia was observed either spontaneously or after the administration of drugs but without any atrial stimulation (Fig. 28-8). Three modes of cessation were observed, sometimes coexisting in the same patient: (1) sudden cessation not preceded by any change in the tachycardia rate (10 times), (2) cessation proceded by a progressive slowing of the rate (9 times), (3) and cessation preceded by the alternance of long and short cycles (13 times).

Introducing premature stimuli in the atrial cycle made it possible in all cases to define three different zones, in the same manner as for A-V junctional tachycardias. The first zone covers a prematurity of 0 to 20 percent of the testing stimulus: the stimulated P wave was followed by a compensatory pause which did not influence the course of the tachycardia. Occasionally it could modify the P-R interval of the cycle following the pause, but not the rate of the tachycardia. The second zone covers about 20 to 40 percent of prematurity of the stimulus test. The tachycardia was reset without being terminated, and the return cycle was always longer than the basic one, but its prolongation was not related to the mode of conduction of the stimulated P wave to the ventricle: occasionally the stimulated P wave could be blocked without interrupting the tachycardia. In the earliest zone (40 to 60 percent of prematurity) the atrial stimulation readily terminated the tachycardia: a single stimulus was sufficient in all cases, provided the stimulation was given in an area not too far from the earliest point of activation of the atrium, and this fact needs further elucidation.

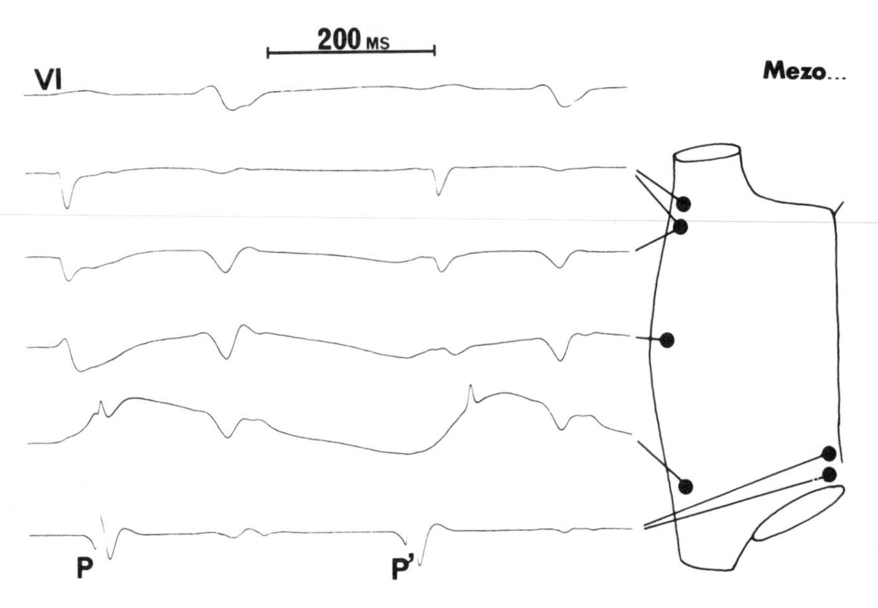

Figure 28–7. Endocavitary mapping. Comparing the last sinus P wave to the first P′ of the tachycardia clearly shows in the different unipolar and bipolar leads (see the diagram) that P′ originates in the lower part of the interatrial septum. In this patient (the same as in Figure 28-5), a type I second-degree A-V block strongly supported the atrial location of the reentry, but a participation of the upper A-V node in the circuit was not completely excluded.

In 17 out of 20 cases, the closer the stimulating electrode to the earliest point of atrial activation, the lesser the prematurity of the stimulus necessary to stop the tachycardia. In other words, all acts as if the "weak" point of the circuit, in which the stimulated impulse penetrates and is blocked, coincided with the earliest activated atrial area: a fact which strongly suggests that the size of the circuit is very limited, possibly or even probably microscopic. On the other hand, in three cases the area of stimulation where a stimulus could stop the tachycardia with the longer coupling interval did *not* correspond with the earliest point of activation. In these cases, it appears that the zone of termination occupied the major part of the cycle, in such a way that a stimulation given in an area activated very late (at the end of P) was able to prevent the next P wave (i.e., to stop the tachycardia) while the activation had already appeared at the earliest point. Of course, in those cases, one should be very careful in excluding the possibility of a coincidental termination; in our cases, the fact was reproducibly observed.

DISCUSSION

With the experience of 40 cases of sustained intra-atrial reentry described in the literature since Narula's[13] first case in man, the clinical pattern of this syndrome appears to be easy to recognize. There is no particular incidence of age or sex, and a good proportion of patients is free of any heart disease. A rather paradoxical fact, probably related to the importance of the basic intra-atrial conduction disturbance, is that patients without heart disease are prone to have other (either spontaneous or provoked) atrial tachycardias like flutter or fibrillation, while patients having a valvular disease or cardiomyopathies do not develop this kind of atrial arrhythmia. The diagnosis of intra-atrial reentry should be suspected in case of rather slow, well-tolerated atrial tachycardia, the episodes of which are either long, or short but recurring. They resemble superficially the recurring form of A-V junctional reciprocating tachycardia,[6,7] except that the rate is slower and that the pattern of the P wave is different.

From an electrophysiological point of view, the diagnosis of this particular arrhythmia should be discussed in four steps: (1) the diagnosis of the reentry mechanism, (2) the differential diagnosis with much more frequently observed A-V junctional tachycardias, (3) the diagnosis of the localization of the circuit within the atrium, and (4) the evaluation of its macro or microscopic size.

The Reentry Mechanism

Cranefield[9] has recently shown that a number of criteria usually employed by clinical electrophysiologists in the diagnosis of reentry should be challenged, since there might be evidence experimentally for authentic automatic foci. This is particularly true for the criteria of initiation and termination of these atrial reentries. Other facts favor reentry and are not difficult to show when the circuit is located within the A-V junction, for the simple reason that it is possible to explore the circuit from different points (atrium, His bundle and ventricle). Data obtained from these different areas allow the macroscopic nature of these circuits to be evaluated. Capture phenomena are very helpful in this task.[5] The problem is much more difficult when the circuit is supposedly located somewhere in the atrium. If the existence of reentry has been shown experimentally in the atrium by Allessie[1] it remains that, strictly speaking, in humans, the diagnosis of intra-atrial "reentry" means only in most published cases that the tachycardia is initiated and terminated by artificial stimuli. The possible role of postpotential phenomena in this

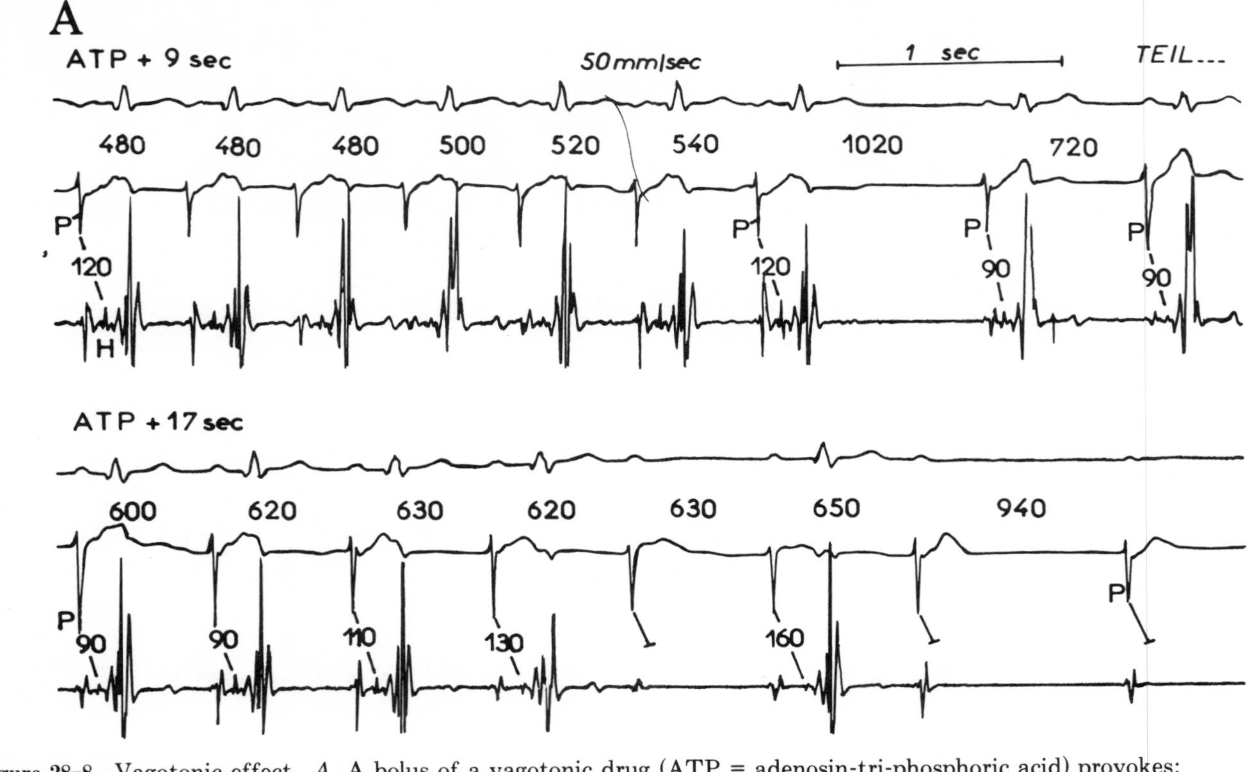

Figure 28-8. Vagotonic effect. *A,* A bolus of a vagotonic drug (ATP = adenosin-tri-phosphoric acid) provokes:
—after 9 seconds the termination of the tachycardia with a short phenomenon of alternation.
—after 17 seconds a type I second-degree A-V block and a sinus bradycardia. *(Continued on next page.)*

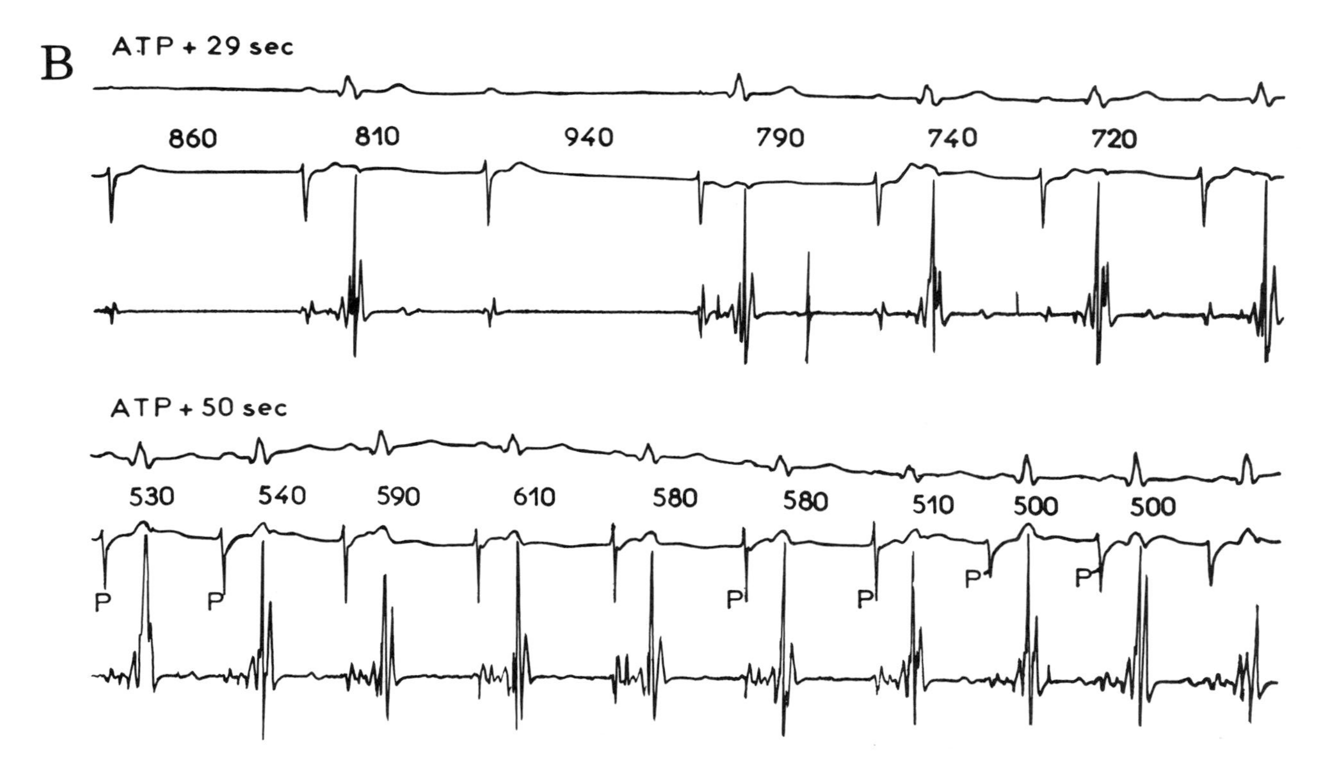

Figure 28–8. *(Continued).* *B,* ATP provokes after 17 seconds a type I second-degree A-V block and a sinus bradycardia, which terminate after 29 seconds.

—and the tachycardia starts again after 50 seconds when the increased sympathetic drive accelerates the sinus rate.

"triggered" activity should be kept in mind. The fact that a progressive acceleration of the pacing rate at moderate frequencies does provoke the tachycardia recalls strikingly the mode of initiation particular to the "permanent" form of reciprocating tachycardia, the reentrant character of which is in no doubt.[6,7] Still, triggered activity related to delayed after depolarizations can be provoked by this form of stimulation.[9] On the other hand, the fact that in some cases the atrial pacing is the best way to *prevent* the tachycardia is probably even more conclusive, as it recalls the mode of prevention of some A-V junctional tachycardias.[8] Finally, the onset of tachycardia after an escape beat arising from the circuit itself, as suggested by its pattern identical to that of the following P waves, though observed in the reciprocating tachycardias secondary to an A-V junctional escape beat in case of W.P.W. syndrome,[8] suggests the possible role of an automatic focus. Added to these criteria, the alternance of long and short cycles is more suggestive of variation of conduction than of excitability[8] even though a simple alternating exit block can always be invoked.

Differential Diagnosis With of A–V Junctional Reentry

As A-V junctional tachycardias are much more frequent, and hence probable in case of supraventricular reentry, obviously the first step in diagnosing an intra-atrial reentry is to eliminate accurately any possibility of A-V nodal tachycardia or latent W.P.W. syndrome, a precaution which is not always followed in the literature.

By definition, this possibility is clearly excluded every time a complete or high-degree retrograde V-A block is present. If a V-A conduction is present at fast ventricular pacing rates, several possibilities should be entertained. The permanent form of A-V junctional tachycardia is rather easy to recognize, particularly the characteristic pattern of the P′ waves and the time relationship between P and R.[7]

But this form has in common with intra-atrial reentry the initiation of the tachycardia by a progressively accelerated atrial pacing, and the absence of a requisite prolongation of P-R at the onset of tachycardia. As far as paroxysmal A-V nodal tachycardias are concerned, the presence of a second-degree A-V block during the tachycardia is not perfectly convincing on theoretical grounds, as some cases, though very rare, do exist.[20] In one case (Fig. 28-7) we cannot completely exclude the possibility, since there is no definite difference of atrial activation during the tachycardia and during ventricular pacing.

Even if an HRA-to-LRA depolarization sequence excludes an A-V nodal tachycardia, the possibility of a latent accessory pathway responsible for the tachycardia could occur if a retrograde conduction is present.

This possibility is not theoretical, particularly in case of right-sided latent accessory pathways, and we did observe it, as did others. Practically, in case of 1/1 reentrant tachycardia, such a diagnosis can never be excluded. Finally, we have observed two cases of dual reciprocating tachycardia, one located in the atrium and one in the junction, a coexistence which must be more than coincidental.

Atrial and Sinus Nodal Reentry

In our opinion, the term of sinus nodal reentry is probably used in excess, based on the fact that the HRA-to-LRA sequence of activation is not sufficient to define it. As stated above, 12 of our cases had this sequence and would have been qualified as such, using only bipolar filtered recordings. Even though this technique is employed, the term should not be used if the time relationships are not strictly the same as during sinus rhythm. Among the cases published in the literature, no more than half a dozen fulfill these criteria and we have observed only one. It is particularly interesting to note that this case was one of the two displaying a spontaneous sinoatrial block. In addition it was not possible to elicit the tachycardia by the extrastimulus technique, and the tachycardia was prevented by atrial pacing. However, it was indeed the most certain case of reentry, as it was possible to prove the macroscopy of the circuit.

Micro or Macroreentry

Determining the size of the circuit of reentry is already rather difficult in the case of A-V junctional tachycardia. It is almost impossible in intra-atrial reentry, and only by chance was it possible in three of our patients, thanks to the slow rate of the tachycardia and the easiness with which the permanent reentry was interrupted. If the tachycardia is actually due to a reentrant mechanism, one must admit that the progression of the impulse is concealed most of the time, because the visible part of the atrial depolarization is only the P wave. Blocking the impulse and stopping the reentrant impulse by stimulating *after* the very beginning of the P wave in a still responsive area supposes that the "equilibrium" of the circuit is very unstable.[7]

Indirect evidence of the macroscopy of the circuit is the dissociation between the site of the earliest activation and weak point of the circuit, i.e., the point where the latest stimulation stopping the tachycardia can be delivered. Determining this point is often difficult because it supposes a mapping of stimulation in the atrium, performed under very stable conditions of rate and permanence of the tachycardia. These conditions are rather infrequent in these patients.

However, our impression is that in most cases, there is a coincidence between the point of earliest activation and the "weak" point of the circuit, suggesting that the reentry circuit is microscopic.

SUMMARY

Twenty cases of sustained tachycardia due to intra-atrial reentry were investigated in patients aged 17 to 80 (mean 47). The average frequency of the tachycardia was 128.6/min (extremes 95 and 180). Three modes of onset of the tachycardia were observed: atrial extra-stimulus (19 times), progressively accelerated atrial pacing (9 times) and atrial escape beat (10 times). The tachycardia was stopped in all cases by a premature stimulation. When spontaneous, the termination was either sudden (10 times) or preceded by a progressive slowing (9 times) or an alternating phenomenon of long-short cycle (13 times). Precise atrial mapping allowed us to localize the first atrial depolarization less frequently in the sinus node area (1 case) than in the mean right atrium (21 cases), the low right atrium (2 cases) the interatrial septum (2 cases) and the left atrium (4 cases). The macroscopic size of the reentry circuit was demonstrated in only three cases. A junctional reentry was accurately ruled out in all cases thanks to the existence of a second or third-degree A-V or V-A block, or by studying the sequence of retrograde atrial activation. A true junctional reciprocating tachycardia was associated to the intra-atrial reentry in two cases.

REFERENCES

1. Allessie, M.A., Bonke, F.I.M., and Schopman, F.J.G.: Circus movement in rabbit atrial muscle as a mechanism of tachycardia. *Circ. Res.* **33**: 54, 1973.
2. Allessie, M.A., Bonke, F.I., and Schopman, F.J.G.: Observations on circus movement tachycardia in the isolated rabbit atrium. In Wellens, H.J.J., Lie, K.I., and Janse, M.J. (eds.): *The Conduction System of the Heart.* Leiden, Stenfert Kroese, 1976, p. 249.
3. Brechenmacher, C., and Voegtlin, R.: Tachycardie sinusale par réentrée. *Ann. Card. Angeiol.* **23**: 535, 1974.
4. Castellanos, A., Aranda, J., Moleiro, F., et al.: Effects of the pacing site in sinus node reentrant tachycardia. *J. Electrocard.* **9**: 165, 1976.
5. Coumel, P., Attuel, P., Motte, G., et al.: Les tachycardies jonctionnelles paroxystiques. Evaluation du point de jonction inférieur du circuit de réentrée. Démembrement des rythmes réciproques intranodaux. *Arch. Mal. Coeur* **68**: 1255, 1975.

6. Coumel, P. and Barold, S.S.: Mechanisms of supraventricular tachycardias. In Narula, O.S. (ed.): *International Symposium on Recent Advances in Clinical Electrophysiology.* Philadelphia, F.A. Davis 1975, p. 203.
7. Coumel, P., Attuel, P., and Flammang, D.: The role of the conduction system in supra-ventricular tachycardias. In Wellens, H.J.J., Lie, K.I. and Janse, M.J. (eds.): *The Conduction System of the Heart.* Leiden, Stenfert Kroese, 1976, p. 424.
8. Coumel, P., Attuel, P., Slama, R., et al.: "Incessant" tachycardias in the Wolff-Parkinson-White syndrome II. The role of atypical cycle-length dependency and nodal-His escape beats in initiating reciprocating tachycardias. *Br. Heart J.* **38**: 897, 1976.
9. Cranefield, P.F.: *The Conduction of the Cardiac Impulse.* Mt. Kisco, N.Y., Futura Publishing Co. 1975, p. 199.
10. Curry, P.V.L., Evan, T.R., and Krikler, D.M.: Paroxysmal reciprocating sinus tachycardia. *Eur. J. Cardiol.* **6**: 199, 1977.
11. Han, J., Malozzi, A.M., and Moe, G.K.: Sino-atrial reciprocation in the isolated rabbit heart. *Circ. Res.* **22**: 355, 1968.
12. Janse, M.J., and Anderson, R.H.: Specialized internodal atrial pathways—fact or fiction? *Eur. J. Cardiol.* **2**, 117, 1974.
13. Narula, O.S.: Sinus node re-entry. A mechanism for supraventricular tachycardia. *Circulation* **50**: 1114, 1974.
14. Pahlajani, D.B., Miller, R.A., and Serratto, M.: Sinus node re-entry and sinus node tachycardia. *Am. Heart J.* **90**: 305, 1975.
15. Paritzky, Z., Obayashi, K., and Mandel, W.J.: Atrial tachycardia secondary to sino-atrial node reentry. *Chest* **66**: 526, 1974.
16. Paulay, K.L., Varghese, P.J., and Damato, A.N.: Sinus node re-entry: an in vivo demonstration in the dog. *Circ. Res.* **32**: 455, 1973.
17. Paulay, K.L., Varghese, P.J., and Damato, A.N.: Atrial rythmus in response to an early atrial premature depolarization in man. *Am. Heart J.* **85**: 323, 1973.
18. Spurrell, R.A.J., Krikler, A.M., and Sowton, E.: Concealed bypasses of the atrioventricular node in patients with paroxysmal supraventricular tachycardia revealed by intra-cardiac electrical stimulation and verapamil. *Am. J. Cardiol.* **33**: 590, 1974.
19. Weisfogel, G.M., Batsford, W.P., Paulay, K.L., et al.: Sinus node re-entrant tachycardia in man. *Am. Heart J.* **90**: 295, 1975.
20. Wellens, H.J.J.: Unusual examples of supraventricular reentrant tachycardias. *Circulation* **51**: 997, 1975.
21. Wu, D., Amat-y-Leon, F., and Denes, P., et al.: Demonstration of sustained sinus and atrial reentry as a mechanism of paroxysmal supraventricular tachycardia. *Circulation* **51**: 234, 1975.

29

Concealed Conduction: Eighty-Five Years After Engelmann

Charles Fisch, M.D.

In 1980, the concept of concealed conduction (CC) is 85 years old and yet continues to fascinate the clinical electrocardiographer and the experimental electrophysiologist alike.

Engelmann[1] working in Utrecht clearly defined this concept when he wrote that "every effective atrial stimulation, even if it does not elicit a ventricular systole, prolongs the subsequent A-V interval." This is more remarkable when one recalls that the electrocardiograph was introduced by Einthoven 11 years later, in 1905.

The now classical work of Lewis and Master[2] and simultaneously that of Drury[3] in London, Ashman[4] in the U.S.A. and Scherf and Shookhoff[5,6] in Vienna is familiar to all.

Beginning some 20 years later, Langendorf, Pick and Katz published an elegant series of papers applying this concept to the human.[7]

Advent of microelectrophysiology, the renewed studies of CC in the intact animal[8,9] and finally development of His bundle electrocardiography added a new and exciting dimension to the concept of concealed conduction. The recording of incomplete penetration at the cellular level by Hoffman, Cranefield and Stuckey[10] and documenting concealed junctional discharge by Rosen, Rahimtoola and Gunnar[11] using His bundle recording gave us the sought after confirmation of the concept. Until the advent of these direct methods of recording from the specialized conduc-

Supported in part by the Hermann C. Krannert Fund, and by Grants HL-06408 and HL-07182 from the National Heart, Lung and Blood Institute of the National Institutes of Health, U.S. Public Health Service, and the American Heart Association, Indiana Affiliate.

tion tissue, a diagnosis of CC was a purely deductive one. The new techniques proved the validity of the elegant, painstaking and time-consuming analysis of the clinical records and observations made in the intact animal, beginning with Engelmann in 1904.

The renewed interest in concealed conduction coupled with the advent of new and sophisticated instrumentation allowed a gradual extension of this concept to tissues outside the AV node. For example, concealment of atrial premature complexes within the perinodal tissue results in first-degree sinoatrial delay. Similarly, by altering the rate of atrial pacing one can recognize concealment of the nonpropagated stimulus by its effect on the subsequent stimulus to P interval.[12] A variety of manifestations of CC within the specialized ventricular conduction tissue has also been described.

The reason for the unusual interest in concealed conduction by clinicians is that this concept is an ideal model for the study of electrocardiography of complex arrhythmias. This is true largely because this model emphasizes two basic facts; namely, that an analysis of complex arrhythmias is frequently one of deductive reasoning, and secondly, that the goal of such deductive reasoning is to describe the behavior of the specialized conduction tissue by analyzing the working myocardium reflected in the P and QRS waves.

DIAGNOSIS

The subject of concealed conduction is currently so broad that any presentation dealing with this concept has to be arbitrarily limited. It is our intent to deal with the specificity of the diagnosis of CC.

In the course of review of our material it became obvious that CC could be grouped in four categories on the basis of available proof of the concept. Examples of each category were selected for one of the following reasons: (1) not previously described, (2) rarely observed, or (3) raised questions about some currently perceived mechanisms of CC.

Electrocardiographic Features

The records demonstrating concealed conduction can be divided into the following four groups:

I. Unequivocal concealed conduction. Such records demonstrate that with a slight change in the temporal relationship of, for example RP-PR, complete conduction can be demonstrated (Fig. 29-1).

II. Concealed conduction is a very likely, if not the only possible mechanism, but complete conduction, thus the proof of the concept, is not

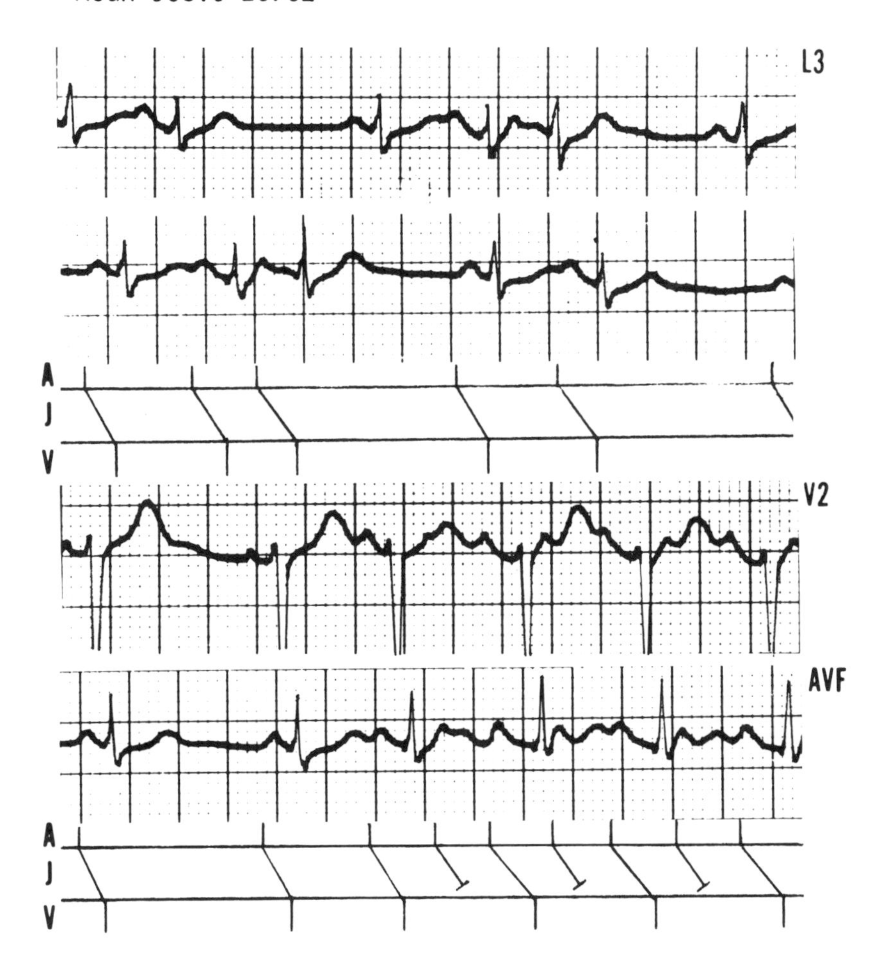

Figure 29–1. Concealed conduction resulting in prolongation of subsequent P-R. See text for details.

demonstrated (Fig. 29-2). A classical example of such a phenomenon is prolongation of the P-R secondary to concealment of an interpolated PVC into the junctional tissue, but without demonstrating a negative P wave, evidence of possible complete retrograde conduction.

III. Concealed conduction is assumed on basis of observation made in the animal but without confirmation in the human. Mechanisms other than CC are equally likely (Figs. 29-3, 29-4).

IV. Concealed conduction appears to be an interesting, sometimes remote, possibility but to date lacking proof either in the human or animal (Figs. 29-5, 29-6).

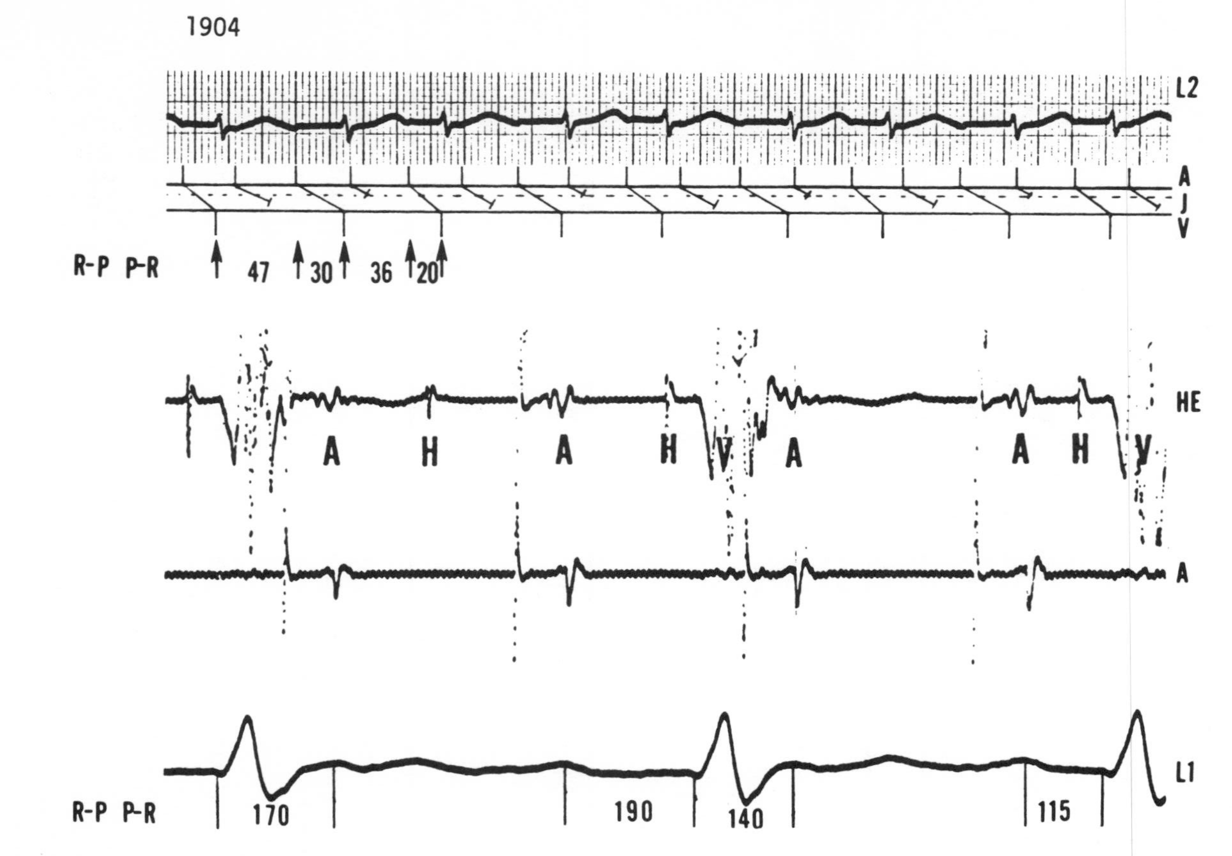

Figure 29–2. A-V alternans due to concealed conduction. See text for details.

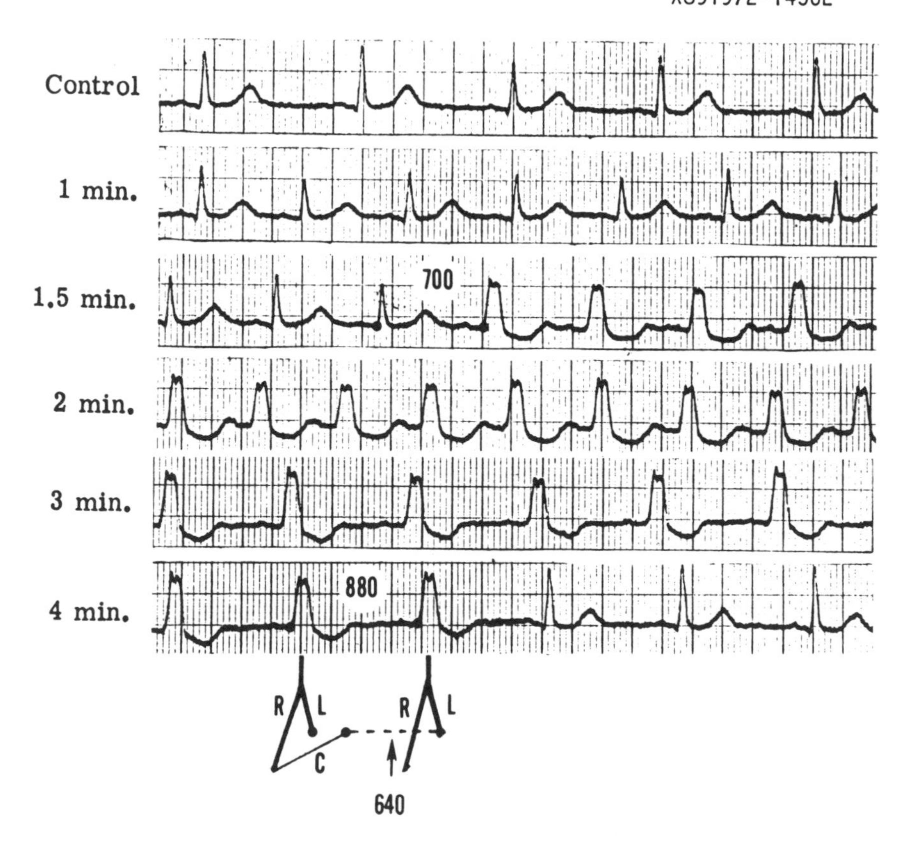

Figure 29-3. Concealed conduction into left bundle branch. See text for details.

Figure 29-1 is a unique, and to my knowledge first demonstration of the same phenomenon which Lewis and Masters[2] induced experimentally in dogs in 1925, but appearing spontaneously in the human.

The basic rhythm is sinus with atrial premature complexes (APC) and a run of atrial tachycardia (AT). A, J, V—atrium, junction and ventricle, respectively. All time intervals are given in hundredths of a second.

The bottom two tracings (V2, AVF) demonstrate two sinus P waves at a P-P interval of 76 and PR of 12 to 14. Following the second P there is a run of AT with a 2:1 AV response. The P-R of conducted P (e.g., P 5, 7, 9) is approximately 16 as opposed to 12 for the third P. This, in spite the fact that the RP of the third P is 34 and that of the fifth P is 36. In any event not shorter. The unexpected prolongation of P-R with onset of AT is ascribed to concealed conduction of the blocked P affecting propagation of the subsequent P wave.

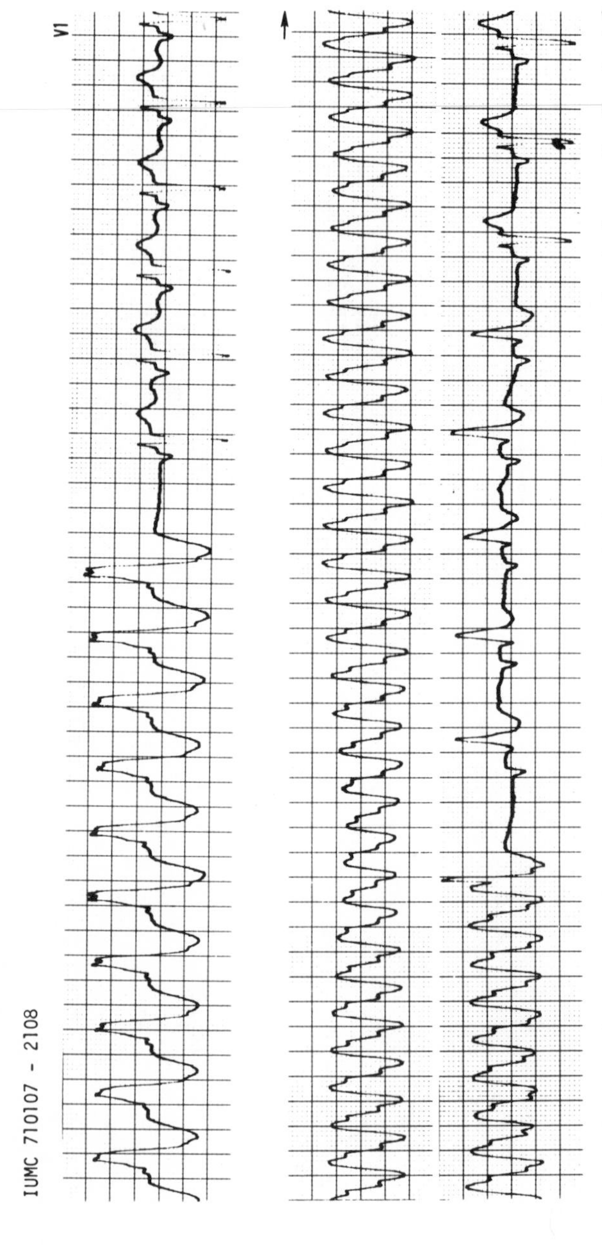

Figure 29–4. Right bundle branch block due to repetitive invasion by impulses of ventricular tachycardia. See text for details.

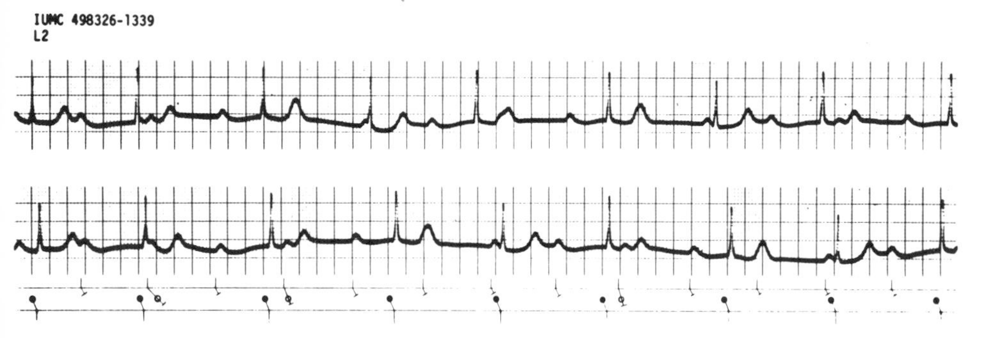

Figure 29–5. Concealed conduction during the supernormal phase of A-V conduction. See text for details.

The proof of this assumption can be seen in L3 where P waves are conducted to the ventricles. Similarly positioned P waves in V2 and AVF are blocked. Extrapolation of the behavior of P in L2 to those in V2 and AVF, allows the diagnosis of CC of the nonconducted P in leads V2 and AVF.

Figure 29-2 gives confirmation, hitherto not described, of concealed conduction as the mechanism responsible for A-V alternans with a paradoxical relationship of their respective RP-PR intervals. Such clinical records have been previously described.[13]

Lead 2 shows AT with 2:1 block and A-V alternans following the alternate conducted P wave. In the Lewis diagram the A-V junction (J) is divided into upper and lower portions by the dotted line. Some of the blocked P waves are shown to penetrate deeply and are followed by prolonged P-R of the subsegmentally conducted P. On the other hand, the P wave blocked high in the AV junction is followed by shorter P-R of the next conducted P. Thus the paradox of the longer R-P (47) of the conducted P being followed by longer P-R (30), while the shorter R-P (36) of conducted P is followed by shorter P-R (20). This an "unphysiological" and unexpected behavior is explained by deep penetration (CC) of the blocked P because of a longer preceding R-P (e.g., P2 has a longer R-P than P4).

The duration of the respective R-P and P-R of conducted P is noted below the Lewis diagram.

The same RP-PR relationship is shown in L1 recorded simultaneously with the His bundle electrogram (HE). The heart is paced at a regular rate. Four atrial (A) complexes are seen, two conducted and two blocked. The V-A (R-P) of the first A (P) measures 170 msec. This A (P) is conducted to the His bundle (H) and blocked below it. Because of the deep penetration (CC in case of the surface ECG) the A-V (P-R) of the

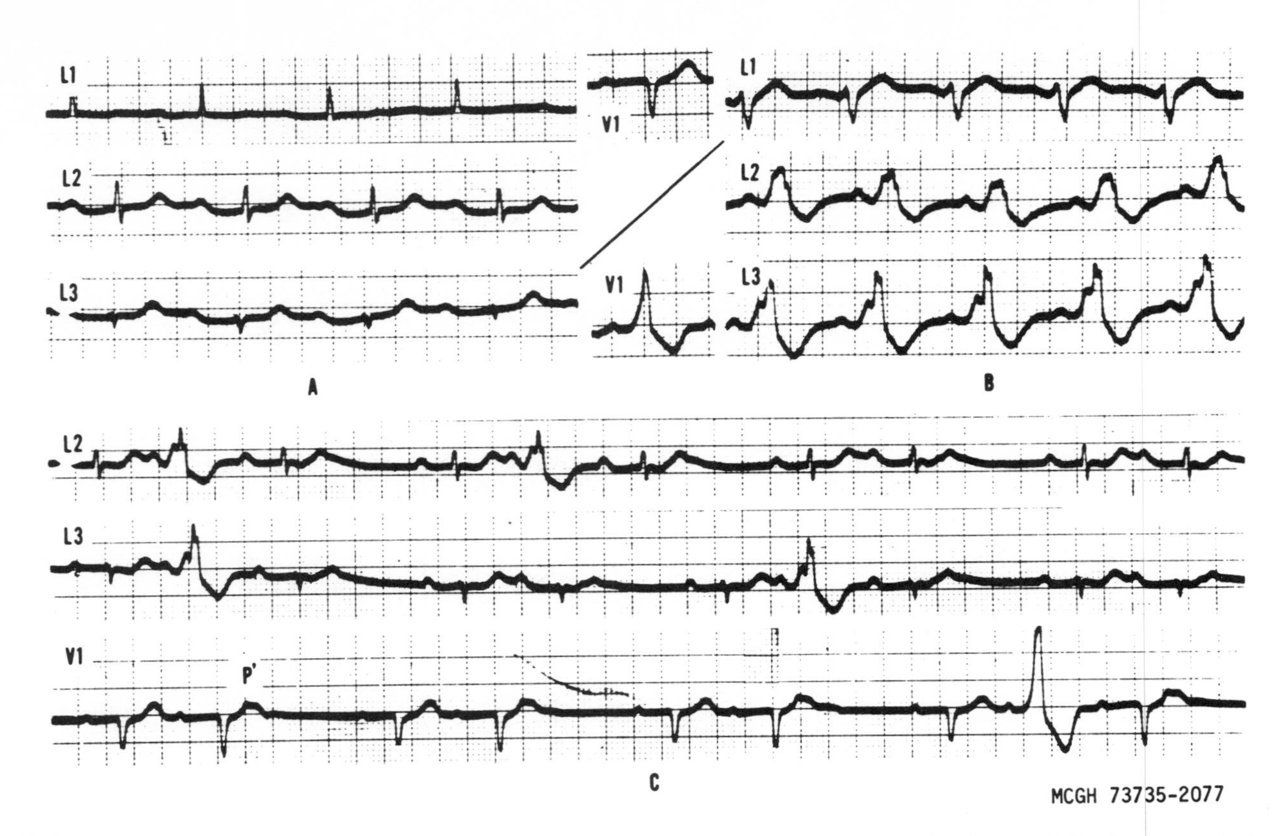

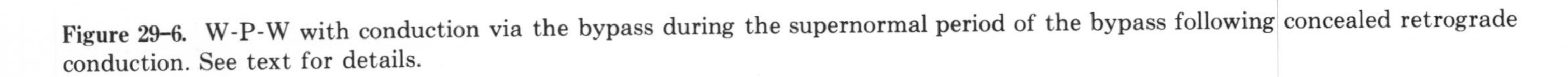

Figure 29–6. W-P-W with conduction via the bypass during the supernormal period of the bypass following concealed retrograde conduction. See text for details.

next conducted A (P) is 190 msec. The third A (P) follows a V-A (R-P) of only 140 msec, is blocked above the H and thus does not interfere with A-V (P-R) of the fourth, conducted A (P). The A-V (P-R) of this fourth A (P) is only 115 msec.

The deep penetration of the first A (P) with recording of the H potential validates the concept of CC. The latter in turn explains the paradox of a long, 520 msec, V-A (R-P) followed by long, 190 msec, A-V (P-R), and a short, 500 msec, V-A (R-P) being followed by a shorter, 115 msec, A-V (P-R).

Figure 29-3 shows sections taken from a continuous record (L1) after administration of amyl nitrate.

The heart rate accelerates gradually from a baseline R-R of 1040. When the R-R is shortened to 700 (1.5 min), the critical interval at which a rate dependent left bundle branch block (LBBB) is recorded. The paradox, however, is the persistence of LBBB with slowing of the rate to an R-R of 880, 180 longer than the critical R-R of 700. The most commonly accepted explanation for this paradox is CC of an impulse from the right bundle (RB) to the left bundle (LB), with delayed activation of the LB and thus a foreshortened LB to LB interval. This delayed activation cannot be demonstrated in the surface ECG, because activity of the LB is not manifest in the ECG. The above concept is illustrated by the diagram in which an impulse from RB (R) conceals (C) into the LB (L) resulting in an arbitrary LB to LB interval of 640, sufficiently short to perpetuate the rate dependent LBBB. The above explanation must assume an effect of the concealed impulse sufficiently long to shorten the LB to LB by at least 180 (880-700). In the normal animal the foreshortening of the cycle due to transseptal conduction is only 40 to 50 msec.[9] This is a much shorter time interval than one has to accept for this tracing, namely 180 msec. Whether concealed delay in activation of LBB of this magnitude is possible in a diseased human heart remains to be seen.

An equally possible explanation is the "fatigue" phenomenon, most likely due to retardation of transmembrane recovery of ionic balance secondary to disease of the conduction system. This is clearly the case when in the course of a regular tachycardia the QRS prolongs gradually to complete bundle branch block. A more interesting manifestation of RBBB persistence, likely due to depression of conduction, a form of fatigue, secondary to rapid and repetitive invasion in the course of ventricular tachycardia (see Figure 29-4).

Figure 29-4 demonstrates ventricular tachycardia (VT), probably right ventricular (Lead V1), followed by QRS complexes, sinus in origin, with a RBBB morphology. The sinus rate shows gradual acceleration with resumption of normal intraventricular conduction. The P-R also shortens from 20 to 14 suggesting, either accompanying LBB delay, or delay in the jucntion secondary to concealed invasion by impulses of the VT. This record suggests that "fatigue" and delay or block of conduction with gradual recovery, can result from repetitive invasion, either concealed as in the case illustrated or without concealment. Such "fatigue" can result in delay or block of an impulse in the intraventricular conduction system without necessarily having to invoke concealed transeptal activation from the opposite bundle.

Figure 29-5 is part of a long record. The rhythm is sinus with a P-P of approximately 760 and complete AV dissociation. The basic cycle length (R-R) of the subsidiary junctional focus is 1000. However, R-R intervals from 1400 to 1440 were also noted. The latter are seen only in association with an R-P of 8 to 16 and rarely an R-P of 20.

It is assumed that the P waves with a R-P of 8 to 20 penetrated, concealed, into the junction and displaced the junctional impulse. This is illustrated by the open circle in the Lewis diagram. The question remains as to the mechanism of the deep penetration of the P waves with an R-P of 8 to 20 and not that of the P waves following longer R-P. Normally, the latter are more likely to penetrate deeply into the junction. The proposed explanation of this paradoxical behavior is that CC of the P waves with an R-P of 8 to 20 is related to the supernormal phase of A-V conduction.

Figure 29-6 is an interesting and unusual example of W-P-W with what appears to be supernormality of the bypass possibly secondary to concealed retrograde penetration of the bypass.[14] This is an example of group IV in which concealed conduction is possible but must be considered purely conjectural and unproven.

A. Sinus rhythm with a P-R of 32.

B. W-P-W, type A and a P-R of 12 to 14.

C. Sinus rhythm with gradual prolongation of the P-R (Wenckebach), each sequence of Wenckebach is terminated by a retrograde P wave (P′), probably via the bypass. The first P with the shortest P-R of a sequence is never followed by P′, probably because of refractoriness of the atrium. However, concealed conduction into the bypass cannot be excluded. Similarly P′ never follows a W-P-W pattern probably because of refractoriness of the bypass per se due to antegrade conduction. Failure to record P′ after antegrade conduction via the bypass suggests that the P′ are indeed due to retrograde activation via the bypass, rather than reciprocation via the A-V junction. Conduction via the bypass is seen only with P waves on the downslope of the R, after an R-P of 24 to 40, suggesting that excitation arrives in the ventricle during its supernormal period and a W-P-W complex is registered. One can suggest that all sinus P waves attempt to traverse the bypass, but only impulses finding the ventricle during the supernormal period of recovery complete the ventricular activation and result in W-P-W complex. The alternate explanation, equally likely, in view of presence of P′ secondary to retrograde conduction via the bypass, is that following each sinus P-QRS there is an attempted (concealed) retrograde conduction via the bypass. This concealed conduction, in turn, induces a supernormal period in the bypass making a successful antegrade propagation of the sinus impulse over the bypass with registration of the W-P-W complex possible.

SUMMARY

Examples of the wide spectrum of concealed conduction, some proven, some yet to be proven were briefly discussed. The focus of the presentation was on specificity of the diagnosis.

Concealed conduction is the best model for in depth study of electrocardiography of complex arrhythmias.

REFERENCES

1. Engelmann, T.W.: Beobachtungen and Versuche am suspendieren Herzen. *Pflüger Arch.* **56**: 149, 1894.
2. Lewis, T., and Master, A.M.: Observations upon conduction in the mammalian heart. A-V conduction. *Heart* **12**: 209, 1925.
3. Drury, A.N.: Further observations upon intrauricular block produced by pressure or cooling. *Heart* **12**: 143, 1925.
4. Ashman, R.: Conductivity in compressed cardiac muscle. *Am. J. Physiol.* **74**: 121, 1925.
5. Scherf, D., and Shookhoff, C.: Reizleitungsstorungen in Bundel. I. Uber Verändurugen des atrioventrikularen Rhythnms durch Extrasystolen. *Wein. Arch. f. Inn. Med.* **10**: 97, 1925.
6. Scherf, D., and Shookhoff, C.: Reizleitungsstorungen in Bundle. II. Leitungsstorungen nach Eingriffen auf die Schenkel. *Wien. Arch. f. Inn. Med.* **11**: 425, 1925.
7. Pick, A., Langendorf, R., and Katz, L.N.: The supernormal phase of atrioventricular conduction. I. Fundamental mechanisms. *Circulation* **26**: 388, 1962.
8. Moe, G.K., Abildskov, J.A., and Mendez, C.: An experimental study of concealed conduction. *Am. Heart J.* **67**: 338, 1964.
9. Moe, G.K., Mendez, C., and Han, J.: Aberrant A-V impulse propagation in the dog heart: a study of functional bundle branch block. *Circ. Res.* **16**: 265, 1965.
10. Hoffman, B.F., Cranefield, P.R., and Stuckey, J.H.: Concealed conduction. *Circ. Res.* **9**: 194, 1961.

11. Rosen, K.M., Rahimtoola, S.H., and Gunnar, R.M.: Pseudo A-V block secondary to premature nonpropagated His bundle depolarization. Documentation by His bundle electrocardiography. *Circulation* **42**: 367, 1970.
12. Sung, R.J., Myerburg, R.J., and Castellanos, A.: Electrophysiological demonstration of concealed conduction in the human atrium. *Circulation* **58**: 940, 1978.
13. Langendorf, R.: Alternation of A-V conduction time. *Am. Heart J.* **55**: 181, 1958.
14. McHenry, P.L., Knoebel, S.B., and Fisch, C.: The W-P-W syndrome with supernormal conduction through the anomalous bypass. *Circulation* **34**: 734, 1966.

Index

N

P

Q

R

S

T

V

W